the Unofficial Guide™ to Smart Nutrition

Ross Hume Hall, Ph.D.

IDG Books Worldwide, Inc.
An International Data Group Company
Foster City, CA • Chicago, IL • Indianapolis, IN
• New York, NY

IDG Books Worldwide, Inc.
An International Data Group Company
919 E. Hillsdale Boulevard
Suite 400
Foster City, CA 94404

For general information on IDG Books Worldwide's books in the U.S., please call our Consumer Customer Service department at 800-762-2974. For reseller information, including discounts and previous sales, please call our Reseller Customer Service department at 800-434-3422.

ISBN: 0-02-863589-2

Manufactured in the United States of America

10 9 8 7 6 5 4 3 2 1

First edition

Acknowledgments

My wife, Anne Jones Hall, M.A., C.N.S., a nutritionist in her own right, is my partner in the pursuit of upgraded nutrition, within a home framework and modern-product world. Over the years, Anne and I have maintained a unique collaboration. Having backed into nutrition from the world of photographic modeling, she went on to pursue nutrition degrees, specializing in energy endurance.

As advocates for better food and nutrition education, we published a nutrition journal for health professionals. This present book is an outgrowth of one issue, Strategy for Wellness. The strategy featured a way of assessing the nutritional quality of food products—the four quality levels.

Anne took the idea of better food choices based on the four quality levels to the field, so to speak. Working with health professionals and world-class athletes, she showed that this simple approach to upgrading nutrition works. Although I take responsibility for the way four quality levels are used in this book, I owe Anne a profound debt for her role in the genesis and fine-tuning of the concept. She also critiqued chapter drafts. The book is the richer for her comments and insight.

I also wish to thank Donald and Martha Hall, Gail and Jim Spring, N.D., and Mary Beth Bezzina for reading chapter drafts and giving me their no-holds-barred views. A special thanks to Kitty Werner, for many years the President of the League of Vermont Writers, who bought the interested parties together. Kitty was instrumental in launching this project.

Finally, I wish to thank all members of my family, which range from the latest grandchild to my century-old mother. Through sharing with them challenges of food shopping, eating on the fly, and navigating a quagmire of conflicting nutritional advice, I gained an appreciation of the practical struggles to improve one's nutrition. This book is dedicated to all of them.

Contents

The *Unofficial Guide* Reader's Bill of Rights

We Give You More Than the Official Line

Welcome to the *Unofficial Guide* series of Lifestyle titles—books that deliver critical, unbiased information that other books can't or won't reveal—the inside scoop. Our goal is to provide you with the most accessible, useful information and advice possible. The recommendations we offer in these pages are not influenced by the corporate line of any organization or industry; we give you the hard facts, whether those institutions like them or not. If something is ill-advised or will cause a loss of time and/or money, we'll give you ample warning. And if it is a worthwhile option, we'll let you know that, too.

Armed and Ready

Our hand-picked authors confidently and critically report on a wide range of topics that matter to smart readers like you. Our authors are passionate about their subjects, but they have distanced themselves enough to help you be armed and protected, and to help you make educated decisions as you go through your process. It is our intent that, after having read this book, you will avoid the pitfalls everyone else falls into and you'll get it right the first time.

Don't be fooled by cheap imitations; this is the *genuine article Unofficial Guide* series from IDG Books Worldwide, Inc. You may be familiar with our proven track record of the travel *Unofficial Guides,* which have more than two million copies in print. Each year thousands of travelers—new and old—are armed with a brand-new, fully updated edition of the flagship *Unofficial Guide to Walt Disney World,* by Bob Sehlinger. It is our intention here to provide you with the same level of objective authority that Mr. Sehlinger does in his brainchild.

The Unofficial Panel of Experts

Every work in the Lifestyle *Unofficial Guides* is intensively inspected by a team of three top professionals in their fields. These experts review the manuscript for factual accuracy, comprehensiveness, and an insider's determination as to whether the manuscript fulfills the credo in this Reader's Bill of Rights. In other words, our panel ensures that you are, in fact, getting "the inside scoop."

Our Pledge

The authors, the editorial staff, and the Unofficial Panel of Experts assembled for *Unofficial Guides* are determined to lay out the most valuable alternatives available for our readers. This dictum means that our writers must be explicit, prescriptive, and, above all, direct. We strive to be thorough and complete, but our goal is not necessarily to have the "most" or "all" of the information on a topic; this is not, after all, an encyclopedia. Our objective is to help you narrow down your options to the best of what is available, unbiased by affiliation with any industry or organization.

In each *Unofficial Guide* we give you:

- Comprehensive coverage of necessary and vital information
- Authoritative, rigidly fact-checked data
- The most up-to-date insights into trends
- Savvy, sophisticated writing that's also readable
- Sensible, applicable facts and secrets that only an insider knows

Special Features

Every book in our series offers the following six special sidebars in the margins that were devised to help you get things done cheaply, efficiently, and smartly.

1. "Timesaver"—tips and shortcuts that save you time.

2. "Moneysaver"—tips and shortcuts that save you money.

3. "Watch Out!"—more serious cautions and warnings.

4. "Bright Idea"—general tips and shortcuts to help you find an easier or smarter way to do something.

5. "Quote"—statements from real people that are intended to be prescriptive and valuable to you.

6. "Unofficially…"—an insider's fact or anecdote.

We also recognize your need to have quick information at your fingertips, and we have thus provided the following comprehensive sections at the back of the book:

1. Glossary: Definitions of complicated terminology and jargon.

2. Resource Guide: Lists of relevant agencies, associations, institutions, Web sites, etc.

3. Recommended Reading List: Suggested titles that can help you get more in-depth information on related topics.

4. Important Documents: "Official" pieces of information you need to refer to, such as government forms.

5. Guides to Nutritional Quality Levels: Facts and numbers presented at-a-glance for easy reference.

6. Index.

Letters, Comments, and Questions from Readers

We strive to continually improve the *Unofficial* series, and input from our readers is a valuable way for us to do that. Many of those who have used the *Unofficial Guide* travel books write to the authors to ask questions, make comments, or share their own discoveries and lessons. For Lifestyle *Unofficial Guides,* we would also appreciate all such correspondence, both positive and critical, and we will make our best efforts to incorporate appropriate readers' feedback and comments in revised editions of this work.

How to write to us:
Unofficial Guides
Lifestyle Guides
IDG Books
1633 Broadway
New York, NY 10019
Attention: Reader's Comments

About the Author

Ross Hume Hall, Ph.D, brings a lifetime of professional experience in fields related to the preservation of good health. A former chairperson of the Department of Biochemistry, McMaster University Medical Faculty, Hamilton, Ontario, Hall graduated from the University of Toronto in chemistry, and earned his Ph.D. in nutritional biochemistry from Cambridge University.

He combines his expertise in human biochemistry, nutrition, food technology, and the health effects of environmental toxicology into a practical approach that gives people new insights into food and how it affects their health. In addition to doing original scientific research, Hall has written over 200 articles for magazines and newspapers. He and his wife, Anne Jones Hall, M.A., C.N.S, published a widely acclaimed newsletter on nutrition and health for health professionals.

Hall's government service has included being an advisor to the Canadian Minister of the Environment and co-Chair of the Human Health Committee of the International Joint Commission.

This committee is concerned with the impacts of pesticide residues and industrial contaminants on the health of the 35 million people living around the Great Lakes. He also served on a National Academy of Sciences committee, studying the health and safety issues of nitrites used in food preservation.

He is author of two nontechnical books, *Food For Naught: The Decline in Nutrition,* and *Health and the Global Environment.* Hall regularly comments on food/health issues on radio and television.

The *Unofficial Guide* Panel of Experts

The *Unofficial* editorial team recognizes that you've purchased this book with the expectation of getting the most authoritative, carefully inspected information currently available. Toward that end, for each and every title in this series, we have selected a minimum of three "official" experts who constitute the "Unofficial Panel." These experts painstakingly review the manuscripts to ensure: factual accuracy of all data; inclusion of the most up-to-date and relevant information; and insights drawn from an insider's perspective so that you are armed with all the necessary facts you need—but the institutions don't want you to know.

For *The Unofficial Guide to Smart Nutrition,* we are proud to introduce the following panel of experts:

Judith E. Brown, Ph.D. Dr. Brown is a widely-published authority on nutrition. Currently a professor and major chair of Public Health Nutrition in the School of Public Health, University of Minnesota, Brown's writings include studies on prenatal nutritional counseling and breast-feeding. Among her books are *The Science of Human Nutrition* (Harcourt Brace Jovanovich, 1990), *Everywoman's Guide to Nutrition* (Univ. of Minnesota Press, 1991), and, most recently, *Nutrition for Fertility, Pregnancy, and Breastfeeding* (Lowell House, 1998).

Brown received her B.S. in dietetics from the Rochester Institute of Technology, the M.P.H. (Nutrition) from the University of Michigan, Ann Arbor, and the Ph.D. in Human Nutrition from Florida State University, Tallahassee.

Michael Janson, M.D. Dr. Janson is a practicing physician and a well-known author and speaker on the topics of nutrition, alternative medicine, vitamins, and other dietary supplements in medical therapy. His books include *The Vitamin Revolution in Health Care, Chelation Therapy and Your Health,* and *All about Saw Palmetto and Prostate Health.* He writes extensively for periodicals and has been quoted in *Time* and many health magazines. A frequent guest on TV and radio, he hosted *Alive and Well,* a Boston area health radio show, and currently is a cohost of *Time for Health,* a daily Boston radio show. He is an expert author for the Web site drugstore.com and runs the health news updates at www.drjanson.com/.

Dr. Janson is past president of the American College for Advancement in Medicine and the American Preventive Medical Association, and a charter member of the American Holistic Medical Association. He completed medical school at Boston University in 1970 and currently practices at Path to Health, in Burlington, Mass.

Dian Shepperson Mills   Ms. Mills is a Cert. Ed. (Nutrition), B.A. (Education and Psychology), Dip. ION (Clinical Nutrition), and M.A. Health Education (Nutrition). She works at the Centre for Nutritional Medicine in Harley Street, London, which aims to use a scientific, evidence-based understanding of nutrition to improve health, maximize performance, and contribute to disease management and prevention. Doctors and nutritionists work together to offer primary healthcare service. She established Lamberts Library Trust in Tunbridge Wells, the largest electronic nutrition library in Europe. Her research interests include endometriosis, male and female infertility, and female endocrine disorders. She is a founder member of the charity SHE Trust (Simply Holistic Endometriosis) and is a Governor of the Institute for Optimum Nutrition in London. She is also the author of *Endometriosis—a Key to Healing through Nutrition* (Element).

Introduction

A ll the wisdom handed out by medical authorities on staying healthy boils down to one simple statement—exercise every day and eat the right food. Easy to say, devilish hard to execute. The exercise part is not so hard. A vigorous walk suffices. Food is where the devil waits.

In this *Unofficial Guide to Smart Nutrition,* we're going to take on the devil. We'll look at a new way of choosing foods in the modern supermarket, delicatessen, takeout, and restaurant. This new way cuts through such controversies as fat in the diet, fast foods, red meat, excess sugar, and why weight-loss diets fail. You'll learn how to reach your health goals without sacrificing your basic food preference, whether hearty meat eater, vegetarian, or any of the regional styles.

Note, we stress the word *modern.* Foods you eat today aren't the foods you ate 10 or 20 years ago. The food industry has undergone a remarkable change, and traditional nutrition advice is not keeping up. Just look at the statistics on food-related health problems—the devil's successes, if you will.

- Health authorities for 40 years have demonized cholesterol and fat. Yet the American Heart Association says the chance of falling victim to heart disease has climbed to the highest peak ever.

- We know that food plays a major role in breast cancer. Yet one woman out of eight contracts the disease (during her lifetime), compared to one in twenty a generation ago.

- Three out of four people know that inappropriate food choice is the main cause of adult-onset diabetes. Yet the American Diabetes Society reports 800,000 new cases every year.

- On any given day, four out of ten adults follow a weight-loss diet. Yet the average American weighs 171 pounds, compared to 160 pounds 10 years ago.

What's going on? Why, in spite of all the advice on food and health, are food-connected health problems skyrocketing? The answer lies in a social revolution that has turned the food-health connection upside down. Traditional nutrition advice about protein percentages, fat grams, vitamin supplementation, and so forth no longer works. People following such advice still make unwise food choices, even with the best of intentions.

Clearly, a new way of looking at and choosing foods is needed, and that's what you'll learn in this book.

Smart nutrition looks at the total food—not just at the protein percentage or number of fat grams, but at the total nutritional value of the food to your body. Smart nutrition looks at the nutrition a food brings, but also at the baggage the food may carry, such as chemical additives and pollutants, which stress the body in some way.

In taking a broad, holistic view of nutrition, this book takes a broad, holistic view of your personal health. We look at the total way nutrition affects your personal well-being. We look at how smart nutrition can:

- Vitalize the body, lifting chronic tiredness and giving you the energy that lasts for the entire day.

- Pump up your immune defenses so you rarely suffer the inconvenience of a cold or the flu.

- Strengthen the inner capacity of the body to resist premature breakdown resulting in such diseases as heart disease, cancer, adult-onset diabetes, and osteoporosis.

- Adjust your weight naturally to match your body type and build.

The social revolution in food

Before discussing smart nutrition, let's look at the social revolution in food and see how it affects you. The revolution is going on all around you. You are part of it, which is perhaps why you haven't noticed it. Home cooking, for instance, is going the way of the horse and buggy. We now have the mobile stomach. People graze through convenience marts, supermarkets, vending machines, delis, and fast-food restaurants rather than eating three sit-down meals a day. Grazing makes it much harder to judge how much you eat, and much harder to balance what you eat.

And when people do prepare meals at home, they cook less from scratch. The American Meat

Institute found that when consumers use their kitchen, they allot no more than half an hour to prepare and cook a meal. They won't use any ingredient or follow any recipe if it means that they can't get the food on the table within 30 minutes of entering the kitchen. In fact, in many families, the 30-minute time slot includes preparing and eating.

According to the NDP Group of Chicago, IL, a survey company that tracks the country's eating habits, the three most popular dinner/lunch entrees are meals that require little time to prepare: pizza (purchased frozen from a supermarket or delivered hot to the door), ham sandwiches, and peanut butter and jelly sandwiches.

If folks want a more elaborate meal, they bring it home from a restaurant or deli takeout. Supermarkets devote a large proportion of their frozen food section to complete meals, a meal ready to eat within 5 minutes of putting it in the microwave oven. This consumer trend of buying complete meals, whether hot from a restaurant or frozen and ready to eat, has become so commonplace that the food industry coined a new term for it—*Home Meal Replacement*.

For the home consumer, it's the equivalent of having a personal cook in the kitchen, someone else to do the work. The social revolution in foods and food preparation can be capsulated in one word—convenience. The time people spent shopping, planning, and preparing for meals in past years has been freed up for other activities.

It's convenient not to have to plan menus and block off time for meal preparation. When hunger strikes just open a box, for example, of Kraft Macaroni & Cheese, a double slotted, microwave-safe tray filled with cheese on one side and elbow macaroni on the other. Add water, blend, and pop in the microwave oven. The personal "cook" in this case is a factory with industrial machinery and technicians skilled in preparing macaroni and cheese by the ton.

In embracing convenience, consumers hand over responsibility for their own nutritional well-being to others. But the factory managers and technicians are not really concerned about nutrition. Their challenge is to design and produce foods that won't wilt or develop strange flavors under the physical stress of factory processing. They chemically treat cheese so it can be cooked at industrial temperatures without collapsing into an unsightly glob. They add special preservatives, artificial colors, and artificial flavors so the product can sit for months in a warehouse and then withstand jouncing coast-to-coast trucking, to say nothing of the destruction caused by freezing and thawing.

In short, the first priority for food manufacturers is having an appealing product arrive on the consumer's table months after it has been produced. Nutrition is secondary.

The unchanging human body, the changing foods

There is one constant amid this social revolution in how we eat—your body. Your body is still the same old human body that has been handed down through ancestral genes since the Ice Age. Food changes, but basic human needs do not. And that's the problem. Those alarming health statistics and the ballooning size of the average American are telltale signs that the body's basic needs go unfulfilled.

In saying that food has changed, we need to recognize that the modern food scene is remarkably diverse. Some delis offer 300 different luncheon dishes. Go into your average supermarket and you find 30,000 different food items. Within that diversity, the range of nutritional values is startling, from wonderful foods that satisfy your prehistoric body to others that provide only bare subsistence. The problem staring you in the face is knowing which is which. How do you judge the new foods in relation to unchanging human nutritional needs?

Traditional criteria of judging foods are no longer sufficient. Take, for example, the United States Department of Agriculture's (USDA) Food Pyramid. This food guide recommends that every day you eat three to five servings of vegetables. Good advice? Partly, but the USDA doesn't give you a clue as to how you should buy your vegetables.

I went up and down the aisles of the local Price Chopper supermarket, and counted 1,750 different items that qualify for the USDA's vegetable category. From the body's perspective, nutritional value ranged from mediocre to excellent.

When the nutrition and health people at the USDA recommended those servings of vegetables, they had in mind health benefits that *fresh* vegetables bring to your body. The advice is sound as far as it goes. But without an understanding of the varying nutritional value among 1,750 vegetable items, you could easily undermine that advice. You could choose vegetable products that do your body little good.

How, then, do you distinguish the mediocre from the excellent?

The four nutritional quality levels

Continuing with the vegetable category as an example, we could give you two ways of judging the nutritional value of a food product. We could bog you down in tables of specific food products, each with a nutritional rating. Or, we could give you a few simple rules, easy to remember.

Naturally, we take the latter course. The items in every food category are ranked in four quality levels; level 1 is top nutritional quality, and level 4 is the lowest nutritional quality. Food products are assigned to each level based on total nutritional quality. Here is the way, for example, that the vegetable products are assigned.

- Quality level 1, fresh (for instance, a salad)

- Quality level 2, fresh, lightly steamed or cooked

- Quality level 3, frozen

- Quality level 4, canned

In assigning quality levels, we avoid the terms "good" or "bad," nor do we use that negative term, "junk food." The idea is that from a nutritional point of view some foods are *better than others.*

The canned vegetables at quality level 4 are not completely devoid of nutrition. But frozen foods nutritionally are better than canned. Similarly, fresh vegetables lightly cooked are better than frozen, and so on. Chapter 2, "Fruits and Vegetables," takes up the vegetable category in detail, explaining the reasons for the category assignments.

By referring to the four nutritional quality levels, you can easily slot, for example, all 1,750 supermarket vegetable items. Part II of the book provides nutritional quality levels for all categories of food.

The concept behind the four levels is that food products in each level are nutritionally better than the products in one level lower. The purpose behind the four levels is to give you smart choices. You eat only so much food, so why not chose the "better-than" item?

That's smart nutrition.

We hasten to point out that with smart nutrition you don't have to give up any of the pleasures of eating. You chose the food you enjoy, food that fits your way of life. Smart nutrition gives you a basis for making better choices within your eating style.

A holistic view of health and the human body

Smart nutrition is more than making food choice; it's a blend of nutrition and personal well-being. The reward of making nutritionally better food choices is "better-than" health.

As mentioned a moment ago, we see health as far more than not being ill. Why settle for a high frequency of colds, or fatigue that strikes early in the day, or ballooning weight that diets don't control? You function, but you could function better. You want your whole body to perform at top level.

This idea of wholeness has spawned the term *holistic.* This book takes a holistic view of the human body, inspired by the belief that all parts and systems work together.

Deep inside your body, all organs and systems (for instance, the immune system) interconnect, each with every other. This communication network ensures that every muscle, organ, and tissue works in concert. Because of this network, all parts of your body experience the same state of health, whether mediocre or wonderful. What you want in life is for every millimeter of your body to be in sync.

We can't stress this point enough. Health rewards flow from the whole body, not from an isolated organ, like the heart, or a system, like the immune. Nature doesn't work in isolation.

To illustrate, consider the case of Marie S., unable to stop the downhill slide of osteoporosis. Well-to-do, Marie easily afforded the best medical advice and treatment money could buy. She took calcium supplements and drank milk with a religious fervor. Yet, it seemed the more she focused on calcium, the more hollow her bones became. She was afraid to go anywhere for fear she'd accidentally hurt herself or fall. Marie knew that diet is a factor in osteoporosis. But she thought all she needed to do was reach for a bottle of calcium pills. She didn't give a thought to her total diet. She ate nothing but quality level 4 foods in every category. Her total diet—definitely not smart—canceled any benefit stemming from calcium supplements and medical care.

Smart nutrition means eating for the whole body, not focusing on a single body part like bones, heart, or, for that matter, weight. Incidentally, with respect to weight, the worse thing people can do is use weight as the sole criterion as to how well they eat. A misplaced focus on weight can result in the very thing the person fears—ballooning weight.

When you eat for the whole body, weight magically adjusts to a healthy size.

Smart nutrition looks at total food

Traditional diet advice focuses on chemical components of foods. You are told, for instance, to eat a certain percentage of protein or avoid sugar or fat. This advice is hardly real life. You don't eat pure sugar, or cholesterol, or protein. You eat food. Your body has to deal with everything that comes in, the good and the bad. Smart nutrition deals with the entire food: the nutrients, the food additives, the pesticidesresidues, the scrapings off the package liner.

Marian Burros, writing in the *New York Times* (January 13, 1999), points out that chemicals from certain brands of cling wrap migrate into foods, particularly fatty foods like cheese. These chemicals have been linked to breast cancer. In Chapter 13, "Food Safety: Avoiding Foodborne Illness," we give you the scoop on how to avoid the health hazards of such migrating chemicals.

Certainly, the traditional nutritional numbers of protein percentage, fat grams, vitamin content, and so on, represents useful facts. Such facts by themselves, however, don't give the full story on how your body responds to a meal of macaroni and cheese, industrially fabricated ages before you take the first bite. Smart nutrition goes beyond the traditional numbers.

Putting food into your social context

Traditional weight-loss diets fail for two reasons: The advice is scientifically unsound and/or the diet is difficult to maintain. The diet doesn't fit into a person's lifestyle. Traditional diets tend to have a single focus, whether it's the amount of fat in the food or some exotic combination of foods. Such diets ignore the fact that people live different lives and are at different stages in life. A single-focus diet doesn't work for everyone.

Take my six grown children, who are all married with families. In five of the families, both parents work. In any given evening, one child is going to band practice, another to soccer, another doing something else. The parents have to squeeze meals into the cracks between work and family demands.

That is an example of social context. Smart nutrition takes into account your social context—

your stage in life (single, family with kids, golden years) and the way you live your life. Smart nutrition is not a rigid diet. It is a way of eating, a way of making better food choices, that offers infinite flexibility.

Healthy bodies have a price tag

Healthy bodies come with a price tag. The health-care system and the modern food system will not deliver a slim body and health to you on a silver platter. You can't afford to be a passive eater accepting whatever food is conveniently at hand. We don't live in a Garden of Eden. We live in an imperfect world, populated by nutritional devils. You have to be alert and take charge.

You think, for instance, when you go into a supermarket with its 30,000 different items, that you have overwhelming choice. Well, you do, but it's not your choice—it's the supermarket's. The aisles and displays of the supermarket are artfully arranged so you pick the most expensive item, the one with the highest markup and often the lowest nutrition. Those expensive items are shelved 51 to 53 inches above the floor, the eye-contact level of the average woman. Other high-cost items (usually nutritional quality level 4) are stacked at the ends of the isles where you trip over them—and stick them in your shopping cart.

The background music beats a funeral-paced 60 beats a minute. Supermarket planners found that by slowing down the music, shoppers walk more slowly—and buy more. In fact, surveys show that shoppers make two-thirds of their purchases on the spur of the moment—"splurchases," as they are known in the business.

This book gives you the ability and confidence to avoid being manipulated by the food system. You'll receive the two things you must have to take charge in the supermarket, deli, or restaurant: knowledge and skills.

This book also gives you insight into the nutritional quality of modern foods and an understanding of how these foods interact with your body. On the practical side, the book gives you the skills to shop the 30,000-item supermarket and order in delicatessens and restaurants on your terms.

Smart nutrition has its rewards

As you'll also learn in this book, smart nutrition is not just an abstract goal; it has tangible, practical payoffs. Here are just a few of the rewards of smart nutrition:

- Natural adjustment of body size
- Immediate rise in your energy level
- Fewer colds and scratchy throats
- Healthier and smarter babies
- Low risk of the six diet-related killer diseases: heart disease, stroke, atherosclerosis, liver disease, adult-onset diabetes, and cancer (especially breast)
- Superior chance of living your golden years, free of disability

In sum, smart nutrition is not a diet; it's a way of choosing foods that fit your lifestyle and stage of life. Smart nutrition embraces your total health. It's more than simply not being sick; it's enjoying a total state of superior physical and mental well-being.

A Cell's-eye View of Nourishment

PART I

The Basics of Smart Nutrition

Chapter 1

Nutrition is all about judgment. Shop an average-sized supermarket, and you are faced with 30,000 different items. Even with a full shopping cart, you can choose only a tiny fraction of the store's selection. Why do you select what you do? Underlying your choices is a gut feeling that certain food items are better than others. Typically, three factors go into your decisions, whether or not you are aware of them:

1. Familiarity with the specific foods, including brand loyalty

2. Your personal tastes, as well as those of your family

3. Nutritional advice you read or heard about concerning the specific products you choose

But it is becoming increasingly difficult to rely on those three factors for making decisions about what foods to buy and eat. The food scene is in a state of flux. In 1998, for instance, the food industry introduced 11,037 new products. A similar number of familiar products vanished. In addition, new ways of presenting foods constantly appear. To take just one example, more of the foods supermarkets sell are in the form of ready-to-eat meals.

Food product advertising also is undergoing radical change. Food manufacturers once were content to advertise their products as simply "nutritious," whether or not the item really was. Now manufacturers advertise their foods with specific health claims. You've probably run across some of these claims on TV ads and on the packaging of some of your favorite foods: "heart healthy," "prevents osteoporosis," "good for regularity," and so on.

It's confusing. The signposts you use for judging which foods to buy might as well have an expiration date. The nutritional advice you read just a few years ago is not necessarily helpful now. Worse, it can even be dangerously misleading. In view of the shifting food scene, we need a better way of judging the nutritional value of foods, a standard that won't go out-of-date.

Smart nutrition is a clear way of judging foods, one that works in any current supermarket, deli, and restaurant. It's all about navigating today's constantly shifting food scene—the new products and new ways of food presentation. Smart nutrition gives you a basis for judging foods that satisfies personal tastes and your body's nutritional needs at the same time. Best of all, there is no expiration date on smart nutrition! It's a way of judging food quality that applies to the current situation and is flexible enough to take into account any future changes in food production and marketing.

The three principles of smart nutrition

This book provides you with a set of easy-to-remember guidelines—nutritional landmarks, if

Bright Idea
Even if you've neglected your diet in the past, it's never too late to start making changes. Use the easy-to-follow advice in this book as a starting point to better nutrition for yourself and your family.

you will. These guidelines will serve you far better than any handbook. It would be easy to list the 30,000 items currently sold in a medium-sized supermarket and rate the food quality of each. But what would you gain? You'd have a dictionary-sized volume, one that is clumsy to use and, with so many changing products, soon out-of-date. In this book, however, you'll learn guidelines you can tuck away in the back of your mind, always ready to use.

As you read the following chapters, you see judgments, not between good and bad foods, but of one *type* of food being a better choice than another. For example, under certain circumstances, a fresh vegetable is a better choice than the same vegetable frozen. Under other circumstances the frozen is the better choice. Why? There has to be a basis for making such a judgment. So before getting into more detailed explanations, this introductory chapter lays out the basis for making such food choices, the foundation on which the concept of smart nutrition is built.

To make smart nutrition work for you, we ask questions about three areas:

1. **Science.** What does science—not just nutritional science but all scientific fields—tell us about right food choices? To the greatest extent possible, we should be led by fact, not wishful thinking or myth. Of course, science cannot tell us everything; there are gaps in scientific understanding. In that case, we fill in the gaps with common sense.

2. **Human genes.** Given your genetic heritage, what food choices will give full expression to that heritage? The genes you carry in your body have traveled down through time, generation after generation, millennium after

millennium, from your prehistoric ancestors to the present. Those genes partially dictate how your body responds—for better or for worse—to the food you eat.

3. **Social circumstances.** Considering your lifestyle and stage of life, how can you best enjoy your food and at the same time satisfy your body's nutritional needs? This question puts your nutritional needs into a human context. After all, you don't exist in isolation like a rat caged in a nutrition lab. You have a life. You belong in a certain age group and have a particular family situation. You may travel, eat out a lot, or eat mostly at home; you may like to cook, or maybe not. You may or may not engage in strenuous exercise. Your nutritional needs vary with all these circumstances. So you need to ask how you can meet those needs, whatever your personal circumstances.

In this chapter, we take up the first two principles. The third principle, social circumstances, will be covered in the next chapter.

> 66
> Eating well to improve our chances for a vibrant, long life is a strategy worth exploring.
> —Mary S. Choate, M.S., R.D.
> 99

Genetic heritage and a cell's-eye view of food

The old adage, "You are what you eat," sounds trite, but it's one of those fundamental truths. Your entire body, from brain to toenails, is composed of the food you ate this morning, yesterday, and even within the last seven years. The reason: Your body is constantly falling apart and has to be rebuilt component by component. Some components, such as cell proteins, last a few minutes before they have to be replaced. Other cell proteins last a day. Many are gone by a week. You, of course, don't *look* any different from day to day because the DNA blueprint in every cell ensures that identical body components are inserted in place as rapidly as the old ones break down. The new are rebuilt from the food you eat, as well as the air you breathe and the water you drink.

Because your body's need to rebuild is ongoing, your nutritional needs are ongoing, too. Every day is a new day for your body, a new day for renewal and fresh nutrition.

Genes do not adapt

Suppose a time machine whisked a person from the Stone Age, 100,000 years ago, into today's world. Given a bath and modern clothing, that individual could pass on the street unnoticed. Human bodies haven't changed much in that period. Our genes and our biology are the same. Put another way, the genes and biology we have today evolved in a Stone Age world. What does this mean for modern nutrition? Our ancestors of that era had a biology suited to the foods of the times. They lived as part of the natural environment, eating whatever nature offered in their immediate habitat or, in the case of hunter-gatherers, what could be found in the wider surrounding areas.

One of the remarkable features of human biology, and one that has great significance today, is that so many of our prehistoric ancestors adapted to diverse environments better than any other animal did. Humans are able to thrive on an incredible diversity of foods. The Inuit (once called Eskimos), living in the Arctic, ate a traditional diet largely comprised of blubber and fish. Indigenous people in tropical lands ate fruits, roots, and the occasional small animal. No matter where humans migrated, they lived off whatever foods existed in that region.

Unofficially...
Good health and long life with less incidence of disease result from a four-cornered interaction between your genes, your personal environment, your habits and behaviors, and your food.

You might conclude from this that humans can adapt to any kind of a diet. Far from it. A common thread runs through all that diversity of our ancestors: The foods they ate, whether tropical or polar, were natural, and freshly gathered or freshly killed.

This fact of prehistoric life has enormous significance for life today. While so much of human existence has changed over the millennia, your genes are the same as your 100,000-year-old ancestors. So you are still genetically suited to thrive best on diverse foods in their *natural* state.

Surprisingly, we can't talk of the human body adapting to modern foods, because human biology doesn't change. You may question that statement—after all, everyone knows people who eat junky foods and yet seem to do just fine, right? Wrong. Everyone's long-term health and vitality diminishes, because their biology refuses to adapt to the food they eat.

We have to turn the food-body equation around. Stuck with 100,000-year-old genes, we have to adapt modern foods to human biology. In the practical sense, this means making food choices in the supermarket and deli that best satisfy those old genes. That's smart nutrition.

A cell's-eye view of food

Most nutrition advice you read in magazines and books is given from the viewpoint of food. You see advice such as "Eat liver because it gives you iron." "Drink milk because it has calcium." "Eat leafy vegetables because they give you the vitamin folic acid." These facts are true, but such advice takes food out of context—that is, the context of you, the eater. When you eat a food, whether it's spinach, lettuce, or chicken pot pie, you eat the entire food. From your body's perspective, the entire food counts, not just an isolated component. Your body responds to the total nutrition the food delivers, not just one or two elements in it. So what's the best way to take into account the whole effect of the food you're eating? Rather than looking at nutrition from the food's viewpoint, so to speak, you get a far better understanding of a food's nutritional value by looking at it from your body's viewpoint—what I call a cell's-eye view.

One of the principal tasks of a cell is to rebuild itself. If a cell could talk, the question it would ask is: "From my perspective, does a particular kind of food deliver the building blocks I need?"

Here's an illustration of how the cell's-eye view works in practice. Your brain consists of some trillion cells. Each cell is connected through 6,000 fibers to other cells—your neural network. The components of the cells—the proteins, the fats, and the thousands of other items of each cell and of the 6,000 connecting fibers—are constantly breaking up and must be replaced.

It's a remarkable phenomenon. A brain cell plugs a brand-new component into cell structures as rapidly as the old deteriorates and is taken out of service. The work of the brain carries on undiminished.

A cell's-eye view tells you that no single food component by itself prevents falloff of brain efficiency. Your food must deliver the diverse set of components, all the building blocks the cell needs for renewal. If food quality shortchanges brain cells, for instance, an individual may expect a whole host of undesirable effects, some as severe as irritability and a decrease in short-term memory.

Watch Out!
Carefully scrutinize advice you hear about food. For example, you probably hear stories that eggs are not so great because they contain cholesterol. Yes, eggs do contain cholesterol, but from a cell's-eye view, the egg delivers a package of diverse cell-building blocks. Put in the perspective of total diet, eggs have much to offer.

What is true for brain cells is true for every other body cell, from skin cells to liver cells to heart cells and so on. The cells of different organs have different needs, but they all require a diversity of nutritional components, and they must have a regular supply of them. Even fasting is no exception to this. During fasting, cell renewal does continue, but the body is then forced, in effect, to cannibalize itself. The body draws upon less critical parts of the body, like muscles and the digestive system, so that nutritional components can be made available to high-priority organs like the brain. This of course reduces efficiency and can leads to other problems, as we'll discuss later.

We are concerned in this book with eating right every day, choosing foods from a cell's-eye view. It's a total perspective of what a food offers—or, to be more exact, what a person's total diet offers.

Why do we eat?

Life would be much simpler if we had a body like an insect's. I don't mean having six legs and a head, thorax, and abdomen. I mean having a normal human body, but, like the body of many adult insects, a body that has to be built only once. The hard exoskeleton of an adult insect's body is only produced once—it doesn't need constant replenishing. It lasts a lifetime, albeit a short lifetime, and during that life the insect needs only a little sugar to supply energy for movement.

If this were true for humans, once our bodies were built during childhood, we could get by solely on sugar water as adults. Simple, huh? We can't do this, of course, because as mentioned, the human body is constantly breaking down and must be rebuilt on a daily basis. Food must do more than just supply energy needs.

Thus, from our body's perspective, we eat for at least two purposes:

1. To supply fuel to be burned for energy
2. To supply the building blocks for cell renewal and for cellular products such as hormones, antibodies, and enzymes

Can a single food serve both purposes? Not necessarily. Most foods supply energy, but not all foods supply cell building blocks. You get energy from the sugar in a soft drink, but no building blocks. In contrast, foods like nuts and fresh vegetables supply nutritional building blocks cells can either burn for energy or use for cell renewal.

From a cell's-eye view, it doesn't make any sense, therefore, to choose a food that supplies only energy. We're not insects. We have to have those cell building blocks. Practical nutrition demands we aim for the second purpose.

Your body needs energy for renewal

Every person expends a minimum amount of energy required to sustain her or his body in a waking state. This amount of energy, termed basal metabolic rate (BMR), is the energy you expend lying down not moving any muscles. The term metabolism refers to the collective chemistry occurring in all cells that generates and uses this energy. BMR includes the energy needed for cell renewal, keeping the body warm, and maintaining body functions, such as heart beat, breathing, and mental activity.

The BMR is measured as calories. For women, the BMR typically ranges from 1,200 to 1,450 calories, the equivalent of the energy of a 60-watt light bulb. For men, BMR typically ranges from 1,600 to 1,800 calories. The total amount of energy you expend in a day is the BMR plus energy used for muscular activity.

Consider an average-sized woman, fairly active, burning 2,000 calories a day. If her BMR is at the top of the range, 1,450 calories, she burns about 70 percent of her daily calories just to maintain basic body functions. The remaining 30 percent fuels daily activities. What's more, the BMR is fairly constant regardless of circumstance. If this average-sized woman engages in strenuous activity and burns 3,000 calories, her BMR remains roughly at 1,450 calories. Those additional calories power the big muscles that move the body.

BMR may seem like an abstract concept, far removed from daily life, but it's actually an important factor in weight-loss diets. If you go on a calorie-restricted diet, for example, your BMR still operates at roughly the same fixed rate. So if you aren't eating enough for both physical activity and BMR, your body starts drawing from its own stores to maintain the BMR. Good, you say. You want the BMR to consume that excess fat. But—and this is a big but—a lot of fad diets cause the body to consume not only fat but vital body components as well. It's sort of like chopping up the furniture to keep the fireplace going.

When we take up the topic of fad diets in Chapter 12, "Sensible Weight Loss Versus Fad Diets," you'll learn how to use BMR creatively to avoid that other nightmare of weight-loss diets—weight rebound.

Watch Out!
Be aware of your basal metabolic rate (BMR). You don't have to know exactly what the value is, but remember its function and what it means for your nutritional needs before you engage in any calorie-restricted diet.

Your body needs food for renewal

Most animals of the world are specialized eaters. Carnivores—the lions, sharks, wolves, and eagles of the world—must eat meat. They can't survive on a diet of grass or grain. Herbivores—the cows, antelope, deer, and rabbits of the world—survive wonderfully on grass. They would not do well eating meat. In each case the animal's teeth, digestive system, and body metabolism match its specialized diet.

As already mentioned, humans have far greater flexibility in their choice of food. As omnivores, we are able to eat vegetables, grains, meats, dairy products, and a whole range of other foods. This dietary flexibility enabled early humans to colonize all parts of the globe, and enables us in a contemporary world to enjoy the vast variety of foods offered in food markets.

But flexibility has a limit, and in the case of diet it concerns the daily rebuilding of the body. The body rebuilds its tens of thousands of different components from a basic set of building blocks. While the body can produce some of the building blocks on its own, most it cannot. Most of these building blocks—vitamins and other nutrients—must come from our diet. Thus, while we have great flexibility in our choice of foods, we are chained, so to speak, to the building blocks we need to get from what we eat.

Cell building blocks

Vitamins, minerals, amino acids, water, and fatty acids are nutrients absolutely essential to cell renewal. Nutrition science has identified 40 of these elements, listed in the following table. Each is necessary for life. That means that if any one of these substances is absent from the diet, death eventually ensues, even though the other 39 are present in abundance. No substitutes: That's how essential each is in the diet.

Sounds grim, but in a practical sense, few people in this modern age are dying because of the absence of one of these nutrients. Even a bad diet can often provide enough to keep a person alive.

But mere survival isn't the whole point. Much of what concerns us in this book centers on avoiding dietary deficits. And health disorders can arise from a partial deficit of any one of these nutrients. So truly smart nutrition doesn't focus on getting enough of this or that vitamin or mineral, but on choosing an overall diet that delivers all 40 nutrients in abundance (though not excess).

TABLE 1.1: IDENTIFIED ESSENTIAL NUTRIENTS FOR HUMANS

Category	Nutrient
The essential amino acids of proteins	Histidine
	Isoleucine
	Leucine
	Lysine
	Methionine
	Phenylalanine
	Threonine
	Tryptophane
	Valine
Vitamins, not stored in body	Ascorbic acid (vitamin C)
	Biotin
	Folic acid (folacin)
	Niacinamide (niacin)
	Pantothenic acid
	Pyridoxine (vitamin B_6)
	Riboflavin (vitamin B_2)
	Thiamin (vitamin B_1)
Vitamins, stored in body	Vitamin A
	Vitamin D

	Vitamin E (d-alpha-tocopherol and the d-beta, d-gamma, and d-delta tocopherols)
	Vitamin K
	Vitamin B_{12}
Minerals, needed in relatively large amounts	Calcium
	Chloride
	Magnesium
	Phosphate
	Potassium
	Sodium
Minerals, needed in minor amounts	Cobalt
	Chromium
	Copper
	Fluorine
	Iron
	Iodine
	Manganese
	Molybdenum
	Selenium
	Zinc
Essential fatty acids	Linoleic acid (omega-6)
	Linolenic acid (omega-3)

Essential amino acids and protein requirement

First of all, what is a protein? You may think immediately of muscles. Indeed, muscles are partly composed of protein, but proteins are the entire body's most versatile component. Your hair and nails are almost pure protein. The connective tissue that holds your body together, collagen, is also mostly protein. By far the biggest class of proteins is the *enzymes*. Enzymes, with minerals, carry out the work of cells. In heart cells, enzymes initiate the signals

Moneysaver
You've probably heard rumors that plant protein is inferior to the protein of red meat. Not so. Plant proteins are made from the same 20 amino acids as the proteins of red meat and the proteins of the human body. You save a lot of money by substituting good sources of plant protein, like legumes, for expensive meat and fish.

that cause heart muscle to contract. In the brain, enzymes help keep the electric messages flashing between neurons. Enzymes digest the food you eat.

Proteins are complex substances of varied size, made from among 20 different amino acids. But there are only nine amino acids listed in the table of essential dietary nutrients above. Why? The body is able to make some of the amino acids, the building blocks of protein, on its own. These are called the *nonessential* amino acid. But essential amino acid can only be obtained from protein in the diet.

Now here's the hitch. If the protein in a diet is insufficient to supply all nine of the essential amino acids, the body stops making its own protein, and the body begins to waste away.

O.K., that's the science. What does it mean for our dietary choices? For people eating meat and other high-protein foods, there is no issue. They get all the essential amino acids they need. On the other hand, some weight-loss diets and vegetarian regimens shortchange the protein. This is a dangerous situation. If the individual is a child, growth is retarded, for example. For adults, core body proteins waste away, leading to weakened immune defenses and a host of other body ills.

We'll discuss essential amino acids in greater detail in Chapter 9, "Vegetarianism: Should You Move Towards a Plant-Based Diet?," and Chapter 12, "Sensible Weight Loss Versus Fad Diets."

Get your nonstorable vitamins every day

The vitamins listed in the table of essential nutrients are divided into those the body stores and those it does not. The vitamins that cannot be stored present an urgent challenge. They are rapidly used up in the body's daily metabolism, as well as being washed out in the urine. The challenge comes in making sure you organize your diet so that the foods you eat over the course of the day deliver these vitamins.

How much is enough? These vitamins were originally discovered as nutrients that prevent disease. Niacin, for example, prevents pellagra, a disease that causes insanity. Vitamin C prevents scurvy, a potentially fatal disease common among sailors of past centuries.

Only a small amount of each vitamin is needed to prevent the disease, and so some scientists concluded that that small amount is all a person needed. Not true! We now recognize that higher amounts are needed if optimum body function and health is a goal. This point receives more attention in later chapters.

A special comment about biotin. It is one vitamin in the nonstorable category you don't have to think about. You may never have heard of this vitamin; in fact, you seldom see it listed on bottles of multivitamins. There's a good reason for this: Friendly bacteria in your intestines synthesize the biotin you need.

Vitamins that can be stored

All the storable vitamins on the list, with exception of vitamin B_{12}, dissolve in fat. The body stores any surplus in fatty tissues, making the vitamins available for times when daily intake falls below a minimal level.

The storage feature is especially important for vitamin D. Skin cells contain a substance that, when hit by sunlight, changes into vitamin D. In the Stone Age, no sun, no vitamin D. So people living in seasonal climates had to rely exclusively on the buildup

Bright Idea
When thinking about nutrition, remember the difference between *minimum* and *optimum*. You don't just want to avoid deficiencies, you want to enjoy the benefits of optimum levels of vitamins, minerals, and other nutrients.

Bright Idea
You improve your chances of getting the full spectrum of "minor" (trace) minerals if you include in your daily diet some organically grown products. Organic farmers engage in practices that enhance these minerals in the soil.

of vitamin D during the summer to last during the winter months. Nowadays, of course, people can get vitamin D in supplements and as an additive in milk. But since most people in advanced societies live indoors, and even when outside, many folk dress to avoid sun exposure, we might get even less vitamin D from the sun than our ancestors did. So dietary intake of vitamin D may become just as important as with the other vitamins.

Vitamin B_{12} is stored in the liver, which has special proteins that capture the vitamin. From a practical viewpoint, as in the case of the fat-soluble vitamins, daily intake is not critical to health—as long as you get sufficient B_{12} on a regular basis.

Minerals

Mineral deficiency is often a greater problem than vitamin deficiency. Minerals like iron, calcium, and so forth are the basic, unchangeable elements of Planet Earth. They cannot be synthesized or destroyed by any organic process. We depend on plants to absorb minerals from the ground, but plants absorb only what is in the soil. Mineral distribution in soil is uneven, varying from region to region. In addition, modern agriculture heavily fertilizes crops with artificial fertilizer, which may not contain the full spectrum of minerals. So the amounts and spectrum of minerals in a food product depend on where the crop was grown and on the amount of processing. Food processing tends to wash out minerals, because most are readily soluble in water. The net result is that a person's diet can easily be deficient in one or more of the minerals.

Your total daily intake of all the minerals is roughly 1.5 grams (a heaping $1/4$ teaspoon), not much compared to the 2 to $2 1/2$ pounds of food (dry weight) you eat every day. But their role is crucial. Minerals are enablers—each enables a part of the complex cell machinery to work. Iron, for instance, is built into hemoglobin, the blood protein that carries oxygen from lungs to body tissues and carbon dioxide back to the lungs. Hemoglobin just doesn't work without iron. And each of the minerals listed in the table of essential nutrients is just as vital as iron. Total absence of any leads to death.

As the table indicates, minerals are grouped into two categories, depending on whether the daily requirement is less or more than 100 milligrams.

To recap, keep in mind the following three points about vitamins and minerals:

1. Ingest necessary nonstorable vitamins every day.

2. Eat a variety of fresh fruits and vegetables to ensure you get the full spectrum of vitamins and minerals. Processing washes them out of foods.

3. Don't worry so much about *individual* vitamins and minerals. The key to smart nutrition is choosing foods from a cell's-eye view. Your body needs every one of the known nutrients—as well as any not yet discovered.

Carbohydrates: Complex and Simple

For most people, carbohydrates supply 50 percent or more of daily calories (protein provides around 15 percent, fat around 33 percent). As the name implies, *carbohydrates* are built from carbon and water. With the exception of lactose in milk, all nutritionally important carbohydrates are produced by plants. Meats, meat products, and dairy products like cheeses (where the lactose is removed) provide insignificant amounts of carbohydrates.

For nutritional purposes, we divide the carbo-hydrates into two categories:

- **Complex.** These are the starches of grains, potatoes, and vegetables.

- **Simple.** These are the sugars. The ones of major nutritional importance are sucrose (table sugar), lactose (milk sugar), fructose (fruit sugar), and glucose (the sugar derived from corn syrup).

Watch Out!
Don't think of carbohydrates simply as a source of energy. Think of the foods they are in. If all you needed were the carbs, you could just eat candy bars all day. But whole grain cereals and fresh vegetables deliver carbohydrate as starch, together with vitamin and mineral cell builders, and fiber.

Carbohydrates are a major source of fuel or energy. Whether complex or simple, the body digests the carbohydrate and converts it to glucose. Glucose is the sugar that circulates in the blood, and for that reason it is often referred to as *blood sugar.* The brain derives over 80 percent of its energy from blood glucose. If blood glucose falls below a certain level, you feel faint. The reason? Not enough fuel reaches the brain to keep you conscious.

A big mistake nutrition advisers often make is to lump all carbohydrates under a single heading. You see this one word on the nutrition labels of many products: *carbohydrate.* True, starches and the simple sugars end up in the body as blood glucose, but the way your body responds to each differs enormously. This is because of the speed of digestion. Starches take time to digest, so glucose trickles into the blood at a rate the body easily handles. Sugars, in contrast, zip through the intestines at a high speed and are dumped into the blood. In some people, the over-load can make a person jittery—think "sugar high."

What about sugars in fruits? Do they cause glu-cose overload in blood? No, because the sugar of fruits is encased in fibrous structures. When you eat a fruit, the sugar is released slowly. This braking action, however, is largely cancelled if the fruit is juiced.

Fat and cholesterol

Nature designed fat as a concentrated energy form. A gram of fat delivers 9 calories, while a gram of carbohydrate or protein delivers only 4 calories. Plant seeds store fat (in the form of oils) as energy to be used when the seed germinates. Animals store layers of fat to serve as insulation as well as emergency fuel in times of food scarcity. We need a minimum of 15 to 25 grams of fat a day to supply sufficient amounts of the essential fatty acids and to aid in absorption of the fat-soluble vitamins (A, D, E, and K).

Chapter 4, "Extracted Fats and Oils" has a detailed explanation of how to get more essential fatty acids in your diet.

Apart from the issue of essential fatty acids, not eating enough fat is hardly a problem for most folks. Americans, on average, get 35 percent of their calories from fat because of the high percentage of animal foods in their diet. Plant foods—the grains and vegetables—contain relatively little fat. Meat, on the other hand, consists solely of protein and fat; it has very little carbohydrates (glycogen). Many people have the mistaken idea that if they trim the visible fat from a piece of meat, they remove the fat. Not at all. In spite of the removal of all this fat, cooked meat (say, a beef roast) delivers 50 percent of calories from protein and 50 percent from fat.

When we talk about animal fat we should also mention cholesterol. This substance occurs only in animals and is always associated with fat. Whole milk contains cholesterol, for example, which is dissolved in the milk fat. Thus when whole milk is separated into cream and skim milk, the cholesterol remains dissolved in the cream. Skim milk is relatively free of cholesterol; the butter made from the cream is where the cholesterol winds up.

From a nutritional point of view, you consume cholesterol every time you eat animal fat in the form of butter, cheese, meat, fish, eggs, and the like. Cholesterol, however, is more than a passenger in animal fat. It is an essential cell building block. Every cell in the body depends on cholesterol to form the cell membrane which envelopes and holds the cell together. Cholesterol is the glue, so to speak, that binds together the membrane that surrounds each cell. Think of it as the stitching in a suit of clothes—if you remove the stitches, the garment falls apart. Similarly, without cholesterol, your brain would stop functioning and your nervous system would collapse. In short, you'd be dead.

Fortunately, your liver makes all the cholesterol the body needs, about 1.5 grams a day, so you don't need any cholesterol in your diet.

Icing on the nutritional cake— fiber and phytochemicals

Traditional nutrition science focused on what the human body needs to survive—a matter of life or death. That focus is turning now to a goal more sophisticated than sheer survival—a quest for optimum well-being. This brings us to two substances that are key to achieving optimum nutrition—fiber and phytochemicals. True, you can survive without them. But new studies show you'll never achieve a healthful nirvana unless you welcome fiber and phytochemicals in your diet.

Fiber and phytochemicals (*phyto* means "plant-related") exist only in the plant world. They are completely absent from meats, meat products, and

Unofficially...
There is a big difference between an adequate diet and an optimum diet, according to J. Bruce German, professor of food science and technology, U.C. Davis. An optimum diet includes a generous amount of fiber which is necessary to keep the cells that line the gut wall healthy. Healthy cells absorb nutrients more effectively.

dairy foods. You've heard the mantra: "Eat your vegetables." Your mother's advice was even more sound than she realized. Eating vegetables helps ensure you get these vital substances in your diet.

Fiber smoothes passage through the digestive system

The traditional definition of fiber is a food substance that is not digested and passes through the bowel—"aiding regularity," to use an advertising phrase. That's a bit simplistic. The term *fiber* covers multiple substances that are on the whole indigestible—that is, indigestible to you. But keep in mind that the lower bowel is full of microbes. The microbial inhabitants are critical to one's health, and one thing that keeps the microbes healthy is the fiber you eat.

The interaction between fiber, microbes, and host—you—is complex and, at this point in time, poorly understood. But we do know that this interaction aids the absorption of important nutrients.

If we graded people on how much fiber they get in their diet, most would fail, for two reasons. First, the standard American diet favors meat and dairy products, neither of which furnishes fiber. Second, much of the fiber of grains is located in the bran, which is discarded during the refining process. Even so-called enriched flour contains almost no fiber. Good sources of fiber are vegetables, unrefined grains, beans, nuts, and fruits.

Phytochemicals, the new wonder substances

Phytochemicals, in a broad sense, refer to any chemical in plants. Technically, that could include vitamins, fiber, and, for that matter, carbohydrates. The term as used in the nutrition world, however, is

Bright Idea
Instead of drinking a glass of orange juice from a carton, peel an orange and eat it. That way, you'll get the full benefit of the orange's fiber.

restricted to a group of plant chemicals that aren't vitamins or other traditional nutrients. Plant cells, like cells of the human body, manufacture thousands and thousands of substances. When we eat a plant food, we ingest all the phytochemicals it contains.

We now recognize their importance to overall nutritional well-being. Consider vitamin A, for example. If you take a vitamin A supplement, the active substance in the pill very likely is beta-carotene. The body converts beta-carotene to vitamin A, and for this reason beta-carotene is often called *provitamin A*. So you might think that as long as you obtain sufficient beta-carotene, you're doing fine, whether it comes from a pill or from yellow vegetables (such as carrots, squash, and sweet potatoes).

In fact, however, plants, particularly the leafy vegetables, produce hundreds of carotenes beside the beta. We don't know exactly what all these other carotenes do in the human body. We do know, however, that a spectrum of carotenes benefits the body more than just the beta alone.

Carotenes represent one type of phytochemicals. There are thousands more. We take up in more detail the issue of phytochemicals in the diet when we talk about fruits and vegetables (Chapter 2, "Fruits and Vegetables") and again when we talk about food supplements (Chapter 8, "To Supplement or Not to Supplement Is No Longer the Question").

The overall message: Balance your diet

The lists of vitamins, minerals, proteins, fats, and so forth nutrition science has given us serves as a backdrop. But they don't help much when we're cruising the aisles of the local supermarket. What foods should we actually select to achieve a balanced diet?

And what is a balanced diet? No single food delivers a complete set of required nutrients. Therefore, you have to eat a variety of foods, which leads to a definition for a balanced diet.

> *All the foods you eat over the course of the day provide an optimum amount of every nutrient, and that includes those important non-nutrients like fiber and phytochemicals.*

This definition still doesn't help in the supermarket, unfortunately. We have to translate the idea of a balanced diet into what foods to actually choose.

Advice on what foods to eat is nothing new. Practically every book and article written on food and eating offers a guide on how to achieve balance in what you eat. But how practical are all these food guides? The three questions you want answered about a guide are:

1. Does the guide work in the modern supermarket and restaurant?

2. Does the guide work within your lifestyle and stage of life?

3. Does the guide work within the way you like to eat?

Most nutrition guides fail these questions. While good on the theory of creating a balanced diet, they are short on practical advice. What should you actually choose in the 30,000-item supermarket? The official nutrition guide of the United States government illustrates the shortcomings of such guides. This guide to a balanced diet, created by the Department of Agriculture (USDA), is called the *Food Guide Pyramid* (see figure on the following page).

> 66
> It's an inescapable reality that most people, nutritionists included, do not wish to count nutrients every time they walk down the aisle of a supermarket or sit down for a meal.
> —Joan Dye Gussow, Ed.D., former chair, Department of Nutrition Education, Columbia University Teacher's College
> 99

The USDA Food Guide Pyramid

The USDA Food Guide Pyramid divides foods into six groups. The pyramid shape is designed to indicate the relative importance of the different categories. Grains form the base, with fruits and vegetables located in the next rank above. Animal products—dairy and meats—are assigned to the third rank. The meat category also includes meat substitutes. At the apex, you see added sugars, such as those in soft drinks, candy, and sweet cakes, and added fats, such as salad oil and butter or margarine.

USDA says that for a balanced diet, you should choose servings from each category every day. The USDA's advice stops short of advising which food products within each category to choose.

The Food Guide Pyramid developed by the U.S. Department of Agriculture (USDA), 1992.

A Guide to Daily Food Choices

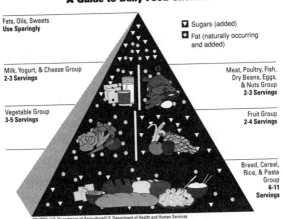

Fats, Oils, Sweets
Use Sparingly

☑ Sugars (added)
☐ Fat (naturally occurring and added)

Milk, Yogurt, & Cheese Group
2-3 Servings

Meat, Poultry, Fish, Dry Beans, Eggs, & Nuts Group
2-3 Servings

Vegetable Group
3-5 Servings

Fruit Group
2-4 Servings

Bread, Cereal, Rice, & Pasta Group
6-11 Servings

SOURCE: U.S. Department of Agriculture/U.S. Department of Health and Human Services

If you look closely at the pyramid, you see that it doesn't answer the previous three questions that would help tailor the guide to your life, and here's why:

1. **The pyramid graphics are unrealistic.** Notice anything odd about the pyramid's graphics? Do

they look like food products you see filling shopping carts in the supermarket? Certainly not. The graphics give no indication that much of the food people eat has been processed; processing, as we'll see in coming chapters, can radically diminish the nutritional value of foods. One can follow the Food Guide Pyramid to the letter while selecting white bread in the grain category, french fries in the vegetable category, canned fruit cocktail in the fruit category, ice cream for dairy, and hot dogs for meat. While satisfying the Food Guide Pyramid, such food choices would horribly unbalance the work of the body's cells.

2. **The pyramid is written by many hands.**
   Government food guides have many authors, and some of the loudest are those of the dairy and meat industries. These industries make sure that a guide sanctioned by the government promotes their interests. Although the dairy and meat categories wound up on the pyramid's third rank, because of the relatively high number of servings, these two categories account for 40 percent of the pyramid's total calories.

There are many roads to a balanced diet

The USDA Food Guide Pyramid is only one way to construct a balanced diet. It is not a realistic guide for people living in areas where dairy products are rarely eaten and meat is eaten only occasionally. Peoples in these areas can eat well-balanced diets constructed quite differently than that indicated by the USDA Food Guide Pyramid. There's nothing magic about the pyramid.

Watch Out!
The federal government has passed laws that say a drug must be effective. A drug marketed to relieve headaches, for instance, must relieve headaches. But the government has yet to pass a law that says a food product has to be nutritious.

There is, in fact, huge flexibility in the way you arrive at a balanced diet. A goal of this book is to show you how to achieve a balanced diet that fits your lifestyle and your stage of life, a diet that suits you personally.

Two views of health

You can see in this introductory chapter that smart nutrition combines nutrition science, common sense, and an eye towards our biological heritage. Our genes govern the nutritional framework within which we must work—something we cannot forget. This is the cell's-eye view.

Finally, why concern ourselves at all about nutrition? The ultimate reward, of course, is health and vitality. But smart nutrition raises the level of what that phrase "health and vitality" means.

The traditional view of health is that if you are not in a doctor's office or don't need medical services, you must be healthy. In other words, you are able to more or less get through your daily life, even if you take heartburn pills, lack energy, sleep poorly, or suffer a sluggish bowel.

Human biology offers far greater potential, more than staying out of a doctor's office. In contrast to this limited view, a holistic view describes health as vital and vigorous living, a style of life exploiting all the wonders endowed by one's human heritage.

This book embraces the holistic view as a goal. Choose foods that, whatever your stage of life, whatever your living circumstances, whatever your taste preference, foster maximum health and vitality.

> " There is an internal urge to be healthy and vigorous.
> —Roger Williams, vitamin pioneer "

Just the facts

- You make better food choices if you look at foods from your body's perspective—a cell's-eye view.

- Don't choose foods solely to give you energy. If you choose foods that give your body the building blocks for cell renewal, energy needs will also be taken care of.

- Don't worry about getting enough of this or that vitamin. Think in terms of total diet, of getting the full spectrum of vitamins, minerals, and other nutrients, including fiber and phyto-chemicals.

- The USDA Food Guide Pyramid, the official government guide to balanced nutrition, is only one of thousands of ways of selecting foods to give you a balanced diet.

Smart Nutrition in Your Basic Food Categories

PART II

GET THE SCOOP ON...
Why fresh is better than frozen • Why frozen is
better than canned • The best way of preparing
vegetables • Nutritional rip-offs in fruit juices •
The advantages of going organic

Fruits and Vegetables

"Eat five servings of fruits and vegetables every day." How often have you seen that command repeated in practically every article and book on food and health? Yet in real life, four out of ten adults eat two or less servings a day of fruit and vegetables—and the "vegetable" serving is usually french fries. Five out of ten people eat only three servings. That leaves only one person out of ten who gets the full five servings.

Why care if you eat fewer than the five servings? Is there something magic about the number five? Not really, but you should consider that number, if anything, a bare-bones *minimum.*

Medical authorities who study the health benefits of fruits and vegetables say that it takes five servings to gain those benefits, such as a lower chance of heart disease, stroke, and cancer. For many young people and those in the prime of life, those deadly or debilitating diseases seem too remote to worry about. But there's also a more immediate reason for eating fruit and vegetables: They affect how you feel this moment, the energy you have, and the smooth trafficking of your mental processes. In this chapter, we'll look in greater detail at the benefits of increasing the number and quality of fruits and vegetables in your diet.

Potassium—what a cell needs most

A cell's-eye view of fruits and vegetables gives us one explanation of why they are so important. It's all about one mineral—potassium. Body cells are full of fluid, distinct from blood. Whereas sodium is the principal mineral in blood, the fluid inside cells is loaded with potassium. The potassium helps prevent cells from collapsing from fluid loss. You've seen what happens when a broccoli stalk or carrot loses moisture: The vegetable goes limp. This is a good metaphor for what happens with people. When cells lose potassium, they lose water. Then they collapse enough to lose efficiency, and *you* collapse, too—you start to feel a lack of pep.

But that's not the only benefit of potassium. It is critical for speedy nerve transmission. In extreme cases, when brain cells have insufficient potassium, efficiency plummets, signals misfire, and one's ability to think straight diminishes. Emotional equilibrium may also suffer.

Here's the nutritional problem. Your body constantly loses potassium in the urine, and therefore you have to eat sufficient potassium to replace the daily loss. Guess what are the best sources of potassium? Fruits and vegetables, of course.

What about sodium? It's a necessary mineral, too. But most people's diets have a high level of salt (sodium chloride), and moreover the human body conserves sodium, and, in fact, not much is needed in the diet. Sodium is not an issue; the real dietary issue is getting enough potassium into your body.

Unofficially...
A goal of five servings of fruits and vegetables is intended for a sedentary woman eating about 1,500 calories per day. Men and active women, with their larger caloric intake, should in fact eat *nine* servings a day.

Look, for example, at the potassium and sodium content of foods listed in the following table.

TABLE 2.1: POTASSIUM AND SODIUM LEVELS IN DIFFERENT FOODS (IN MG PER 100 CALORIES OF FOOD VALUE)

Food	Potassium	Sodium
Apple	189	2
Asparagus	1,069	8
Banana	435	1
Green beans	760	21
Apple pie	31	121
Pork and beans	172	380
Frankfurter	71	356

(*Source:* USDA Handbook No. 8)

As this table suggests, while processed foods provide some potassium, they also deliver excessive sodium, which in some people leads to high blood pressure. You can see from the table that fruits and vegetables deliver high levels of potassium without the high level of sodium.

Don't make excuses

Why is it so hard for the average consumer to eat the recommended complement of fruit and vegetables? Ask a random group of shoppers why they don't buy and eat more fruits and vegetables, and they give two stock answers:

- They are too expensive
- They are too much trouble to prepare

But how compelling are these reasons?

"Too expensive"

Of course, like any other food, fruits and vegetables cost money. But you should look at expenses beyond the immediate cost of the food. Suppose, for example, that you take medication for a chronic

Watch Out!
Thinking of taking a potassium supplement to make sure you get enough of this essential mineral? Think again. Unless you do so under advice of a doctor, you risk overloading. Stick to fruits and vegetables—with them, it is impossible to overload.

condition such as high blood pressure or adult-onset diabetes. Adding more fruits and vegetables to your life may enable you to take less of the drugs, or eliminate them altogether (after consulting with your doctor, of course). That's a savings. More importantly, fruits and vegetables erect a first-line defense against disease, reducing the likelihood that chronic, diet-related disease will start in the first place. More savings.

And compared to another food you might eat, the actual cost of fruits and vegetables may be less. Say you're hungry and want a snack. Compare the price of an orange or apple with a bag of potato chips or a candy bar. Your pocketbook wins with the fruit, and your body wins with a spectrum of cell builders.

"Too much trouble to prepare"

Supermarkets sell many fresh vegetables washed, shredded or sliced, and bagged. They are ready to be cooked or eaten right from the package. Lettuce, for example, is washed more thoroughly than you can at home. There is a downside to the sliced vegetables, because slicing exposes surfaces to air oxidation and a loss of certain vitamins. If, however, the choice is between the bagged, fresh vegetable and no vegetable at all, take the bagged.

Finally, you can always open a package of frozen vegetables. They are not as nutritious as fresh, as we'll discuss later, but if you're strapped for time, go for the frozen.

What's a serving?

Government officials and nutritionists love to talk about servings—as in the phrase "five daily servings of fruit and vegetables"—but they seldom explain

Bright Idea
If you want to have ready-to-eat fruits and vegetables on hand without a lot of preparation, pick up fresh salad from your supermarket salad bar when you do your grocery shopping. Just be sure to choose items that are really fresh, not canned items.

what they mean by the term. Here's a quick guide. Each of the following items represent one serving:

- 3½ asparagus spears
- 1 small beet
- Boston lettuce (¼ head)
- green beans (10)
- 1 medium-size carrot
- 1 smallish potato
- 1 medium-size parsnip
- Swiss chard (2 leaves, stems removed)
- 1 small turnip
- 1 medium apple
- 1 medium banana
- 1 medium orange

Appendix D includes a table that further explains these serving sizes.

Let's say you want to eat five servings of vegetables. Sounds overwhelming, doesn't it? But let's look at how that amount might look on a dinner plate. Two servings of cooked squash, two of carrots, and one of green beans covers about one-third of a 10-inch-diameter dinner plate, with plenty of room left for other items.

Here are some simple tips for bringing more fresh fruit and vegetables into your diet:

- Snack on fruit instead of potato chips.
- Add fruit (such as raisins, sliced bananas or apples, or fresh blueberries) to your morning cereal.
- Use the salad bar at a supermarket or restaurant.

- Drink freshly squeezed juice instead of soft drinks.

- Buy prewashed and prepared vegetables.

A quick guide to fruits and vegetables

The mantra "Eat five servings of fruits and vegetables daily" doesn't help you understand which form of these foods you should eat. Not all fruit and vegetable products are created equal. Processing can markedly lower the nutritional quality of fruit and vegetables; for example, peas and carrots in a can have less dietary value than fresh peas and carrots. So if you're trying to improve your diet by boosting your intake of fruits and vegetables, it doesn't make sense to eat products of lesser quality.

To help you understand what ranks as better and worse quality, take a look at the following table.

TABLE 2.2: A GUIDE TO THE NUTRITIONAL RANKING OF FRUITS AND VEGETABLES

Quality Scale	Fruits	Vegetables
1st Rank	Raw	Fresh, raw
2nd Rank	Frozen	Fresh, lightly cooked
3rd Rank	Dried	Frozen
4th Rank	Canned	Canned

The Quick Guide is meant to give you an easy-to-understand rule of thumb when you have to make quick decisions about what to buy and eat. It has no complex rules or tables of specific products. Just remember: Canned is better than nothing at all; frozen is better than canned; for vegetables, fresh, lightly cooked is better than frozen; and fresh and raw is best of all. You also need to use common sense. You wouldn't eat potatoes raw, but most vegetables can be eaten this way.

Unofficially...
Have you ever tried to delude yourself that a cherry roll-up counted as a serving of fruit? You're in good company. In 1981, in a budget-cutting move, the USDA declared that ketchup counted as a serving of vegetables for government-funded school lunch programs. Luckily, outraged nutritionists and parents forced the USDA to reverse its decision.

This guide works whatever your location and lifestyle. You may live in an area where fresh produce is readily available, or you may not. Perhaps you shop only once a week. So instead of trying to follow a one-size-fits-all guide, just select a fruit or vegetable product as high up as possible on the quality scale, whatever your life circumstances. If you like peas but simply don't have time to shell fresh peas, choose frozen over canned.

Of course, you'll still have to exercise some judgment. Wilted, "fresh" string beans kept too long in the refrigerator aren't necessarily going to be better than frozen string beans. So, to help you sharpen your common sense and understand the principles behind the guide, let's run through the four levels—first for the vegetables, then the fruits.

Vegetables: Canned, frozen, and fresh

Keep in mind that a harvested vegetable is still a living organism, composed of cells. Life doesn't cease when a carrot is dug up or a lettuce head separated from its roots. Harvested lettuce heads, carrots, and string beans breathe just like we do. Not with lungs, of course, but each cell consumes oxygen. Enzymes work and life processes continue, all necessary to keep the vegetable tissue firm and fresh. The stronger those post-harvest life processes are, the higher the nutritional value will be. Once harvested, however, the vegetable's living processes start slowing down.

Here's the practical problem: How do you conserve nutritional value between the time of harvest and the time of consumption? In particular, how do you do it when the consumer lives 3,000 miles from the grower? The common solution is canning,

Moneysaver
If you are trying to lose weight, fruits and vegetables will help you achieve your goal *and* save you money. They deliver solid nutritional value with a minimum of calories. Eat more fruits and vegetables and your chances for weight loss are excellent, and it's much cheaper than going to a weight-loss clinic or buying expensive (and potentially harmful) pills.

freezing, or refrigerated trucking. Each method of preservation presents challenges for the consumer.

When is "fresh" fresh?

For storage purposes, vegetables fall into two main categories—the short-keepers and the long-keepers. *Short-keepers* are the aboveground vegetables, such as lettuces, broccoli, green beans, and so on. *Long-keepers* are generally the belowground vegetables, such as turnips, carrots, potatoes, and parsnips. (One exception is winter squash, which also keeps well.)

Short-keepers present a serious challenge. Within 24 hours of picking, broccoli and other green vegetables lose about one-third of their vitamin C, even when refrigerated. Unless you grow your own vegetables and rush them from garden to plate, there's no point worrying about this initial 24 hours—you can't do anything about it. The good news is that after that initial free fall, the rate of vitamin C loss decreases. And while vitamin C is sensitive to post-harvest loss, other vitamins, phytochemicals, and minerals are more stable. Still, the faster the vegetables travel between field and plate, the better.

For people living on the East Coast and Midwest, vegetables from California and Mexico can take 5 to 7 days to truck. Local distribution adds at least 2 more days. Of course, there's no way to determine exactly how long vegetables have been in transit, or whether they've sat unrefrigerated on a sunny loading dock. You'll have to use your best judgment when you go to purchase them.

Keep in mind these four points when choosing and using fresh produce:

- Check for appearance, crispness, and color.

- On warm days, take a large cooler in your car to keep produce cool on the way home.

- Don't plan to store the short-keepers long in your refrigerator. Use them within a few days.

- Buy local produce in season.

Root vegetables present less of a problem. Commercial warehouses closely control humidity and temperature and can store these vegetables several months with minimal deterioration. Your home refrigerator, unfortunately, is not as well controlled. The big enemy is moisture loss. Minimize the loss by putting vegetables in your refrigerator's crisper, the box or drawer that helps retain moisture. And use your root vegetables within a week or two of purchase, before they show signs of softening or mold. (Mold itself is not necessarily dangerous; it's just a sign of deterioration.)

Eat raw vegetables every day

That admonition to eat five servings of fruits and vegetables daily includes raw vegetables, preferably leafy ones. The leaves of a plant are its biological engines, where it produces a range of vitamins as well as phytochemicals by the thousands. You can take full advantage of this nutritional cornucopia by eating a freshly made salad. Caution: When choosing lettuce, choose a dark, leafy variety over iceberg lettuce. This lettuce, the result of industrial craftsmanship, is designed to keep—seemingly, forever. *Iceberg*, as the name implies, is mostly water, with very few living cells and therefore less nutrients than its more robust neighbors on the produce counter. Supermarkets now stock a variety of densely green, tasty, and nutritional lettuces. Choose those and enjoy!

Bright Idea
When you buy fresh beets from a produce stand, don't discard the leafy-green tops. They are highly nutritious. Steam the tops lightly 2 to 4 minutes the day of purchase—they won't stay fresh long. The beet roots keep much longer, however.

(Incidentally, one way to judge a restaurant's quality is to observe the house salad or salad bar. If you see iceberg lettuce, thumbs down.)

Safe handling of fresh vegetables

We often pay little attention to how we prepare vegetables, but by following these tips, you'll have safer, tastier, and more satisfying dishes:

- Wash hands with warm water and soap for at least 20 seconds before and after handling food. Clean under your fingernails, too. And wash your hands between preparing raw meat and fish and preparing fresh fruits and vegetables.

- Rinse raw produce in warm water. Don't use soap or other detergents. If necessary and appropriate, use a small scrub brush to remove surface dirt.

- Use smooth, durable, and nonabsorbent cutting boards that can be cleaned and sanitized easily. Wash with hot water, soap, and a scrub brush to remove food particles. They can also be washed in an automatic dishwasher.

- If you prefer wood boards, keep the fruit and vegetable board separate from the one you use to cut raw meat. Rinse immediately after use. Don't let juices soak into the wood.

- Store in the refrigerator cut, peeled, and broken-apart fruit and vegetables (such as melon balls) at or below 41°F (5°C).

- When buying from a salad bar, avoid fruit and vegetables that look brownish, slimy, or dried out. These are signs that the product has been stored at an improper temperature.

Watch Out!
Red hot chilies contain capsaicin (pronounced *cap-SAY-sun*), the chemical that makes them hot. While capsaicin doesn't bother the tough interior of the stomach, it can burn your eyes and face. Wear plastic or rubber gloves when handling chilies.

Don't overcook fresh vegetables

Heat destroys living tissue. In fact, that's the very reason we cook vegetables, to break down tissue and make the vegetables softer. Unfortunately, heat also destroys delicate vitamins. And if you cook in boiling water, minerals, vitamins, and phytochemicals will leach into the water. Cooking is therefore a balancing act between softening the vegetables and minimizing nutrient loss. Of all cooking methods, steaming provides the best control with minimal leaching. And the water can be used for soups or other purposes.

The nutritional value of the vegetable, once cooked, goes downhill in a hurry. Cooked vegetables should be eaten immediately. A baked potato loses 60 percent of its vitamin C within an hour of coming out of the oven. And, no matter what your mom told you about not wasting food, don't bother to keep leftover vegetables. They continue to lose nutritional value in the refrigerator and, worse, are rapidly colonized by bacteria. Uncooked vegetables, while alive, have natural defenses against bacterial infection. Cooked vegetables have no defense.

Does freezing retain nutritional value?

Why are frozen vegetables listed one step lower in the Quick Guide? In theory, they should be as good as fresh. Processing plants are generally located in the areas where vegetables are grown and harvested, so the vegetables are processed within a few hours of picking. In theory, their nutritional quality would be preserved. Right? Well, freezing, like cooking, is destructive. The trick is to minimize that destruction.

Vegetables to be frozen are first blanched for about 2 minutes by immersion in boiling water or

Bright Idea
Expand your repertoire of vegetables. Try celeriac, a starchy root also called knob celery or celery root. It looks like an angry squid, but once peeled the flesh can be grated into a salad. It can also be steamed and mashed like potatoes or braised alongside a meat. However prepared, celeriac livens a dish.

steam. Blanching is done to deactivate enzymes that would cause the vegetable to go soft and mushy. But this cooking, brief as it is, causes tissue destruction. Cell walls are breached and water leaks out, carrying with it some of the vitamin and mineral content.

Following blanching, the vegetables are frozen, generally with a blast of air at a temperature equivalent to Antarctica in winter. This flash-freezing minimizes further tissue destruction that would result from the formation of ice crystals.

There are nutritional losses to this point, but probably no more serious than home cooking of fresh vegetables. But the transportation of frozen vegetables from the frozen food plant to you, the consumer, creates further opportunity for nutritional losses.

First, there is the problem of time. You may think of frozen foods as being in a state of suspended animation. This is not true. The same natural processes of deterioration you see in fresh vegetables operate in the frozen state, albeit slower. Frozen vegetables contain a number of powerful enzymes that escape blanching. These enzymes keep on working, causing slow degradation and creating unpleasant odors, just as fresh vegetables can go bad. The longer frozen vegetables are stored, the more they degrade.

Second, there's human nature. In a perfect world, frozen vegetables would be transported to your local supermarket, kept in Arctic cold the whole way. But the world of frozen food transport is not perfect. Frozen vegetables move though several warehouses on the way to the supermarket. Careless handling allows the frozen packages to thaw and then be refrozen—often several times. Every time the vegetable cycles through thawing and refreezing, the tissue breaks down further. More minerals and vitamins leak out, and taste flattens.

When you see the frozen package in the supermarket, however, you have no way of knowing how long the food has been stored or whether or not it has been thawed and refrozen. What's more, freezers in many supermarkets operate above optimum storage temperatures. The result is yet more deterioration.

In spite of all this, frozen vegetables still offer good nutritional value, just not as much as quality fresh vegetables. Note the word "quality." Always exercise common sense. If the choice is between a slightly wilted fresh vegetable and the same vegetable in a frozen package, the frozen may be the wiser choice.

Remember these five tips when selecting a frozen vegetable:

1. Select firm packages. Avoid packages that are limp, wet, or sweating—these are signs that the vegetables are in the process of defrosting.

2. Avoid packages stained by the contents or with ice on the outside. They may have been defrosted and refrozen at some stage during transport. The contents may be safe to eat, but refrozen vegetables will normally not taste as good as freshly frozen vegetables.

3. Use vegetables immediately after defrosting to avoid loss of quality.

4. Pass up vegetables that come in a sauce. The sauce can mask poor vegetable quality.

5. If you store frozen vegetables for any length of time in a home freezer, label the package with the date you bought the item. If your freezer

Watch Out! Avoid letting frozen foods thaw before you're ready to prepare them for eating. When in the supermarket, buy frozen items last. Plan to get them home and into a freezer as fast as possible. Have a cooler in the car.

operates at 10°F, discard the item after 3 months. If your freezer maintains 0°F, discard after 1 year.

Canned vegetables—the bottom quality level

Canning is the oldest of modern food preservation methods. It goes back to the beginning of the 19th century, when Napoleon sought a way to preserve food for his troops. The canning-factory equipment may be modern, but the process hasn't changed much in 200 years. The food is sealed in a can and cooked at a temperature far above the boiling point (240°F/116°C) for 30 to 90 minutes—the equivalent of boiling vegetables on the stove for 2 hours. The vegetables' tissue collapses. Vitamin C, thiamin, niacin, and riboflavin levels are reduced severely, and flavor is lost.

Manufacturers don't apply all this heat to make the vegetables tender. Rather, prolonged heating is used to destroy canning's arch villain, the bacterium *Clostridium botulinum.* This bacteria thrives in the airless cans, so every last spore must be eliminated. If the bacteria grows in the can it creates a toxin, the cause of the fatal disease botulism.

Heating destroys the toxin, so if contaminated food is cooked after opening the can, no problem. Manufacturers worry, however, that people often eat the contents cold, hence the extraordinary high processing temperature. In any case, a can with a bulging end plate warns you of bacterial action. Discard it.

After canning, vegetables continue to deteriorate slowly, particularly if stored above 75°F. The taste of the vegetables diminishes, to say the least. The vitamins mentioned above continue to disintegrate, protein quality diminishes, and fat oxidizes.

You'd be wise not to store canned vegetables longer than a year. It's a question of taste, not safety. Canned vegetables recovered from a ship wrecked a hundred years ago were sterile, but not very appetizing.

Although canned vegetables rank at the bottom of the Quick Guide, keep circumstances in mind. Tomatoes are a case in point. Tomatoes arriving in the northern states during the cold months are generally rock-solid and tasteless. In that case, canned tomatoes may be the better choice. But in the summer, fresh, locally grown tomatoes win hands down.

Don't count fries as a vegetable serving

Since we're talking about vegetables, you might be wondering about that highly popular potato dish, french fries. They are in a class by themselves. In fact, they are off the quality scale completely. Fries are cooked in a hot bath of fat. A substantial amount of the fat penetrates and coats the potato sticks. As a result, 40 percent of the caloric value of fries comes from added fat. A serving of french fries delivers about 20 grams of fat, about four teaspoons. Eat them for pleasure if your wish, but from a cell's-eye view, they offer little nutrition benefit.

Fruits are nutritional powerhouses

All fruits are nutritional powerhouses and can be eaten fresh. You may have seen tables where fruits are ranked according to their levels of vitamin C and other vitamins. If vitamin C was the criterion for selecting a fruit, the kiwi would win over all others. But every fruit offers much more than vitamin C— a spectrum of other vitamins, minerals, fiber, and those all-important phytochemicals by the thousands.

Bright Idea
When possible, store vegetables in the basement or some other cool area of the home. Kitchens tend to be warmer.

In a nutritional sense, any fruit is a superior food, and you should eat fruits you like. It doesn't hurt, however, to eat a variety, especially as fruits come and go with the seasons. Included in Appendix D is a list of the peak harvesting seasons for fruits grown in North America.

Pick unbruised fruit

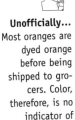

Once ripe, fruits don't last long, even under the best of circumstances, though they last a few extra days if you refrigerate the ripe fruit. A fruit's tendency to rot is accelerated by even a small bruise or cut. The injury does not stay localized—the whole fruit bursts into self-destruction, and the fruit fades into mush. So when you buy fruit, it pays to carefully examine it for scuffs, bruises, or other damage.

The fast deterioration of ripe fruit presents a serious marketing problem. Fruits, like tropical fruits that spend a long time in transit, are picked before they ripen. They may soften, but that is not a true ripening in the sense of full development of sugars and flavor. Bananas are an exception. They continue to ripen after picking. In fact, you are wise to buy bananas that have a slight green color. They will turn yellow as they ripen at home.

Processed fruits: Mushiness is a problem

Texture plays an important role in enjoying a fruit. Who likes biting into a mushy piece of fruit? People seem more tolerant of mushy vegetables—we don't mind mashed potatoes. Most fruits don't freeze well, turning into unappetizing slush, although some fruits, like blueberries and cranberries, hold up reasonably well.

The issues of slow deterioration mentioned above regarding frozen vegetables apply to the frozen berries as well.

Drying is one of the oldest ways of preserving fruits. Drying is effective because bacteria cannot grow in the absence of water. Sun drying was once the common way to remove water, particularly for raisins. Now fruits are dried in a blast of hot air. Light-colored fruits are dipped in a solution of sulfur dioxide and other sulfur compounds to prevent browning. This is done for cosmetic reasons only—browning does not degrade nutritional value.

It is difficult to can fruits without breakdown. When a fruit is heated, its cell walls break down and the inner fluid gushes out. The cell structure collapses. (That is a technical description of how fruit goes mushy.) Manufacturers of canned fruit prevent fluid leakage by adding sugar to the canning water; the syrup prevents the fluid from draining out of the fruit pieces. The benefit of this process is that the canned fruit retains its firmness; the downside is that the fruit pieces swim in a thick syrup. The sugar boosts calories without adding nutritional benefit.

The fact that canned fruit pieces are firm to the bite doesn't mean the fruit has retained its original nutritional value. Although phytochemicals and fiber remain, nutritional losses are severe, as with vegetable canning. The advantage of canned fruit is that the fruit may be closer to the peak of ripeness when it is processed.

In light of these considerations, canned fruit should not be considered one of the five servings of fruit and vegetables. Think of it as pleasant dessert.

Fruit juice quality varies widely

By drinking 6 ounces of fruit juice, half the size of a soft drink can, you consume one official serving of fruit. The official guide to eating fruits and vegetables, however, says nothing about the quality of

Bright Idea
Eat an apple a day. The pectin—the apple's fiber—sweeps through the bowel, carrying with it toxins that can cause headaches. Think of the money you can save on headache pills!

juice. A wide variety of juices are on the market, and their nutritional quality varies enormously. In fact, some juice products offer no more nutrition than a soft drink. The accompanying table presents a Guide to the nutritional ranking of fruit juices.

TABLE 2.3: A GUIDE TO THE NUTRITIONAL RANKING OF FRUIT JUICES

Quality Scale	Fruit Juice
1st Rank	Freshly squeezed juice
2nd Rank	Premium juice in a dated carton or bottle (not from concentrate)
3rd Rank	Juice reconstituted from frozen concentrate
4th Rank	Juice drinks

The fruit offers more nutrition than the juice

If the choice is between eating a whole fruit and drinking juice, choose the whole fruit because it offers the better nutritional value. However, there are times when a glass of juice is welcomed. If the choice is between juice and a soft drink, definitely take the juice.

Juicing a fruit exposes the nutrients to air. Deterioration starts the instant the juice drips through the squeezer. That is why freshly squeezed juice ranks first in the Guide. Most of the nutrients are retained, although fiber is usually lost. In the case of oranges or grapefruit, you can avoid losing so much fiber by adding the fiber caught in the squeezer into the juice.

Packaged fruit juices

Even if juice is packaged in a tight carton, deterioration—as measured by loss of vitamin C—continues. So if you buy juice this way, look for cartons with the furthest expiration date. Premium juices that have never been concentrated, while more expensive, deliver more nutritional value than juice reconstituted from concentrate. The same goes for juice you make at home from frozen concentrate.

The reason is that the juice factory heats and exposes the juice to air in order to drive off water. Nutritional value can plummet during this process. Frozen concentrate you buy in the supermarket slowly deteriorates during storage, the same way frozen fruits and vegetables do. You don't know how long the frozen concentrate has been in storage, or if it has remained frozen 100 percent of the time.

Many juice concentrates are imported from other countries, like Brazil. There is a lengthy time between when the product leaves the foreign factory and arrives in your kitchen.

Mixed juice and sugared juice drink rip-offs

You see juices labeled "vitamin C added." You may wonder why the manufacturer adds this vitamin, since most fruits juices contain vitamin C already. Well, the moment fruit is juiced, its juice begins to lose vitamin C as well as a host of other sensitive nutrients. If the manufacturer adds vitamin C, it may mean the product has undergone severe nutritional loss. And remember, adding back vitamin C does not restore the losses of other nutrients.

Beware of mixed juices. You pick up a carton with a flashy picture of a featured fruit, generally an expensive fruit. The label says, for example, "Mango with Other Juices," giving you the impression that the product is mostly mango juice. Not at all. The product's main ingredient is probably white grape juice, a product manufacturers use to fill the can or bottle.

To be sure, some products containing a mixture of juices are quality products. Check the label to

Unofficially...
The quality of fresh fruit varies immensely. Your own senses are as good a judge of quality as a scientific instrument. How the fruit feels when you bite into it and its flavor and sweetness are all guides to nutritional quality. As with fresh vegetables, you have to use common sense and rely on your own judgment.

make sure the juices are those featured on the main label.

Finally, anything called a drink, blend, beverage, punch, or juice blend contains hardly any genuine fruit juice. The main component is water and sugar. These products are ranked at quality level 4, but as far as nutrition is concerned, don't even bother with them. They are in the same category as soft drinks.

Looking for quality in store-bought fruit juice? Remember these tips:

- For juices in dated cartons, buy the furthest expiration date.

- Once you've opened a carton or made up juice from concentrate, store in a tight container in the refrigerator no more than 2 weeks.

- White grape juice on the label of mixed juices is a tip-off of low quality.

- If you see added sugar on the label, except for tart juices like cranberry, consider the drink not much better than a soft drink.

- Go for the nutritious rich juices, such as grape-fruit, pineapple, orange, and prune.

Fiber, phytochemicals, and health

Study after study has shown that people who eat fruits and vegetables have substantially lower risks of cancer and other serious diseases. While this fact was known for decades, it wasn't clear why. Now the answers are coming in. Traditional nutrition science focused only on vitamins and minerals, forgetting about other things. Those other components of fruits and vegetables, fiber and phytochemicals, are now proving to be as important to good health as vitamins and minerals.

As mentioned previously, you don't obtain fiber or phytochemicals from meats or animal products. Your only source is the plant foods you eat. Don't be fooled by the thought of getting fiber or phyto-chemicals in a pill. While a pill can provide you with added fiber, it is technically impossible to capture the diversity of the phytochemicals in a pill. Eat a tomato, for example, and it is estimated that you eat over 10,000 different phytochemicals. Scientists have identified only a fraction of the 10,000. They don't know which ones or which combinations are the most important to the human body. And for the time being, you don't need to know. Just eat the tomato!

Fiber sweeps out cholesterol

The principal value of fiber is that it regularizes intestinal action and helps feed the some 500 species of bacteria that live in the lower bowel. An added fiber benefit is its ability to grab and hold tox-ins. As it moves down the intestinal tract, fiber sweeps out toxic materials.

The body also uses the fiber sweep as a key way of ridding itself of cholesterol. The liver converts the cholesterol to bile salts and these are excreted into the intestinal tract. The fiber then helps sweep the bile salts out of the body. In short, dietary fiber is an important tool in eliminating excess cholesterol. Maybe that's one reason eating fruits and vegetables helps lower the risk of heart disease. Eating fruit is certainly cheaper and safer than buying cholesterol-lowering drugs, with their risk of negative side effects.

Here are other ailments associated with insuffi-cient fiber in the diet:

Watch Out!
Add more fiber to your break-fast. Throw a sliced banana or chopped apple or some dried fruit onto your break-fast cereal.

- Constipation
- Varicose veins
- Hemorrhoids
- Diverticulitis
- Cancer of the colon
- High blood pressure

Phytochemicals fight cancer

As body cells go about their business of metabolizing food, they generate substances called *free radicals*. Free radicals are like cannon balls bouncing around inside the cell. They can trigger processes destructive to the cell wall and DNA that lead to cancer. Body cells destroy free radicals with native antioxidants, but only to a limited degree. The body relies heavily on additional antioxidants it gets from food. Yellow and green vegetables, as well as melons and citrus fruits, are loaded with phytochemicals that are strong antioxidants to fight free radicals.

Here is a partial list of fruits and vegetables loaded with antioxidants:

- Apricots
- Blueberries
- Broccoli
- Cantaloupe
- Carrots
- Flaxseed
- Garlic
- Kale
- Mango
- Pumpkin
- Red bell peppers

- Spinach

- Strawberries

- Sweet potato

- Tomato

Cruciferous vegetables also fight cancer

Broccoli belongs to the *cruciferous* family of vegetables because their flowers are shaped like a cross. The botanical name of this family is *Brassica*. These vegetables contain antioxidants and phytochemicals such as indoles and isothiocyanates that are strong anticancer agents. They help stop a cancer before it grows to dangerous size. So between the antioxidants and the anticancer agents, you are smart to include cruciferous vegetables in your meal planning. Here are common crucifers:

- Broccoli

- Bok choy

- Cauliflower

- Brussels sprouts

- Cabbage

- Kale

- Swiss chard

- Turnip

Pesticide residues: A hazard to kids?

Children aren't small adults. In ratio to body weight, they drink more, eat more, and breathe more than adults. This means that, proportionally, they are more vulnerable to the poisonous substances in foods, such as pesticide residues. In addition, a child's body is less able than an adult's to defend against poisonous substances.

Watch Out!
Don't overcook broccoli. Broccoli sprouts contain a cancer-fighting substance, but it is largely destroyed by excessive heat. Consider eating it raw, such as mixed with leafy greens in a salad.

In spite of these well-known facts, however, the federal government sets legal tolerances for pesticide residues in foods as if the population were composed of adults—adult *males,* for that matter. The tolerance levels are based on what a healthy midlife male is expected to tolerate.

Should this matter concern you, or is it just something for government bureaucrats and medical people to argue about? Yes, it should concern you. Commercial agriculture in the United States depends heavily on chemical pesticides to control insect and weed infestations. Only a fraction of the tonnage of pesticides sprayed and dusted on food crops remains in the food, but it is enough to raise concerns over safety, especially children's safety.

The Food Quality Protection Act

This concern surfaced officially with the 1993 release of a National Academy of Sciences report, *Pesticides in the Diet of Infants and Children.* According to the report, levels of pesticides considered safe for adults could cause diminishment of brain function in fetuses and children. What sort of diminishment? Learning disabilities and hyperaggression, says toxicologist Warren Potter of the University of Wisconsin. Other researchers have found that children exposed to high levels of pesticides don't have the eye-hand coordination of children with less exposure.

Scary? It was enough to compel members of Congress, who in 1996 passed the Food Quality Protection Act. This act adopts two features designed to protect children:

- First, the legal levels of pesticides in foods must be reevaluated to take into account the lower tolerance of children.

- Second, the total pesticide burden of a food must be taken into account. Thus, if an apple has residues of five different pesticides, the toxic effect of all five together has to be evaluated.

This legislation, intended to prevent exposure of children to harmful pesticide levels, also benefits adults. An earlier National Academy of Sciences report criticized safety testing of the currently licensed pesticides used on food crops. None of them has been tested for all its toxic effects in humans—children or adults. The message here is that adults as well as children could be harmed by the current levels of pesticides in foods.

In any event, don't expect the 1996 act to be implemented with speed or vigor. The scientific issues are complex, and agricultural interests have many reservations about the act. The arguments could go on for years before any real action is taken.

Washing your fruits and vegetables: Is that enough?

So where does all this leave you, a consumer concerned about minimizing exposure to pesticide residues? There are three strategies for minimizing your exposure to pesticides in and on fresh fruits and vegetables. First, washing and scrubbing removes 50 to 90 percent of pesticide residues lodged on the surface. Peeling potatoes and fruits such as apples and pears also effectively removes surface contamination, but peeling has a downside. It may remove some of the phytochemicals and nutrition located in and just under the skin.

Washing may not remove all the pesticide residues, however. Commercial growers use dozens of different pesticides. While some lodge only on

Unofficially...
If you are a woman, according to George Lucier of the National Institute of Environmental Health Sciences, you can be up to 1,000 times more sensitive to a poison than a man. Your more complex hormonal and reproductive system is particularly vulnerable.

the surface, others penetrate the flesh of fruits and vegetables, as much as a quarter of an inch. So ordinary washing or peeling doesn't remove these residues. Unfortunately, the government doesn't require producers to put a list of the pesticide residues on the label, so you won't know whether or not the fruit or vegetable is contaminated with residues deep inside its flesh.

The best you can do, therefore, is to thoroughly wash all fresh fruit and vegetables. Incidentally, fruits and vegetables destined for freezing or canning are washed (and peeled) at the factory before processing.

The second strategy for minimizing pesticide exposure is to avoid fruits and vegetables with known high levels of pesticide residues. Some crops, because they are more susceptible to insect attack, receive high doses of pesticides.

Using FDA data, the Environmental Working Group on the Community Right to Know, a Washington, D.C.–based nonprofit research organization, compiled the following list of the 12 most-contaminated fruits and vegetables. These are listed in decreasing order of contamination, strawberries having the dubious honor of being the dirtiest:

- Strawberries
- Bell peppers
- Spinach
- U.S. cherries
- Peaches
- Mexican cantaloupe
- Celery
- Apples

Moneysaver
When you buy organic vegetables and fruits, don't just compare the purchase price against non-organic produce. Also compare their value in terms of long-term vitality. You save money and suffering by remaining healthy.

- Apricots
- Green beans
- Chilean grapes
- Cucumbers

The Environmental Working Group on the Community Right to Know also listed the 12 least-contaminated fruits and vegetables, beginning with the cleanest:

- Avocados
- Corn
- Onions
- Sweet potatoes
- Cauliflower
- Brussels sprouts
- U.S. grapes
- Bananas
- Plums
- Green onions
- Watermelon
- Broccoli

We don't suggest you not buy and eat the 12 fruits and vegetables in the top list—the dirty dozen. Take extra care in washing them. That will remove most of the pesticide, but as already mentioned, washing doesn't remove any pesticide residue that has penetrated the flesh. There is a third and better strategy that eliminates issues of cleanliness—go organic.

The third strategy: Go organic

Farmers can grow crops without applying heavy doses of chemical pesticides. In fact, prior to the

1930s, organic farming—that is, farming without chemical pesticides—was the norm. That form of farming, however, came to be seen as old-fashioned and fell into disrepute as commercial agriculture embraced pesticides and artificial fertilizers. There were also economic pressures—pesticides helped farmers control crop loss.

Organic farming, however, is making a comeback. Organic farmers have developed new and sophisticated methods of crop rotation, natural insect repellents, and interplanting to control insects and weeds. They use natural fertilizers instead of chemicals.

Importantly, from the consumer's viewpoint, the distribution system now blankets the country. You find organic produce in mainstream supermarkets. Most medium-size towns have natural food stores and co-ops that feature organic produce.

Farmers who practice organic farming methods and sell their crops as organic must comply with strict rules. In some regions, states set the rules. In other regions, organizations of organic farmers set the rules, inspect the farms, and give permission to use that organization's seal. (The produce or product should state "Certified organic," followed by the name of the certifying agency.) The federal government may one day issue a nationwide set of rules for organic farming; it remains to be seen how that will work out.

In any event, the current way of monitoring organic farms works to the consumer's advantage. The crops are grown more naturally. And while taste is a personal matter, many consumers claim that organic produce tastes better than produce grown with the aid of chemicals.

Watch Out!
When buying organic produce, exercise the same judgment as when buying commercial produce. Is it fresh? A wilted or tattered head of lettuce, even if organically grown, does not offer a high level of nutrition.

Just the facts

- Although health authorities talk of five servings of fruits and vegetables, aim for twice that number. Eat a variety of fruits and vegetables, including a salad and fresh fruit every day.

- Not all fruit and vegetable products are created equal. Fresh is better than frozen (or dried), which is better than canned. When choosing between two products, choose the "better than" product.

- The following items cannot be counted as a fruit or vegetable serving: french fries, jams, jellies, and sugared fruit drinks. They may seem like treats, but are too highly processed to retain any of the nutritional values you expect from fruits and vegetables.

- Individuals concerned about pesticide residues on foods should seek out organic fruits and vegetables. Mainstream supermarkets, as well as natural food stores and farmers' markets, sell organic foods.

GET THE SCOOP ON...
Legumes as a meat substitute ▪ Textured
vegetable protein ▪ Peanut butters ▪ Pasta ▪
Organically grown grains and legumes ▪ Frozen
dough and other bakery tricks

Grains, Legumes, and Nuts

Why eat grains? Our prehistoric ancestors ate relatively little grain. Our human biology evolved in a nutritional world largely without grains. So why do grains form the base of the USDA Food Guide Pyramid? Why make grains the foundation of your diet? There's a bit of history here. Grains as a major dietary component appeared on the human scene about 10,000 years ago when early agriculturists began to cultivate them. They were a convenient food, easily raised in abundance and easily stored (dry grains keep well). Human civilization as we know it today became possible because of grain. One half the calories of the six billion people now living on Planet Earth come from three grains—wheat, rice, and corn.

Yet from a cell's-eye view, grains offer no inherent nutritional advantage over other plant foods. The USDA recommendation to eat 6 to 11 servings of grain a day is, from a human biology perspective, almost excessive. Instead of worrying about a grain

Chapter 3

Unofficially...
Each American
consumes, on
average, 200
pounds of grain
every year. Only
10 pounds of
that, however, is
whole grain.

quota in your diet, think in terms of total diet. As pointed out in the previous chapter, plant foods offer nutritional support impossible to obtain from the animal food categories. So be smart: Upgrade the importance of plant foods in your diet. Depending on your food preferences, choose foods from among the five plant categories—or better still, from each one of them: fruits, vegetables, grains, legumes, and nuts.

Plant foods should underpin your diet. Whether you emphasize fruits, vegetables, or grains or other combination among plant foods, is up to you.

That's theory. But what do you do in the modern supermarket and bake shop to make plant foods work for you? For starters, keep two critical things in mind:

- **Variety.** No single food supplies all the complex nutritional needs of the human body. Within each category, seek variety.

- **Modern processing.** Most grain and legume foods are processed, with varying degrees of nutritional loss. Seek those products that suffer the least drop in nutritional value.

With those two principles in mind, let's get down to practical issues. What information do you need to make superior nutritional choices that fit your personal lifestyle? Let's start with the grains.

Wheat is the number one grain

Wheat flour contains a protein, gluten, that few other grains have. Mixed with water and kneaded, the gluten in the dough develops an elastic texture, forming the dough. Add yeast to the dough, and the living cells of this microorganism convert the carbohydrate of the flour to alcohol—yes, that's right, alcohol! But you'll never become intoxicated from eating bread, because baking drives off alcohol. This is part of fresh-baked bread's wonderful aroma. Yeast is not added to the dough to make alcohol, of course. It's added because it produces carbon dioxide, bubbles of which are trapped in the dough, giving leavened breads their familiar bubbly appearance.

Leavened breads (breads with yeast) come in as many varieties and shapes as there are bakers. Leavened breads include bagels and flatbreads, such as buns, rolls, focaccia, and pizza crusts. From a nutritional standpoint, the bread's shape is unimportant. What makes the difference is what goes into the flour mix, and that is what you should note in judging bread quality.

A note on hard and soft wheat: The difference lies in protein content. Hard spring wheat is 12 to 14 percent protein and is used in making leavened breads. Soft winter wheat is 7 to 9 percent protein and is used for cakes and pastries. All-purpose flour has a protein content somewhere in between.

A Guide to the nutritional ranking of breads

Breads come in many combinations of refined and unrefined flours, but for the purposes of ranking they can be grouped in four quality levels.

TABLE 3.1: A GUIDE TO THE NUTRITIONAL RANKING OF BREADS

Quality Scale	Breads
1st Rank	Whole wheat, whole wheat with other whole grains.
2nd Rank	Whole grain mixed with unbleached white wheat flour.
3rd Rank	Frozen-dough breads containing whole wheat and/or other whole grains. Breads made from 100 percent unbleached white flour.
4th Rank	Commercial white and brown breads, the squeezable kind. Frozen-dough breads made with enriched, white flour.

Watch Out!
Beware of bread labels that scream "low fat," "low calorie," "good source of...," "reduced...," and so forth. These terms are nothing more than advertising gimmicks—they conform to government regulation but give you no real understanding of the nutritional value of the food. Ignore them and read the nutrition label.

First level: Whole-wheat bread is tops

When we talk of wheat kernels as a food, we call them wheat berries. The farmer calls them seeds. The wheat kernel is just that, a seed that contains a living embryo, packed with nutrients, vitamins, and minerals. The bulk of the berry consists of starch (about 86 percent), which is a complex carbohydrate, mixed with protein (about 14 percent). These energy stores feed the embryo while it germinates and before it pushes above ground.

Whole-wheat flour is simply the whole berry, crushed. Nothing is lost. Everything that was in the berry—the vitamins, the special nutrients packed with the embryo, the bran, the starch and protein— is all there, ground together. So when you eat whole-wheat bread, you benefit from the whole nourishment designed for creating a living plant.

What goes for whole-wheat flour goes for other grains. Breads made with a mixture of whole-grain flours rank at the top level.

Second level: Refining reduces wheat's nutritional value

If the wheat berry were a house, it would consist of three distinct parts. A small room houses the embryo with nutrients packed around it. A huge room houses the energy stores, the starch and the protein. The third part, a shell of bran and fiber, envelopes the two rooms. The shell contains the vitamin and mineral stores necessary for germination. They are like pictures hung on the inner walls of the shell.

To continue the house analogy, here is what happens when the flour is refined. The little room with the embryo and its packed nutrients is thrown out. That's the wheat germ. The walls—the bran and fiber—are also thrown out, along with all the vitamins and minerals. All that is left is the starch and protein.

In fact, 30 percent of the wheat berry is discarded during refining to be used as animal feed. Animals get the most nutritious part. At this point the flour has a yellowish cast, due to flecks of pigments such as the carotenes. It is called *unbleached white flour.*

Some people consider unbleached flour superior to ordinary bleached white flour, but it is still a refined flour. Its only superiority is that it has not undergone the changes caused by chemical bleaching. If bread is made from 100 percent unbleached white flour, quality drops to the third level. But bakers often mix it with whole wheat and flours of other grains to make a variety of breads. These mixed flours, because of a whole-grain content, rank at the second quality level.

Third level: Frozen dough, factory to you

Have you ever look closely at the in-store bakery of a supermarket? Generally you see ovens but no mixing equipment. Where do they mix the dough? They don't. It is a specially engineered dough, mixed in large, central factories, and frozen in loaf sizes. Frozen-dough loaves are shipped to bakery locations where they are popped into the oven. Within a half hour or so, out come "fresh-baked" loaves. Well, they *are* fresh baked, but the dough could have been mixed months ago.

More traditional bakeries mix the dough and give it hours to rise. During this period the live yeast works away, creating not only gas to cause the rising but also aromas and flavors. This natural process is shortchanged in the preparation of frozen dough. Chemical additives and dough conditioners replace part of the work of the yeast. Special aroma and flavor additives augment natural aromas and flavors created by the yeast.

Every imaginable baked good, including donuts, Danishes, and bagels, can be manufactured as frozen dough and shipped to small bakeries and supermarket bake shops.

Frozen-dough bread containing whole grain ranks at the third level. But all other frozen breads drop to level four.

When you go into a bakery, how do you know if all those appealing loaves and buns have been baked from frozen dough or baked from scratch? If you can see the actual baking area and you don't see any mixing equipment, as in most supermarkets, you can assume the breads are made from frozen dough. If you see mixing equipment, there's a good chance the breads are made from scratch. But, admittedly, it is a bit of a lottery. Ask the shopkeeper and hope you get an honest answer. If nothing else, you'll impress the bakers with your sophistication about commercial baking.

Fourth level: Soft loaves

Although unbleached white flour ranks below whole-wheat flour, it is still better than the next step millers take—bleaching. Most of the refined flour produced in this country is bleached to get rid of those "unsightly" carotenes. From a nutritional point of view, bleaching makes as much sense as bleaching carrots white. Nevertheless, that is what bread makers do, claiming that people like their bread white.

The chemical agents that destroy the carotenes leave residues of altered substances in the flour. These side products have never been studied to determine their effect on human consumers.

Germany, worrying about the lack of knowledge of what bleaching does to the starch and protein, banned these chemical bleaching agents as long ago as 1958.

Bleaching creates another problem for bakers. It causes some breakdown of the gluten, the protein responsible for the dough's sponginess. Bakers use chemical dough conditioners to make up for this destruction.

You won't see "bleached white flour" anywhere on the label. Instead, you'll see the more friendly term, "enriched flour." Bleached white flour is indeed enriched with iron and four vitamins—thiamin, niacin, riboflavin, and folic acid. The iron and niacin are added to an equivalent level in whole wheat. Thiamin and riboflavin are doubled, and folic acid is tripled.

Although enrichment sounds healthy, this bleached, refined flour by no means regains its whole-grain goodness. The entire spectrum of vitamins and minerals has been degraded during refining. To harken back to the house analogy, all the pictures have been thrown out; only five have been added back. For example, enriched flour has one quarter the potassium as whole-wheat flour. Fiber content drops 80 percent. Phytochemicals, including those yellow carotenes, are destroyed.

Of course, this doesn't mean that enriched flour is bad. Keep in mind that the Guide to Nutritional Ranking is a "better than" scale. When you go into a bake shop or supermarket and you have a choice, pick the "better than" item.

Try a bread machine

Now you can have the aroma and pleasure of eating freshly baked bread right in your own kitchen. Well, you always could if you baked your own bread, but

Unofficially...
British bakers have developed what they call no-time bread. Instead of adding yeast to the dough, they whip air into the dough with an industrial-strength beater. Using this process, it takes 2 minutes to produce a "risen" loaf.

few people seem willing to do that. Bread machines, however, are easy to use. You can load a machine in 5 minutes and leave it alone. Within 2 to 4 hours you have a freshly baked loaf.

Best of all, you have full control over what goes into the loaf. You know exactly what flour or flours you use.

A lot of people like these advantages. One in five households owns a bread machine. Here are tips on getting the most out of it:

- Use the automatic timer. You can load the machine at night and set the timer for a fresh loaf first thing in the morning.

- Keep a variety of flours on hand, such as barley, millet, oats, quinoa, rye, and spelt. Mix in with wheat flour for variety.

- Buy a grain grinder. This way, you can grind your own flour just before loading the bread machine, getting maximum nutritional value and taste from the grain.

Watch Out!
Bakers add caramel color to give white bread a brown look— so-called brown bread. It's no more nutritious than white bread. Those dark browns of pumpernickel and peasant breads are also artificially produced.

- Wheat allergy? If the allergy is caused by a wheat protein other than gluten, substitute spelt flour. Like wheat, spelt has sufficient gluten to make a spongy dough that rises with yeast.

Don't be ripped off by trick labeling

The variety of breads on the market is huge, and no shorthand guide can cover them all. The Nutritional Guide is just that—a guide. Read the labels. See what flours are listed and in what order (they are listed in descending order of quantity). Don't be fooled by terms like "multi-grained," "stone-ground," "pumpernickel," "seven-grain" (Siebenfeld), "rye," or "wheat flour." Unless the word "whole" appears in front of the flour or grain (e.g., whole-wheat flour), then assume the flours are the equivalent of refined white flour and rank at the fourth level.

Beware of a favorite advertising gimmick. You might see the words "whole wheat" or "whole grain" emblazoned in big letters on the bagel or bread package. In fact, whole-wheat flour may be only a lesser component of such a product. The item is mostly refined flour.

Are sweet cakes "grains"?

One of the pleasures of going into a bake shop is looking at all those pastries, cakes, and cookies. Perhaps that's all you should do—look.

These baked products do contain flour, so can they be considered part of the grain group? USDA nutrition guidelines don't make any distinction, which means you could satisfy their recommendation for grain servings by eating only sweet cakes.

Smart nutrition, however, does make a distinction. Pastries, cakes, Danish, and croissants are off the Nutritional Guide. They rank below the bottom level. Why? Flour is only one part of these foods. The rest is fat and sugar, the bulk of the calories. The exception might be a muffin or pastry made with whole-grain flour. Then, depending on the fat and sugar content, it ranks at level 4.

This comment refers to commercial products. You can make muffins and scones at home, using whole-wheat flour with little or no added fat and sugar. That pushes quality level up to the second or first rank.

To sum up, remember these seven things when choosing and keeping breads, rolls, and bagels:

1. Keep bread tightly wrapped at room temperature. Refrigeration speeds up staling.

Moneysaver
People who eat large quantities of white bread, regular pasta, and potatoes risk adult-onset diabetes. Avoid the illness by eating whole-grain products, and save on drugs and treatment costs.

2. Bread can be frozen, but wrap it extraordinarily well in moisture-proof plastic wrap. The bane of frozen bread is freezer burn, due to loss of moisture. In any event, don't keep frozen bread more than three months. (Don't trust your memory: Write the date on the package.)

3. Thaw frozen bread at room temperature, not in a microwave. The microwave dries out the bread.

4. Use a bread machine to enjoy fresh-baked bread. You'll have absolute control over what goes into the bread, and the machine is easy to use.

5. Don't be fooled by the artificial brown color of many breads. The brown color in no way enhances the nutritional quality of the bread.

6. Enjoy cakes, pastries, and muffins as fun foods, but don't count them as part of the grain group. The negative effect of the fat and sugar cancels any positive value due to the flour content.

7. When choosing food products of the grain group, choose those made with whole grains. For top nutrition, every item should be made with whole grain. At the minimum, half the items should be whole grain.

Eat wheat berries directly—bulgur wheat

When we think of wheat we think of bread, but there are other ways to enjoy wheat berries. Add them whole to soups and stews. Cooked and cooled, they can be added to salads or made part of your breakfast cereal. They have the same nutritional value as whole-wheat flour.

Bulgur wheat consists of hard or soft wheat berries that have been boiled, dried, and then cracked into coarse pieces. The result is a pre-cooked, cracked whole wheat. Ancient Romans ate bulgur, calling it *cerealis* after Ceres, the goddess of harvest. The Israelis call it *dagan,* meaning "bursting kernels of grain." People throughout the Middle East consumed a lot of bulgur, including the cold dish now well-known in Western countries, tabouli.

Bright Idea
Bulgur doesn't require cooking. Soak in twice the volume of liquid for half an hour, or refrigerate overnight.

Breakfast cereals

Americans have traditionally eaten cereals, hot or cold, for breakfast. Dozens of cereal products flood the market. The question: Which ones offer whole-grain goodness? Finding them can be tough because of the confusing advertising claims. For example, is a cereal that advertises itself as "high in fiber" whole grain? Not necessarily.

For top level nutritional value, check these two things on the product label:

- Look for the word "whole," e.g., whole wheat or whole oats.

- Look for low or no sugar. Most ready-to-eat breakfast cereals have added sugar that diminishes the amount of grain in the product.

Rolled oats and shredded wheat are whole

Rolled oats contains the entire content of the oat berry. Hot cereal prepared from rolled oats offers the complete spectrum of the grain's nutrition. Rolled oats require very little cooking, the less the better. Bring the water to boil, add the rolled oats, and immediately turn off the heat.

Shredded wheat, which retains all the components of the wheat berry, was first made in Niagara Falls in 1892. In terms of nutrition, shredded wheat continues to lead the ready-to-eat breakfast cereal parade.

How do you sort out advertising puffery?

You often see claims such as the following. They are not false, just misleading:

- **"Fat free."** Cereals contain relatively little fat, and what there is consists largely of the highly desirable essential fatty acids. If they have been discarded during refining, then the claim is true. From a cell's-eye view, however, it means inferior nutritional value.

- **"High fiber."** Whole grains contain a variety of fibers, all of which contribute to the grain's nutritional value. Manufacturers, however, take a refined cereal from which the natural fiber has been partially or wholly deleted and add fiber from another source. The added fiber, however, in no way restores the total nutrition of the grain.

- **"Meets American Heart Association criteria."** The product's manufacturer pays a fee to the heart association for the right to put the association's logo on the package, if the product meets a particular criterion. Other products of equal or superior nutritional merit don't carry the logo, simply because their manufacturers don't pay the fee.

- **"Contains 10 essential vitamins and minerals."** Twenty-nine vitamins and minerals essential for survival have been identified. From the manufacturing standpoint, it is technically difficult and expensive to add all 29. The manufacturer includes those that are cheap and easy to add. More to the point, added vitamins and minerals, like added fiber, don't restore all the

Watch Out!
Beware of a breakfast cereal merchandising trick. Supermarkets often position the least nutritious, highly sugared (and highly profitable) cereals to the right as you face the shelf. Most shoppers are right-handed and are less likely to reach across to the more nutritious cereals.

nutritional goodness that has been degraded in the process of refining the cereal product.

Don't fall for sugared cereals

If you wish to sweeten your breakfast cereal, that's fine, but at least you control the amount of sugar or honey you add. You can't do this with presweetened cereals. Manufacturers add sugar for three reasons, none of which has anything to do with nutrition. First, the flakes are coated with a sugar glaze to protect the cereal from "wilting" due to moisture. This extends shelf life. Second, sugar is cheaper than the processed grain. Third, a sugary flavor masks stale odors, and the sweetness attracts eaters (some, anyway).

Sugar shows up in cereals where you might not expect it. Corn flakes has 7 percent sugar by weight. All-Bran is 20 percent sugar. Other cereals are getting into the range of candies. For example, raisin bran and oat bran are almost one-third sugar (30 percent).

Pasta makes you fat?

"Pasta makes you fat." You've heard that statement, but what really are the facts? Pasta is usually made from semolina, a highly refined flour of durum wheat. Semolina has two things in common with bleached white flour. It may be "enriched," and it has the same nutritional profile and quality rank. So what has this to do with fatness?

If you eat a meal consisting only of pasta—or white bread, for that matter—the starch (carbohydrate) is rapidly digested and converted into sugar (glucose) which enters quickly into the blood stream. The body in response to the resulting high blood glucose level releases insulin. Insulin tells the

Timesaver
Choose fresh pasta, not dried. It cooks within three to four minutes. You also get a higher nutritional benefit. Fresh pasta hasn't gone through a hot air drying and the loss of some of the nutritional value.

body to lower the blood glucose by converting it to fat. That's what happens if you eat white bread or pasta by itself. But in practice, you're unlikely to eat pasta by itself. You eat pasta with a sauce, and in the context of the complete meal, the pasta's carbohydrate is more slowly digested, with the result that glucose enters the blood more slowly. Thus there is less likelihood of an insulin response with rapid conversion of carbohydrate to fat.

If you are really worried about weight gain, enjoy your pasta meal, but don't eat so much.

There is another way to enjoy pasta without worrying that it goes straight to your midriff. Eat whole-grain pastas. Whole-grain pastas, like whole-wheat bread, retain the complete nutrition of wheat, including the fiber. An added plus: The whole grain, whether from bread or pasta, does not gallop through your digestive system like refined flour.

Find whole-grain flavor too strong? Mix whole-grain pasta 50-50 with regular pasta. You (or the kids) won't notice the change.

Here are other tips for extending your range of pasta eating:

- Go organic. A variety of pastas made from organically grown wheat and other grains are available, generally in natural food stores.

- Try pastas made from a mixture of semolina and other flours, like Jerusalem artichoke.

- Be exotic. Eat pasta made from the ancient grains—kamut, quinoa, or spelt.

Brown rice tops the quality scale

All grains have the three-part structure we described for the wheat berry: the embryo or germ, the large starch stores, and the outer coat of bran containing the vitamins and minerals. White rice is manufactured by polishing, which throws out the embryo and bran—along with vitamins, minerals, and essential fatty acids. The nutritional value of white rice plummets to the same quality level as enriched wheat flour—level 4.

From a cell's-eye view it makes no sense to polish rice. You get the starch (carbohydrate) for energy but diminished amounts of the cell building blocks. Unpolished rice, or brown rice, has a full, nutty taste, carrying the full nutritional value of the grain—first rank. If you want to raise your nutritional sights, buy organically grown brown rice. You get the nutrition without the pesticide residues.

Minute rice is a precooked rice in which the grains are slashed. When you put the rice in boiling water, water penetrates the cuts and the rice cooks in a hurry. The nutritional value of this overprocessed rice doesn't even rate being on the Guide to Nutritional Ranking. It ranks below white rice.

Tortillas and corn chips: Look for masa

Tortillas are the fastest-growing segment of the baking industry. On average, every baby, child, and adult consumes four a week. Tortillas are a Mexican food and were traditionally made from corn. Central Americans were growing corn 3,000 years before Columbus arrived.

Mexicans make a corn flour called *masa* which is more nutritious than the corn flour used to make America's tortillas. Why? First, let's sort through the ins and outs of corn products.

Moneysaver
Served rice in a restaurant? Minute rice, because of its shape and bland, mushy texture, is easily recognized, a tip-off to low quality. Save your money and look for a restaurant that at least serves white rice or, better still, brown rice.

TABLE 3.2: A GUIDE TO THE NUTRITIONAL RANKING OF CORN FLOURS AND CORN PRODUCTS

Quality Scale	Corn Product
1st Rank	Sweet corn on the cob
2nd Rank	Masa, unbolted corn flour, blue corn flour
3rd Rank	Corn flour (cornmeal), degermed; grits
4th Rank	Corn flakes

Eat sweet corn on the cob

Corn, also known as maize, can be classed both as a vegetable and as a grain. Sweet corn is a variety that produces sugar as well as starch. In its immature stage, we eat it as corn on the cob. Because this corn is eaten whole with minimal processing—just boil and eat—it ranks above the corn flours. However, if sweet corn is frozen or canned then it drops in rank, as with any other vegetable.

We are interested here in corn as a grain. Corn varieties used in flour-making have kernels filled with starch, as do wheat, rice, and other grains. Like other grains, the vitamin and mineral goodness of corn resides in the embryo (germ) and the outer bran layer.

The dried corn kernels are ground into flour. Depending on the milling process, corn flour loses a little or a lot of its original nutritional value. Knowing the differences in milling, you can check the labels of products, like tortillas, and select the more nutritious brands. Incidentally, the terms *corn flour* and *cornmeal* are interchangeable.

Look for tortillas made with masa

Masa, or Mexican corn flour, is made by boiling the corn in a 5 percent lime solution. This trick goes back to Aztec and Mayan civilizations, when the natives boiled corn with wood ashes. The lime treatment changes the nutritional value in two positive ways.

Bright Idea
Like tortilla chips? Look for those baked instead of deep fried. They have less fat and taste just as good.

First, lime releases the vitamin niacin, which otherwise remains locked in an unusable form. Second, it alters the amino acid composition in a more favorable way.

The boiled corn is then ground into a flour. Look for the words "masa" or "Mexican flour" on the label of tortillas and other corn products.

Incidentally, the word *masa* doesn't always appear on the label of products using this corn flour. The label, however, may describe the flour-making process, and you do see the word *lime,* which indicates the masa process.

Nutritionally, masa ranks below corn on the cob, because it undergoes more processing. On the practical side, fresh sweet corn is seasonal, while corn flours are available year-round. Along with unbolted corn flour, masa ranks above other corn flours.

Look for unbolted and blue corn flour

The corn kernel, like the wheat berry and rice, consists of the three components, the germ (embyro), the starch, and the bran coat. The bran contains most of the vitamin and mineral content. Unbolted corn flour (cornmeal), like whole-wheat flour, is the whole kernel ground into a flour.

Blue corn is a variety in which the blue pigment is embedded in the bran coat. Thus, when blue corn is ground into flour, the flour remains blue only if the bran, and all those vitamins and minerals, are left in the flour.

Corn flour and grits are highly refined

Corn flour or cornmeal is the ground grain that has the embryo (germ) and bran removed. It has lost at least half of the original nutritional value of the corn. Grits, as the name implies, consists of coarse particles of this degermed and branless corn flour.

Unofficially...
Bolting is an old-fashioned term for sieving. Sieving or bolting the flour removes the bran, so unbolted flour retains the bran.

Sometimes you see the word "degermed" added to the label, as if this were a positive attribute!

Finally, a word about corn flakes. The manufacturer rolls grits into flakes and toasts them. Since they are made from an already nutritionally inferior product and since they go through yet another heat process with exposure to air, corn flakes rank lower than the grits.

The legumes

People seeking a meat alternative often look to members of the legume family. The seeds of this family of beans and peas have as much protein as a beefsteak. All the advantages to health, daily energy, and vitality that can be said about vegetables apply equally to legumes. Legumes provide fiber, phytochemicals, and the whole range of vitamins and minerals. The large amount of water-soluble fiber helps lower cholesterol in those with high cholesterol and helps keep cholesterol low in those with normal levels.

The string beans and garden peas that we eat fresh are also legumes, but protein content is lower, in the same range as other fresh vegetables. The high protein level occurs in the seeds, that is, the dry legumes. This section deals with dry beans, lentils, and peas.

What is a legume?

The table below lists some of the common legumes—dry beans, lentils, and peas—you find in the grocery store.

TABLE 3.3: COMMON DRY BEANS AND PEAS

Aduki	Kidney
Black-eyed peas (cow peas)	Mung
Black turtle beans	Navy (white beans)
Cannellini	Pinto
Garbanzo (chick peas)	Red lentils
Great northern	Soldier
Green lentils	Soybeans
Green split peas	Yellow split peas
Fava bean (broad bean)	

Timesaver
Cooked beans freeze well. Save time by cooking a large batch at once. Put whatever you won't eat right away in airtight containers and freeze.

From the botanist's point of view, a legume is a plant that uses nitrogen directly from the air. No other type of plant does this. All other plants must use nitrogen fertilizer added to the soil. The legume has nodules on its roots filled with a special bacteria that do the work of converting nitrogen of the air to soluble nitrates the legume plant can use. This is a symbiotic relation, because the legume supplies nutrients the bacteria need.

Legumes take advantage of this rich source of nitrogen by filling their seeds with protein, which is made from nitrogen. The seeds become the dry beans, lentils, and peas that we enjoy.

How do I eat dry beans?

So you're interested in cutting down on meat consumption and would like to substitute legumes to ensure you get enough protein. But what do you do with these dried things? How do you eat dry beans? You can't eat them raw. They are too hard, but more to the point they contain natural substances that interfere with digestion.

These substances, however, disappear if the legume is sprouted. Keep in mind that a dry bean or pea is a seed. When sprouted, the living embryo

changes the dynamics of the seed. Dangerous substances disappear, vitamin content increases, and
the sprout becomes edible. Nevertheless, we don't
know everything about legume sprouts. We don't
know whether or not there might be residual toxic
substances that, if eaten in quantity, could be harmful. The smart thing is to eat sprouts in moderation,
part of a salad or stir-fry.

Cooked dry beans can be eaten in quantity and
have the versatility to be prepared in hundreds, if
not thousands, of ways. The first step in making a
bean dish is to cook the beans yourself or buy them
in a can. Here is a Guide to the nutritional ranking
of cooked beans.

TABLE 3.4: A GUIDE TO THE NUTRITIONAL RANKING OF COOKED DRY BEANS (OR LENTILS OR PEAS)

Quality Scale	Item
1st Rank	Organic beans, home cooked
2nd Rank	Regular beans, home cooked; organic beans, canned in water
3rd Rank	Regular beans canned in water
4th Rank	Regular beans, canned in brine (salt), molasses, tomato sauce (pork and beans)

Since dry beans, lentils, and peas have to be
cooked, heating causes some nutritional losses.
Although the heat-sensitive vitamins will degrade,
components like fiber, phytochemicals, protein, and
minerals are stable. Nevertheless, at home you have
full control over how much heat you need to apply,
which should be enough to obtain soft, chewable
beans.

Basically, soak beans 8 to 10 hours and cook anywhere from 30 to 90 minutes. A pressure cooker
halves the time. Peas and lentils have shorter cooking times.

For canned beans, pick the ones in water

Many folks find preparation time for cooked beans onerous and prefer the canned variety. Manufacturers can beans in various liquids: plain water, salted water (brine), and sauces. In terms of nutritional quality, water-canned beans are better than brine-canned, which, in turn, are better than those canned in sauces. The sauce-canned ones rank at the bottom, because the sauce generally includes things you don't need, like salt, sugar, and chemical additives.

Again, remember, the Nutritional Guides are just guides. Read labels and make your own informed judgment.

A number of canners use beans grown without chemical pesticides (organic). These products move a rank up the quality scale. For example, organic beans canned in water move up from third to second rank.

A delicate topic: What about gas?

This topic is bound to come up when we talk about dry legumes. Beans and the other legumes contain substances that in some people cause gas. The substances are not easily digested and pass into the lower bowel, where friendly bacteria convert them to acids and carbon dioxide, an odorless gas. But you can solve the gas problem—if indeed it is a problem. Do the following four things:

1. Discard the soaking water and use fresh water to boil the beans.

2. If dry beans or other dry legumes haven't been part of your regular diet, ease them in. The gas problem could be a problem of quantity. Eat small servings at first and then gradually increase serving size.

Bright Idea
Cooked beans can be eaten as such, or put into a variety of dishes such as casseroles, soups, and the popular Mexican dish, refried beans. They also can be chilled, marinated, and put into salads.

3. Try different beans. Not all beans cause a gas problem. Navy, lima, and soy beans are particularly bad offenders.

4. Bacteria in the bowel eventually adjust to the legumes and stop making gas. So if you plan to make dry legumes a frequent component of your diet, gas may become a nonissue.

5. Try taking a digestive aid. A variety of over-the-counter aids containing enzymes that help break down the legume carbohydrate are available.

The soybean, in a class by itself

Watch Out!
Soy flours are used in protein-enriched baked goods, infant foods, cereals, and diet foods. The flours add protein to the products, but keep in mind they are a highly processed food.

You are not likely to eat soybeans in the same way as you eat kidney or navy beans. They are hard to cook—taking 3 to 5 hours of boiling—and they don't taste very good compared to other beans. Nevertheless, you may be eating the soybean in some form without realizing it. Practically unknown prior to World War II, the soybean has become a dominant agricultural crop, for two reasons. First, about 20 percent of the weight of the soybean is oil, which is extracted to make margarine, cooking oils, and other fat products (see Chapter 4, "Extracted Fats and Oils"). Second, the residual mash consists of about half protein and half carbohydrate. This oil-extracted mash is sold as defatted soybean protein flour. If the oil is not extracted and left in the flour, the product is called full-fat soybean flour.

Further refining yields a product that consists almost entirely of the soy protein, called *isolated soy protein* or *soy protein isolate.*

Soy protein mimics meats

Soy protein is a great mimicker. By itself soy protein looks white and has no taste. The secret of mimicking is soy protein's ability to absorb dyes and flavors. You can have any color you want, any flavor you want. To top off this unusual mimicking ability, soy protein can be textured. The resulting product is called textured vegetable protein, TVP. With eyes closed, take a morsel of TVP and you could easily be fooled into believing you are chewing a piece of meat.

To make TVP, manufacturers take soy protein isolate and spin it into threads, which are bundled and cemented together. Flavors and dyes, plus various additives and flavor enhancers, MSG, and hydrolyzed vegetable protein are added. The products can be textured and flavored to resemble pork, beef, lamb, or sea bass. On a nutritional ranking scale of one to four, TVP ranks at the bottom.

Try other soybean products

People who don't like or are allergic to cow's milk often drink soy milk. This product is prepared from soybeans soaked in water, which are then ground into a slurry. The slurry is cooked, strained, and diluted with more water.

Asians have a long history of eating soybean products, but not TVP or soy protein isolate. Tofu, a traditional Asian product, is a soybean curd, made in a similar way to making cheese. The protein is precipitated from a hot-water extract of soybeans.

Natto, miso, and tempeh are fermented products, which means microorganisms have acted on the curd. The microorganisms markedly change the nature of the product, improving protein quality and digestibility. In general, because all these soy products haven't undergone the rigorous industrial production of TVP and are not laced with additives, they rank higher on a nutritional quality scale.

Moneysaver
The protein of a beefsteak costs seven times as much as the same amount of protein from cooked dry beans. Save money with the legumes, as long as you remain aware of how to combine foods for complete protein.

Soybeans lower cholesterol, but are they practical?

You may have heard of one study where soy protein lowered blood cholesterol by about 10 percent for a group of subjects. Remember, however, that they ate a lot of soy protein—47 grams a day. For you to achieve the same cholesterol-lowering benefit, you'd have to eat one and three-quarter pounds of tofu a day. Try stomaching that!

Eating soy protein to gain a single benefit, of course, doesn't make sense—which brings up a principle of smart nutrition. Eat foods for their taste, pleasure, and nutrition, not because they have some druglike action. Certainly, a low blood cholesterol level may be desirable, but you can reach that goal easily by eating an overall, balanced diet, not by eating any single food.

Phytoestrogens: Good or bad?

Another health claim: Soy products influence female hormonal cycles. The fact that soybeans can do this is true. But is that a benefit?

To explain, soybeans contain *isoflavones,* substances that have the same physiological activity as the female sex hormone, estrogen. For this reason, isoflavones are one type of *phytoestrogens.* Isoflavones are stable and carry through into all soy products. Thus, eating a soy product is like taking an estrogen pill; how strong a pill depends on how much soy you eat.

In one experiment, a group of women age 21 to 29, ate soy protein at about the same high level as in the cholesterol-lowering experiment mentioned above. They experienced a lengthening of their menstrual cycles. This result, although not necessarily harmful, illustrates soy's power over normal hormonal function, possibly the result of isoflavones.

Because of their estrogenic activity, soy isofla-vones have been touted as relieving the hot flashes of menopause, relieving symptoms of PMS (pre-menstrual syndrome), and reducing the risk of breast cancer in postmenopausal women. But before you reach for the TVP, a word of caution:

- Estrogen, if taken at all, is a better choice if taken as a pill: It has been investigated and, moreover, the pills should be taken only under the guidance of a health professional. The effects of eating soy phytoestrogens have not been studied extensively. And by eating them in large quantities, you are basically self-medicating.

- The estrogenic effects of soy isoflavones may be beneficial at certain stages of life. But for all we know, they may be harmful at other stages.

Nuts and seeds

Nuts resemble cereals in two ways: They provide the spectrum of B vitamins, and they offer a good reserve of protein. They differ in their high fat con-tent. Unlike meat and dairy fats, nut and seed fats are the heart-friendly mono- and polyunsaturated fats. (These terms are explained in the next chapter.)

Nuts generally serve as side dishes or as condi-ments, with perhaps the exception of peanut butter, a child's staple. Before talking about peanut butter, let's take a quick look at nutritional quality of nuts sold in grocery stores.

There are nuts and there are nuts

Because of nuts' high fat (oil), their content is sus-ceptible to oxidation and turning rancid. They keep best in the shell. If you buy shelled nuts, look for nuts in heavy plastic bags or in vacuum-packed cans.

Watch Out!
The uncertainty about the health benefits of the soy isoflavones is compounded by lack of precise knowledge of the degree of destruction and changes in prop-erties of isoflavones dur-ing the making of soy protein flours, TVP, and so forth. Think of soy products as foods, not as drugs.

TABLE 3.5: A GUIDE TO THE NUTRITIONAL
RANKING OF COMMERCIAL NUTS

Quality Scale	Nuts
1st Rank	Nuts in the shell, raw
2nd Rank	Nuts, shelled, raw
3rd Rank	Nuts, dry roasted
4th Rank	Nuts roasted in oil

If you like roasted nuts, dry roasted are better than ones roasted in oil. Nuts naturally have a high enough fat content. Besides, the roasting oil is often a cheap, nutritionally inferior oil.

Pick peanut butter that is just the peanuts

Although peanuts are classed as a nut, they actually are legumes. Whatever the botanists call them, peanuts are the most widely consumed of the nut family. Peanut butter has to be one of the all-time favorite foods. Here is a quick guide to the nutritional ranking of peanut butters you find in grocery stores.

TABLE 3.6: A GUIDE TO THE NUTRITIONAL
RANKING OF PEANUT BUTTERS

Quality Scale	Peanut Butter
1st Rank	Peanuts freshly ground, nothing added
2nd Rank	Peanuts freshly ground, nothing added, packed in jar, oil separates
3rd Rank	Peanut butter, homogenized
4th Rank	Peanut butter, homogenized with added sugar, peanut oil replaced with cheap oil

We start at the bottom. The FDA in its wisdom declared that peanut butter need contain only 90 percent peanuts. This rule gives manufacturers license to manipulate the product. They remove the peanut oil (which is a higher grade) and substitute lower grade, partially hydrogenated oils. They add sugar (which can mask taste), artificial colors, chemical preservatives, and salt.

The listing of a nonpeanut oil on the label tips you off to this kind of product.

Peanut butters without additives are the better buys. This includes peanut butters that have not been homogenized. (You have to stir up the oil yourself.) In order to homogenize peanut butter, the manufacturer has to add an emulsifying chemical. You don't need to burden your body with this chemical. But more to the point, homogenized peanut butter usually disguises other additives, added sugars, and the fact that the peanut oil has been replaced with a cheap, hydrogenated oil.

Raw peanut butter, freshly ground, ranks at the top. You can go even one step further and use peanuts, organically grown. Natural food stores generally offer the grinding service.

Without question, the bottom-ranked, sweet, silky-smooth peanut butter appeals to kids. But why addict a child to a low-ranked product? From the cell's-eye view, it's better to go for a peanut butter higher up the scale.

Bright Idea
Making a peanut butter sandwich? When you upgrade the quality of peanut butter, why not upgrade the quality of the bread? Switch to a whole-grain bread.

Just the facts

- Include whole-grain breads in your diet. They offer superior nutritional qualities compared to breads made with refined flours. Whole-grain products retain fiber, vitamins, and minerals.

- Vary choice of grains—wheat, barley, rye, oats, quinoa, kamut, amaranth, and spelt.

- Vary your pastas. Try whole-grain pastas as well as pastas made from other grains.

- Expand your legume horizon beyond soy products. Try other legume varieties and other ways of preparing legume dishes.
- Eat nuts raw and peanut butter that is simply freshly ground peanuts.

GET THE SCOOP ON...
Omega-3 fats and heart disease ▪ Saturated,
monounsaturated, and polyunsaturated fats ▪
Avoiding hydrogenated fats ▪ Butter versus
margarine ▪ Olestra ▪ Cold-pressed oils

Extracted Fats and Oils

Try this quiz. Here are five fats: saturated fat, margarine, flaxseed oil, olive oil, and safflower oil.

1. Which type of fat is believed to protect against heart disease?

2. Excessive consumption of which fat is linked to heart disease?

3. If one fat were the only fat in your diet, it would keep you alive. Which one?

4. Which product may contain harmful fats not found in nature?

5. Which of the five fats goes rancid the fastest?

The answers are

1. Olive oil.

2. Saturated fat.

3. Flaxseed or safflower oil.

4. Margarine. (May contain artificially produced trans fats.)

5. Flaxseed oil.

Obviously, there are fats and then there are fats. Not all fats are created equal, and what we do in this chapter is show why. This chapter gives you the expertise to understand terms such as polyunsaturates, saturated fat, and cold-pressed oil. Labeling of products with fats is often unclear. This chapter gives tips on clues to what's really in salad oils, cooking oils, and the fats in a wide range of food products, from baked goods to snack foods and frozen diners.

Fat is a big-ticket item in the American diet. People on average obtain 35 to 40 percent of daily calories from fat from all sources. Some of that fat comes from dairy products and meats. But the bulk of daily fat comes from fats extracted from vegetable sources, such as soybeans, corn, and cottonseed. Extraction strips away the proteins, fiber, minerals, and vitamins that cradle fats in their natural plant home. Subsequent refining alters the fat's makeup. Essential fats may be destroyed. Normal fats may be converted into unnatural forms. The net result: Extraction and refining creates a fat product displaying a set of nutritional values different from those of the original food.

In judging nutritional value of extracted fats, we have to look not only at the vegetable source, but also at how the fat has been manufactured.

The big switch from animal to vegetable fats

Let's start with a little background. Did you know that until well after World War II, stores sold margarine in its natural color—white? Laws promoted by the dairy industry forbade the sale of colored margarine. Not many people bought it. They preferred butter and the other common animal fats,

Watch Out!
Because of a shortage of butter in 19th-century France, Emperor Napoleon III offered a prize for a substitute. A pharmacist, Hippolyte Mège-Mouriés, won the prize in 1869 with flavored beef fat, which he called *margarine*. Forty years later, chemists invented the hydrogenation process that converts liquid vegetable oil to a solid. This process is used today to make margarine.

lard and tallow. All that has changed. Margarine now looks like butter and today outsells butter three to one. And as for lard and tallow, who ever hears of them nowadays?

The big switch to margarine and cooking oils derived from corn and other plant sources was driven partly by economics. The food industry found plant sources to be cheaper and more versatile. But economics by itself wasn't enough. The switch required consumer acceptance. The biggest factor driving the change in consumer tastes was the health claim that vegetable fats and oils are healthier than animal fats. That claim continues to play a big role in how people perceive fats and how they choose products.

Do animal fats cause heart attacks?

The idea that corn oil and margarine are healthier than lard and butter started in the 1950s. Researchers, studying the connection between fat and heart disease in Europe, found a high rate of heart disease in northern European countries compared to the rate in Italy, Greece, and other Mediterranean countries.

The postulated dietary difference: Populations of England, Scotland, Germany, and Scandinavia ate fat obtained mostly from animals. In contrast, Mediterranean populations ate scarcely any butter and other animal fats. Instead, they ate vegetable oils—mainly olive oil.

This link between a diet high in vegetable fat and rare heart disease led to the conclusion that vegetable fats are heart-healthy, while animal fats are not. This finding was highly publicized in the 1950s and became a major factor in public willingness, even eagerness, to buy the new brands of

Watch Out!
General rules
have exceptions.
Residents of the
Netherlands eat
a diet including
dairy and meat
which delivers 48
percent of daily
calories from all
sources of fat.
Yet the Dutch
have the highest
life expectancy
in Europe.

margarine and vegetable cooking oils arriving in supermarkets.

Put health issues in perspective

Keep in mind that the observations about type of fat and heart disease are correlations, not cause and effect relations. Moreover, what about other aspects of a population's diet? Scottish men have the highest rate of heart disease of Europeans. Their consumption of fresh vegetables is almost nonexistent. Peoples of the Mediterranean, in contrast, eat a variety of fresh vegetables.

Put diets in perspective. The total diet is more critical than any one component. This point comes up again in Chapter 9, "Vegetarianism: Should You Move Towards a Plant-based Diet?," when we focus on the virtues of the Mediterranean diet.

Yes, fat plays a role in heart disease and other health issues like weight. But calling animal fat the "bad" fat and vegetable fat the "good" fat overlooks a more fundamental point. What matters most for health is not the source of the fat but the type of fat. Vegetable fats, depending on how they are manufactured, can aid or hinder health. So as we sort through the nutritional issues of margarines, salad oils, and shortenings, we will keep the health issues before us.

To begin, let's clarify the terms fat and oil. An *oil* is a liquid fat—that is, liquid at room temperature. (We call olive oil an oil, even though it freezes solid in the refrigerator.) *Fats* by definition are solid at room temperature—for example, margarine, butter, and the visible fat around a cut of beef. Speaking more generically, however, the word "fat" includes both fats and oils.

All vegetable oil products are processed, some more, some less. The following table ranks nutritional quality of vegetable oils based on degree of processing. Reasons for the rankings are explained in the following sections.

TABLE 4.1: A GUIDE TO THE NUTRITIONAL RANKING OF FATS AND OILS

Quality Scale	Vegetable Oil
1st Rank	Mechanically expressed oils (e.g., olive)
2nd Rank	Cold-pressed oils (e.g., safflower, sunflower)
3rd Rank	Refined oils (e.g., canola, corn, soybean), margarine (nonhydrogenated)
4th Rank	Blended cooking oils, hydrogenated oils, margarine with hydrogenated oil, vegetable shortening

Extracted and refined vegetable oils

Are you looking for a vegetable oil for cooking or for salad dressing and confused by terms such as "cold-pressed," "unrefined," and "cholesterol-free"? The vegetable oils you see in the market have been prepared by a variety of means, all of which change the nutritional profile of the oil. The label terms refer to these different means, but not always accurately. The following information helps cut through the labeling fog.

Vegetable oils start life as part of a seed, stored food for nurturing the germinating seed. From a nutritional point of view, the oil—or to be more exact, the seed—has maximum nutritional value at this stage. You have to eat the seed, however, to benefit: That's practical for some seeds, like sunflower, pumpkin, and flax, and impractical for others, like soybean, rapeseed (canola), and cottonseed. Thus extraction is necessary.

Watch Out!
A ladle of salad dressing gives you as much as 48 grams of fat and 450 calories. For a woman eating 1,500 calories a day, that one ladle delivers the entire day's limit of fat and almost a third of the day's calories.

The oil is packed in microscopic, fibrous cells within the seed together with protective agents like vitamin E. This vitamin prevents the oil from being oxidized by air. Extracting the oil from these tough cells within the seed is difficult. Manufacturers subject the oil-bearing seed to severe measures that destroy some of the nutritional value and also create unhealthy products. The trick is to minimize damage.

Mechanical (expeller) extraction

Before extraction starts, the seeds are often cooked at about 250°F (120°C) and transformed into a mash. The mash is transferred to a press and squeezed. The pressing may be done in a batch press or continuously in a press called an expeller. Either way, a pressure of several tons forces the oil out of the seed, at the same time raising the temperature to 185 to 200°F (85 to 95°C).

High temperature is an oil's enemy. A combination of high temperature and exposure to air causes the fats to start breaking up. The first to go are the essential fatty acids, the ones your body needs. Some companies run cooling water through the expeller, thus protecting the delicate essential fatty acids. This method is called *cold pressing*. Unfortunately for the consumer, this term is not defined by law. An oil can be labeled cold pressed even though the actual pressing temperature is quite high, to say nothing about prior cooking.

Solvent extraction

Mechanical pressing of oil seeds is done on a relatively small scale. For vegetable oil production on a large scale, manufacturers use a petroleum solvent, usually hexane, which dissolves the oil. The solvent is evaporated at about 300°F, leaving the hot oil behind. Traces of solvent may remain in the oil, but in indetectable amounts. If the label on the bottle doesn't say anything about mechanical or expeller pressing, you can be sure the oil was solvent extracted.

Is solvent-extracted oil less or more nutritious than expeller-pressed oil? The answer depends on the amount of heat and exposure to air the oil has suffered. The solvent-extracted oil has been heated, but then so has the mechanically pressed oil (unless it has been genuinely cold pressed). In the end, the choice for some folk comes down to the fact that they don't like the idea of putting a solvent-extracted oil on their salad.

Unrefined and refined oils

Following extraction, the manufacturer may simply filter the oil and sell it as unrefined. But as you see, despite the word "unrefined," at this stage the oil may or may not have been exposed to harsh treatment.

The unrefined oil contains the vitamin E, phytochemicals, and other components, all of which contribute to the oil's taste and nutritional value. The oil may be cloudy and have a strong flavor. This does not detract from the oil's nutrition, but some people like a clear, odorless, taste-free product that doesn't go cloudy in the refrigerator. The oil companies oblige by refining the oil.

The oil can go through as many as 40 steps during refining. A series of chemical and heat treatments (temperatures of 500°F/270°C) remove gums (natural components), colored materials (the colored materials include valuable antioxidants), and aroma-causing substances. The oil is winterized, which means a removal of natural components of the oil that precipitate when the oil is refrigerated.

Bright Idea
Store your oils in the refrigerator. For oils that solidify, like peanut and olive, keep small amounts in dark-colored bottles on the kitchen counter, so you always have some ready to use.

Needless to say, at every step nutritional value degrades. It is a tradeoff with consumer preference for a highly refined oil. Regrettably, from the standpoint of a consumer's right-to-know, oils that have gone through this high-temperature refining may still be sold as "cold pressed."

Pick a product that gives you information

Obviously, when you buy an oil you have to accept some compromise. The oil undergoes some degree of processing. Since labeling information can be spotty, the best bet is to buy a product from a manufacturer who provides information on how the oil was prepared.

If the label provides no information except the dubious phrase "cold pressed," assume the worst: The oil has been subjected to the full refining treatment.

Pick extra virgin olive oil

Vegetable oils are packed in their tiny seed cells together with other valuable nutritional components such as vitamin E, phytosterols, magnesium, and potassium. Extraction and refining strips these substances away. The one oil on the market which retains these components is extra virgin (meaning first pressing) olive oil. Perhaps retention of vitamin E, the phytosterols, and other substances is part of the secret of this oil's health benefit.

Olive oils come in a variety of brands and grades. The extra virgin oil retains the greenish color and intense flavors of the olive. The more refined the oil, the less flavor it has and the less the benefit from other components of the natural olive. The following table ranks the nutritional quality of the oils based on the amount of refining they undergo. Regardless of the amount of refining, all grades of olive oil deliver 120 calories per tablespoon.

Watch Out!
Beware of the term *cholesterol-free*. It's an advertising gimmick used in promoting vegetable oils. Cholesterol does not occur anywhere in the plant world, so the term has no significance. What's worse, the term is often used to draw attention away from the fact that the oil has been highly refined.

TABLE 4.2: A GUIDE TO THE NUTRITIONAL RANKING OF OLIVE OILS

Quality Scale	Olive Oil
1st Rank	Extra virgin. Mechanically expressed, acidity less than 1.0 percent.
2nd Rank	Virgin. Blend of extra virgin and solvent-extracted oils. Acidity no more than 1.5 percent.
3rd Rank	Pure. Solvent extracted and industrially refined.
4th Rank	Pomace. Extracted from the cake left over from higher quality extractions.
	Light. Intense refining removes flavor and color components.

Remember these tips when buying a cooking or salad oil:

- Avoid oils sold in plastic bottles. The oil leaches the chemical plasticizer out of the bottle. Why burden your body with a foreign chemical you don't need?

- Look for oils sold in dark bottles. Light is an enemy of oils. It causes breakdown with the formation of toxic substances. At home, store bottles of oil in cool, dark places or refrigerate.

- If the label says nothing about mechanical pressing, assume the oil is solvent-extracted.

- Is that olive oil you bought too bitter for your taste? Store it tightly bottled for 1 to 2 years. The bitterness will disappear.

Moneysaver
Looking for a less expensive olive oil? Buy a cheap extra virgin oil instead of a pure olive oil.

Understanding the four basic types of fats

When discussing fat and heart disease, overweight, and general good health, you'll often hear talk about the four types of fat: saturated, monounsaturated, polyunsaturated, and trans. You see these terms on nutrition labels and in product ads. What do they mean? How do they relate to health? Some of these fats spell danger; others heal. By understanding the differences between the types of fat, you can make superior choices in your food purchases.

We'll consider the four types of fat one at a time. First, saturated fat.

Potato chips deliver saturated fat

The following table gives information about fat taken from the nutrition label of a popular brand of potato chips.

Watch Out!
A large order of fast-food french fries, like a ladle of salad dressing, delivers 470 calories and 20 grams of fat. About 8 grams of that fat is the undesirable trans type.

TABLE 4.3: FAT CONTENT OF REGULAR POTATO CHIPS

Fat content of 1 serving (1 ounce, 28 chips)	Weight in grams	Percent of daily value*
Total fat	10	15
Saturated fat	3	15

*The daily value is a limit set by the U.S. government. Based on a caloric intake of 2,000 calories, total fat limit is 65 grams; total saturated fat limit is 20 grams.

For the moment, focus on the potato chips' saturated fat. Saturated fat, to say the least, evokes a poor public image. You've seen phrases associated with it, such as "artery clogger." Indeed, research has identified saturated fat as a culprit in the fat link to heart disease. But to be fair, saturated fat is not a poison. The link to heart disease is based on eating too much of it.

How much is too much? The U.S. government sets a limit of 20 grams a day, the value you see printed on nutrition labels. That limit is for a person consuming 2,000 calories, which is what an average-size, active woman consumes. The 20-gram limit is only an estimate, however. No one knows for sure the safe limit. Besides, it varies with the individual and other foods in the diet. But if cutting back on fat in your diet is a goal, the government's 20-gram limit is a benchmark to shoot for.

Your body doesn't need saturated fat for any nutritional reason except for the energy it supplies. Other foods supply energy. Regardless of the exact limit, therefore, it is a matter of prudence to cut back on those foods with a high amount of saturated fat.

Look at the amount of saturated fat in those potato chips, 3 in 1 ounce. If you consume the whole bag (6 ounces) you consume almost your entire 20-gram limit for the day. That doesn't leave room for the saturated fat in dairy and meat products you might eat.

What does the term "saturated" mean?

What does saturated mean? Saturated with what? A fat contains fatty acids, each of which is built from a string of carbon atoms. Hydrogen atoms are attached to the carbons, and, when all possible hydrogen atoms are attached, chemists say the fatty acid is *saturated*. That is, every fatty acid in the fat is saturated with hydrogen.

The term *saturated fat* is a convenient way of describing a broad class of solid fats. Animal fats, on average, have a higher proportion of saturated fat than vegetable fats. Beef fat and butter, for instance, are solid by reason of a high percentage of saturated fat. Butter consists of about 67 percent saturated fat. Potatoes contain a negligible amount of fat. So where does all that fat in the potato chip come from?

The chips are made by slicing the potato and immersing the slices in a vat of very hot vegetable

Unofficially...
You often see the term *triglyceride*. Triglyceride is the scientific name for fat. Technically speaking, a fat consists of three fatty acids joined to glycerol. There are many different fatty acids in nature, so the number of different triglycerides is also enormous. Fortunately, from the point of view of nutrition, we need concern ourselves only with a few classes of fat.

fat. The chips cook and, because of the large surface area, absorb a large quantity of the frying fat. In this particular chip brand, 3 out of 20 grams or 15 percent of the fat consists of saturated fat, all from the frying oil.

Olive oil delivers monounsaturated fat

Why has olive oil acquired a positive image compared to butter and beef fat? It began with the discovery that Mediterranean peoples with their olive oil diet had few heart attacks. Recent medical research continues to favor olive oil. A special fat, rich in olive oil, is believed to help protect against plaque buildup (plaques are fatty deposits on the interior wall of an artery) in coronary arteries, a cause of heart disease.

What is this special fat, and do other cooking oils contain it? This fat is called *monounsaturated* fat. A little chemistry explains what the term means. As mentioned, saturated fat is completely saturated with hydrogen. Hydrogen atoms can be removed from saturated fatty acids of fat in pairs. Removal of one pair of hydrogen atoms creates a *monounsaturated fatty acid*. We often say monounsaturated fat and sometimes just monounsaturate. All the terms mean the same thing.

The key monounsaturated fatty acid is called *oleic acid*. Thus, you often see an oil referred to as a high-oleic oil, which means it contains a high percentage of monounsaturated fat.

All fats of natural origin contain most of the types of fat in varying proportion. Olive oil happens to have a high content of oleic acid. Other vegetable oils also contain monounsaturated fat. The following table lists the fat composition of unrefined vegetable

Bright Idea
Check the grams of saturated fat listed on product labels. Don't be misled by a small serving size. Do a quick calculation to see if the amount you actually eat pushes your daily intake of saturated fat to the government's limit. Keep in mind that the 20-gram benchmark is for all foods you eat in a day.

oils. As you can see from the numbers, olive, canola, and palm kernel oils are the top three with respect to monounsaturated fat.

TABLE 4.4: PERCENTAGES OF FATTY ACIDS IN UNREFINED OILS*

Oil	Polyunsaturated (Linolenic)	Polyunsaturated (Linoleic)	Monounsaturated (Oleic)	Saturated
Corn	59	24	13	
Canola	9	20	56	7
Cottonseed	52	18	26	
Flaxseed	53	3	20	9
Olive	1	8	73	14
Palm kernel	2	11	82	
Peanut	32	45	17	
Sesame	41	39	14	
Soybean	3	45	30	18
Safflower (high linoleic)	74	12	9	
Safflower (high oleic)	14	73	6	
Sunflower (high linoleic)	66	20	10	
Sunflower (high oleic)	40	45	10	
Walnut	5	51	28	16

(Source: U.S. Department of Agriculture, Nutrient Database)

*The percentages don't necessarily add to 100, because other fats not listed are present.

Polyunsaturated fat—the body builder

Fifty-five percent of the substance of your brain is fat. Ever been called a fat head? Take it as a compliment. It's the fat that makes your brain work. The

Watch Out!
The term "polyunsaturated fat" covers a broad class. It includes fats which are essential to good health but can't be produced by the body, and thus essential to the diet. The term also covers fats that are not essential and in fact may be harmful, called trans fats. Beware of products that promote the term "polyunsaturated" without explanation.

impulses flashing along neural fibers—composed of fat—turn you into a thinking person. Not just any fat does this job. The brain is built from a fat in a class by itself—*polyunsaturated fat.*

Polyunsaturated fat plays a key role in the body, not just in the brain, but in all organs and muscles. Every organ and muscle builds polyunsaturated fats into semi-liquid membranes which fold into each cell. The membranes give each tissue a characteristic function. Heart membranes time the beat. Liver membranes cleanse the blood of toxic chemicals. The membranes of muscles guide precision movements. In short, the most vital happenings of your being depend on polyunsaturated fats.

The definition of a polyunsaturated fat is straightforward. Removal of more than two pairs of hydrogens from a saturated fatty acid creates a polyunsaturated fatty acid, or fat. Some fats in animals have five or six pairs of hydrogens removed, but for the sake of discussion we lump them all under the term "polyunsaturated fat."

Estimate the degree of saturation of vegetable oils

The nutrition label of a cooking oil or fat may not indicate how much unsaturated fat it contains. Here is a handy rule of thumb. The higher the percentage of unsaturation in the product, the more liquid it becomes. Vegetable shortening and butter with their saturated fat are solids. Oils rich in monounsaturated fat are liquid at room temperature but freeze in the refrigerator. Oils containing a large amount of polyunsaturated fat remain liquid in the refrigerator.

The following table summarizes these differences.

TABLE 4.5: DEGREE OF SATURATION OF FATS

Fat	Pairs of Hydrogens Removed	Solid or Liquid	Examples
Saturated	None	Soli	Beef fat, butter, shortening
Monoun-saturated	One	Liquid, room; solid, refrigerator	Olive, peanut oils
Polyun-saturated	Two or more	Liquid in refrigerator	Canola, corn, saf-flower, sunflower oil

The lowdown on essential fatty acids

Neither saturated nor monounsaturated fat is essential to your diet. Your body makes these two types of fat from sugar, pasta, grain, potatoes, and other vegetables. But a curious twist of nature leaves humans unable to make key polyunsaturated fats—or to be more exact, fatty acids. These fatty acids must come from plant sources. The entire animal kingdom, from fish to birds to mammals, is in fact hostage to the plant kingdom for the *essential* fatty acids.

The two key fatty acids are *linoleic* and *linolenic*. Nutritionists call the two fatty acids essential because they are just as necessary to the diet as vitamins and minerals. Thus, you must get these dietary essentials either from plant foods or from animals that eat plants.

The essential fatty acids, built into the structures of brain, heart, muscles, and all other organs, are unstable. They are constantly destroyed and must be replaced. If you don't eat enough, tissue membranes gradually deteriorate and body efficiency erodes.

Insufficient linoleic and linolenic acids in the diet can cause a variety of symptoms:

Unofficially...
The names for linoleic and linolenic acids come from the Greek word for flax, *linon*. The word "linen" also comes from that Greek name.

- Muscle weakness
- Vision impairment
- Tingling in arms and legs
- Nervous disorders
- Depression
- Arthritis-like conditions
- Miscarriage
- Heart disease
- Male sterility

Should you be concerned about such symptoms? Is essential fatty acid deficiency an issue with modern foods? The answer is both no and yes. With the massive shift to eating plant-based fats, most people probably obtain sufficient linoleic acid. The problem: How do you get enough linolenic? You need both. The problem is growing worse, because of more intensive processing of vegetable fat which eliminates linolenic acid.

Linolenic acid's disappearing act

Linolenic acid has disappeared from food products made from vegetable fat. The reason has nothing to do with nutrition. It's economic. Linolenic acid—more so than linoleic acid—is highly susceptible to air oxidation. Oxidation causes breakup of the fatty acid, forming poisons, which also give a characteristic rancid odor and flavor. This is nature's way of telling you not to eat rancid foods. Makers of baked goods, potato chips, and snack foods obviously don't want to use a fat product with the slightest tinge of a rancid odor. So oil refiners remove the offending linolenic acid before it goes rancid.

In addition to the tricks of refining, the varieties of soybeans and other oil-producing plants are being changed through gene modification (genetic engineeering) to favor low-linolenic acid content. The net result is that food products with less linolenic acid reach the consumer.

Know the difference between omega-6 and omega-3

Linolenic and linoleic acids are critical to the normal functioning of brain and heart, even more so in the developing bodies of children. The reason is that these fatty acids belong to two broader series of essential fatty acids, called *omega-3* and *omega-6*. Each series consists of several members. Plants make one member each of the two series: linolenic acid (omega-3) and linoleic acid (omega-6). Once eaten, linoleic and linolenic acids are converted by your body biochemistry into other members, respectively, of the two series.

For optimum health, you need both omega-6 and omega-3 fatty acids in the diet. Why? They are two essential building blocks, each playing a unique role in the constant remodeling of body tissues. Your brain, for example, uses the omega-3s in most of its structures. The omega-6s won't do. For instance, you might have a surplus of the omega-6s and a deficit of the omega-3s in your diet, but the human body is unable to convert them to the needed omega-3 fatty acids.

The critical omega-3:omega-6 ratio

Evidence that omega-3 fats are critical to health first surfaced in studies of the Inuit (Eskimos) of northern Canada and Greenland. Eating a traditional diet of fish and seal blubber, these peoples obtained up to two-thirds of daily calories from fat. Yet heart disease was rare. Investigators believe that the high level of omega-3 fats in the fish protected the Inuit against heart disease.

Bright Idea
A baby's neural networks are created beginning at the first trimester and continuing for 6 months after birth. Most of the fat going into the networks is the omega-3 and omega-6 fatty acids. So mother should make sure she eats foods rich in both, but especially the omega-3s. After 6 months it's too late.

Moneysaver
The ratio of omega-3 to omega-6 fats in the brain is 1:1. Save your cash on supplements like ginkgo biloba, which are advertised as improving memory. A better way to sharpen your brain is to ensure you have enough omega-3 fats in the diet to maintain that 1:1 ratio.

The absolute amount of omega-3 fats in the diet, however, may be less important. More critical is the need to balance the amount of omega-3 with the amount of omega-6 fats. The ratio of omega 3: omega-6 fats in the Inuit diet was about 1:2.5. The corresponding ratio in the average American diet is about 1:20.

Nutritionists don't know the best ratio for optimum health, except that the 1:20 ratio seems unbalanced. Since Americans get sufficient omega-6 fatty acids in their diet, the practical challenge is to eat more of the omega-3 fatty acids.

Boost omega-3 fatty acids in your diet

Fresh fish is an excellent source of omega-3 fatty acids. Because of expense and possible chemical contamination, however, you may not wish to eat more than one fish meal a week (see Chapter 5, "Meats, Fish, Poultry, and Eggs"). Meat also provides both omega-3 and omega-6 fats. The problem with meat is that the large amount of saturated fat can overwhelm the two essential fats. Eat the leanest cuts possible.

Plant sources are your best bet. Of the common cooking oils, canola and soybean contain the highest percentage (see the table earlier in this chapter on the percentages of fatty acids in unrefined oils). As already mentioned, changing varieties of canola and soybeans used in oil production as well as harsh refining processes can result in oils on the supermarket shelf with very little omega-3 fatty acid (linolenic).

The following foods are especially rich in the omega-3s:

■ Algae

■ Beans

- Chia
- Fish oil
- Flax seed and flax seed oil
- Grains
- Kukui (candlenut)
- Leafy vegetables
- Purslane
- Tofu (if made from high linolenic soybean oil)
- Walnuts

Should you buy omega-3 supplements?

A word about supplements. Fish oil and flax seed oils are extremely sensitive to light and air oxidation and so aren't good practical sources of omega-3. If you do buy them, choose a store that keeps them refrigerated and buy in small quantities.

Flax seed is an excellent and practical source of linolenic acid. The iron-hard seed coat naturally protects the oil from deterioration but also protects the seed from digestion. You can grind the seed in a coffee grinder. A tablespoon of ground flax seed delivers 1.5 grams of linolenic acid. Sprinkle the freshly ground flour on your cereal or bake in bread or muffins.

A final word about omega-3 fatty acids and the diet–heart disease connection. The omega-3 fatty acids deserve as much attention as the idea that excess saturated fat and cholesterol contribute to heart disease. The food-manufacturing industry, taking advantage of public fears, provides foods lower in saturated fat and cholesterol. Ironically, at the same time, the omega-3 fatty acids are disappearing from manufactured foods.

Watch Out!
Don't go overboard buying omega-3 supplements. An overabundance of omega-3 fatty acids in the diet can tip the omega-3:omega-6 balance in the wrong direction. Also, don't be fooled by supplements sold as gamma-linolenic acid. Despite its name, this fatty acid is an omega-6 not to be confused with alpha linolenic acid, which is in the omega-3 series. (The alpha is generally omitted from the name.)

The lowdown on trans fats

Denny Lynch, vice president for communications for Wendy's restaurants, voiced his exasperation to a *New York Times* reporter in 1993 regarding research on beef fat versus vegetable fat. The fast-food industry had just completed an expensive changeover of the fat used in deep-fat fryers, from beef fat to vegetable fat. They changed to vegetable fat under pressure from health and nutrition activists who claimed that beef fat with its high saturated content damaged peoples' hearts. Later, other research established a link between the vegetable fat in the fryer and an increased risk of heart disease. According to the *New York Times* (March 5, 1993), Lynch was exasperated by the conflicting research. He wished someone could give him the right piece of research to go with.

The vegetable fat used in deep-fat fryers contains *trans* fat, a type of fat linked not only to heart disease but to breast cancer. A study of European women found that women eating a diet high in trans fats had three times the rate of breast cancer as women eating a diet low in those fats.

As with all studies, keep in mind that this observation is a correlation, not necessarily a cause-and-effect relation. Nevertheless, this is troubling issue. Deep-fried foods are popular and eaten in huge quantities. People love the deep-fried taste. But with the taste, they get a lot of fat. Forty-four percent of the calories of french fries comes from absorbed fat. Up to half of that absorbed fat can be the trans, a fat now declared dangerous to one's health.

What's going on? Is the new research right? Is vegetable fat with trans fat as harmful as beef fat (mostly saturated fat)? We look at the issue from two perspectives: that of the food industry and that of the consumer.

Hydrogenation produces trans fats

Restaurants run their deep-fat fryers from morning to late at night, day after day, without changing the oil. The temperature, a searing 355°F (180°C), creates what can best be described as a chemical reactor. The hot fat, exposed to the air, breaks down, producing toxic byproducts that affect taste and discolor the food being cooked. If you are a restaurant operator, discolored oil in the fryer is a major headache. To minimize breakdown and discoloration of the cooking oil, the vegetable oil industry changed the makeup of the vegetable oil by a process known as *hydrogenation.*

Hydrogenation, as the name implies, adds hydrogen back to the unsaturated fatty acids of the oil. The technical result is a fat that resists breakdown in a deep-fat fryer. The industry can run deep-fat fryers longer between oil changes.

Deep-fried foods are not the only source of trans fats. Hydrogenated vegetable oils have a long shelf life, a factor important to the food industry. The hydrogenated fats are therefore used extensively in cooking and salad oils, shortenings, crackers, baked goods, and frozen meals. Because trans fats occur in so many food products, Americans eat anywhere from 11 to 28 grams a day. For some people that amounts to about 20 percent of their total fat calories.

Trans fat linked to health problems

The trans fats produced by hydrogenation are unnatural. From your body's viewpoint, they are misshapen molecules. They offer none of the life-sustaining power of the monounsaturated and polyunsaturated fats in the original vegetable oil.

> **"**
> Trans fatty acids do occur in nature, principally in the rumen of cows. Small amounts of these trans acids may find their way into the fat of cuts of beef. The trans fatty acids produced in commercial processing of vegetable oils are quite different. They are artifacts, not found in nature.
> —Scott Grundy, in the *New York Times*
> **"**

The health issue, however, is murky. Trans fatty acids don't poison—they don't make you sick to the stomach. Bodily harm may come over the long term and is related to how much of the trans fat a person consumes. But no one knows what amount, if any, is safe.

Mary Enig, a respected researcher formerly of the University of Maryland, has studied the effects of trans fats on health. In addition to heart disease and breast cancer links, she and coauthor, Sally Fallon, list the following negative effects of trans fats in two articles published in *Nexus* magazine (Nov./Dec., 1998 and Feb./March, 1999). The trans fatty acids:

- Interfere with the normal function of essential fatty acids.

- Decrease testosterone and increase the level of abnormal sperm (in animals).

- Interfere with pregnancy.

- Lower quality of breast milk.

- Decrease insulin response (not good for diabetics).

- Change the fat makeup of adipose tissue.

Trans fats add to your saturated fat load

How do you know if a food product contains trans fats? Nutrition labels do not help. The FDA requires that the label list amounts of total fat and saturated fat. The manufacturer, as an option, may list monounsaturated and polyunsaturated fats, but is under no obligation to list trans fats. And in view of the unfavorable public image of trans fats, manufacturers are unlikely to voluntarily advertise its presence.

Thus, the presence of trans fats remains hidden— well, not exactly. Let's go back to the fat listed on the label of a bag of potato chips in the table earlier in this chapter. According to the label, the chips contain 10 grams of total fat per serving, of which 3 grams are identified as saturated. What are the mystery 7 grams? Since the chips were deep fried in hydrogenated vegetable oil, we can plausibly assume that as high as 40 percent of the mystery 7 grams is trans—about 3 grams.

Let's do simple addition. In terms of health impact, trans fat has a similar effect as saturated fat. Thus, the potato chips deliver not just the 3 grams of saturated fat per serving but, from your body's viewpoint, 6 grams of the equivalent of saturated fat. We noted earlier that the whole bag delivers your daily limit for saturated fat; more accurately, the bag of chips delivers double that. As a result, the trans fat content of foods, hidden in the label, can easily put your saturated fat intake well over the 20-gram limit.

The Center for Science in the Public Interest in Washington, D.C., analyzed the trans fats in commercial food products and calculated the total burden of trans plus saturated fat, as seen in the following table.

Bright Idea
Avoid trans fatty fats. Buy baked potato chips and tortillas instead of fried. They taste just as good, deliver overall less fat, and, best of all, don't have the trans fats.

TABLE 4.6: TRANS AND SATURATED FAT IN FOODS

Food	Calories	Total Fat (g)	Saturated Fat (g)	Trans Fat (g)	Saturated + Trans Fat (g)
Burger King french fries	470	22	6	7	13
KFC chicken dinner	1,160	52	12	7	19
Red Lobster Admiral Feast	2,020	97	26	22	48
Nabisco Triscuits (7)	140	5	1	1	2
Entenmann homestyle pie 1/6	410	17	5	2	7

TABLE 4.6: TRANS AND SATURATED FAT IN FOODS (CONT.)

Food	Calories	Total Fat (g)	Saturated Fat (g)	Trans Fat (g)	Saturated + Trans Fat (g)
Starbucks blueberry scone	420	15	4	4	8
Cinnabon	670	34	6	6	14

Copyright © 1996 CSPI Adapted from Nutrition Action Healthletter, (1875 Connecticut Ave. NW, Suite 300, Washington, DC 20009-5728. $24 for 10 issues.)

Although the food industry doesn't label trans fats, you don't have to be a chemist to spot them. Here are two easy ways:

- Any food that has been deep fried contains trans fats.

- The code word on product labels for trans fats is "hydrogenated" or "partially hydrogenated." Scan the ingredient list for either term.

Margarine: better than butter?

Margarine deserves special comment. Margarine gained its reputation as a health food because manufacturers make it from vegetable oil containing polyunsaturated fats. But the manufacturing process converts the liquid vegetable oil to a solid fat by hydrogenation. Thus, most margarines contain trans fats, in the range 0 to 30 percent of fat content.

Consumers are often confused by promotions for margarine. They see claims—"rich in polyunsaturated fat"—which imply that eating margarine is good for one's health. Technically, the advertising is correct, because trans fats can be classed as polyunsaturated fats. But as pointed out above, they don't behave in your body like natural polyunsaturated fats. They behave like saturated fat or worse. Thus hard margarine, from your body's viewpoint, contains almost as much saturated fat as butter. The following table lists the percentages of trans plus saturated fat of different types of margarine.

Eat Olestra, stay thin?

The ads tell you that an ounce of potato chips made with the fat substitute Olestra delivers 75 calories compared to 150 for regular chips. For individuals concerned about fat intake, that sounds too good to be true. Is it? The answer is yes and no.

Procter and Gamble created Olestra (brand name Olean) by taking a mixture of fat and sucrose, two natural substances, and combining them in an unnatural way. Olestra molecules are huge, too big for the normal digestive enzymes to handle. So Olestra passes unscathed through the gut. As a technical feat, Olestra is a superior fat replacer. Unlike other replacers on the market, Olestra can be used in deep-fat fryers to fry potato chips, tortillas, and crackers.

Olestra gives the mouthfeel and taste of soybean or cottonseed oil, the fats used to manufacture it. So consumers have a desirable fat taste without the calories.

Is this the dream of being able to enjoy the pleasure of eating without paying a penalty of excess calories? Well, there is, in fact, a penalty. When normal digestion is thwarted, negative things happen. One of the most unpleasant is diarrhea.

Not everyone is affected in this way. A Procter and Gamble spokesperson says that potato chips made with Olestra are no more likely to cause abdominal distress than regular potato chips. Nevertheless, products containing Olestra bear the warning: "May cause abdominal cramping and loose stools."

Unofficially...
European food manufacturers, sensitive to the health issues swirling around trans fats, have long produced margarines without using hydrogenated vegetable oils. American manufacturers have been reluctant to follow suit. Nevertheless, margarines made from nonhydrogenated vegetable fats are entering the American market.

Unofficially...
An editorial in the University of California at Berkeley *Wellness Letter* (February, 1999) suggests that, because of all the unresolved issues surrounding Olestra, the world is better off without it.

Then there's the matter of fat-soluble vitamins. Vitamins A, D, E, and K are normally absorbed in the gut by dissolving in the fat you eat. They also dissolve in Olestra, which sweeps them out of the body. This fact could be a serious matter for those already on the edge of vitamin deficiency.

Finally, people who eat reduced calorie chips made with Olestra may feel liberated from dietary restraint. They wind up eating more calories than they would get eating regular chips.

Choose organic?

Individuals concerned about pesticides in their food should be aware that soybeans and canola (rapeseed) are two crops heavily dosed with pesticides during the growing season. If the oil goes through the refining process, most of the pesticide residues are likely removed. But if you buy unrefined oils, consider those products made from crops grown organically.

Nearly all the commercial soybean and canola crops grown in the United States and Canada have been genetically engineered in some way. Such crops are often referred to as transgenic. The genetic makeup of the plants has been altered to favor production goals.

Soybeans are engineered so that they resist application of the herbicide, Roundup. Formerly, the farmer sprayed herbicide on the field to eliminate weeds before planting the soybeans. The soybeans themselves were not sprayed. Farmers now are able to spray the Roundup-resistant soybeans with the herbicide after planting. The herbicide kills noxious weeds, leaving the soybean crop untouched. The downside for the consumer is that the soybeans may be contaminated with the herbicide.

Genetic engineering is also employed to alter the fat makeup of oilseeds, particularly reducing the amount of linolenic acid (omega-3). From the viewpoint of producers, linolenic acid is a nuisance. It rapidly reacts with the oxygen of air, forming unusual flavors and odors. Plant geneticists have engineered new strains of soybean and canola plants that have reduced amounts of linolenic acid.

From a consumer's standpoint, the issue is knowing which strain of soybean or canola is the source of the oil in the store. For highly refined oils, the issue is not so important. The linolenic acid is partially or totally destroyed during refining. But purchasers of unrefined oils expecting the oil to contain linolenic acid won't know which strain of soybean or canola is used to make the oil. FDA requires no indication on the label if the oil is produced from transgenic plants, unless there is a foreign protein that might cause allergies.

Just the facts

- Fear of fat started with the idea that diets high in saturated fat and cholesterol are linked to heart disease. We should take a broader view. A lack of the essential fatty acid, linolenic (omega-3), a common problem in the average American diet, is just as critical.

- Extraction and refining of vegetable oils can cause sevre nutritional degradation. Less is more: The less processing, the greater the nutritional value.

- Manufactureed foods based on vegetable fats may contain unnatural fats, called trans. Overconsumption of the trans fats has been linked to a number of health problems. The biggest source of trans fats is deep-fried food.

■ Although the fat substitute, Olestra, is not digested—it passes through and out of the body—people may overeat Olestra-containing products, getting more calories than they would from a regular product.

GET THE SCOOP ON...
Why a steak is nutritionally better than
hamburger ▪ Chunked and formed ham ▪ "Fresh"
chicken, frozen in the warehouse ▪ Omega-3
eggs ▪ Farmed versus wild fish

Meats, Fish, Poultry, and Eggs

It's hard to relate those pink-and-red-cellophane–wrapped steaks, fillets, breasts, and ground meat to living animals. Yet meat starts out on the hoof or feet. What happens to the meat between then and the supermarket has a huge impact on whether meat consumption is positive, indifferent, or a drag on the body.

About 80 percent of Americans eat red meat (beef, pork, and lamb) and poultry (chicken and turkey) on a regular basis. On average, each person, young and old, obtains about 500 calories daily from meat, about half of that from fat. This meat represents one-quarter of the daily intake of a woman on a 2,000-calorie diet. It's a big chunk of the day's nutrition, and worth seeking top quality.

Worth how much? A long-term study of some 100,000 female nurses in their middle years found that those who ate red meat suffered two-and-one-half times the rate of colon cancer as those who ate mostly chicken. Is red meat therefore less healthy than chicken? Not necessarily. We need to put the link between meat and colon cancer in perspective. In order to trigger a cancer, a lot of negative things related to nutritional quality must occur. The issue is not so much a difference between eating chicken and red meat, but how to gauge nutritional quality.

We don't know exactly the cuts of meat those 100,000 women ate over a period of years, but it's safe to assume they ate what Americans on average eat. On a nutritional quality scale of one to four, most red meat people eat ranks at the third and fourth level, whereas most poultry products people eat rank at about the second level.

Apart from the cancer issue, there are many reasons related to general health and body weight for upgrading the nutritional quality of the meat in your diet. If you have growing children in the family, upgrading choice is particularly urgent. Each day of growth is like putting one brick in place towards a complete house. Once in place, it is there for good. Why stick in a lower quality brick?

This chapter provides you with a behind-the-scenes look at the meat and fish industries, bridging the gap between hoof and fin and the supermarket. The chapter gives you the know-how to move your choices up a rank or two.

Nutritional ranking of red meat, poultry, and fish depends on two factors: how the animals are raised and how the meat is processed. As far as fish are concerned, the first factor is becoming equally critical to quality, because an increasing percentage of fish is raised in cages or ponds—farmed fish.

Upgrade the rank of your meat choices

The accompanying guide ranks commercial meats on a scale of one to four. Explanation of the rankings follows.

Unofficially...
Congress in 1990 passed a law that exempts nutrition labeling of fresh meat, poultry, and fish. Stores are supposed to post the information in the meat and fish sections, but in many stores posters with small print are positioned behind counters. You need binoculars to read the information.

TABLE 5.1: A GUIDE TO THE NUTRITIONAL RANKING OF COMMERCIAL MEATS

Quality Scale	Meat
1st Rank	Free-range animals; meats, broiled, grilled, or roasted
2nd Rank	Lean steaks; pork chops, broiled or grilled; beef and pork roasts, baked
3rd Rank	Commercial hamburger, broiled; baked ham; frozen meats
4th Rank	Bacon, wieners, sausages, luncheon meats, flaked and chunked meats, low-fat meats

First rank: The advantage of free-range meats

Meat production has become highly industrialized. The aim of the cattle, hog, or chicken producer is to grow the animal as big and fat as possible, and as quickly as possible. A calf following the natural course of nature takes 2½ years to reach a market weight of 1,100 pounds. In industrial settings, that time is compressed to 1 year and 3 months. How is this possible?

Only by manipulating the animal's physiology. Animals are confined to tight pens, allowing little movement. This is done to save space and to prevent the animals from using their muscles. Under these conditions stagnant muscles become layered (marbled) with fat, making the meat more tender. However, confinement breeds disease, which can ripple through the stock. As a preventive measure, animals are fed antibiotics, including ones commonly used in human medicine, like tetracycline and penicillin. The antibiotics have an added feature. They help accelerate the animal's growth. In addition, five different sex hormones are used to tone the animal's flesh into a softer texture, as well as speed maturity.

On top of drugs and hormones, cattle eat a diet of about 90 percent grain, a food not natural to them. Cows, being ruminants, normally eat grass or hay. Their intestinal tract is designed for bulky foods. Grain, in contrast, is an energy-dense feed that overstokes the animal's physiology, accelerating growth with fat-marbled flesh.

Hogs are raised in a similar way, confined to tight pens and given drugs and concentrated feed.

It is hard to imagine that under these production methods the nutritional value of the animal's meat doesn't alter. Just think if your own physiology had been forced so that you reached full adulthood at age 8. Unfortunately, we don't know for sure what happens with meat, because the question of altered nutrition has not been studied. Government agencies such as the USDA and FDA assume a piece of meat is a piece of meat.

Probably 99.5 percent of the meat sold in supermarkets and deli comes from accelerated-growth animals. The remaining half percent of meat comes from animals allowed to mature at a normal rate—organically raised. Here are four rules organic cattle producers follow:

- The animals eat a diet suited to their physiology.
- The animals are pasture-fed. Roaming open fields, they are less susceptible to disease.
- The producers follow good husbandry to keep the animals healthy, using drugs only as last resort.
- The animals are not given sex or growth hormones.

Organically raised meat is generally done on small, family-owned farms. If you are interested in purchasing organic meat, you may have to seek out such farms, although many supermarkets now offer organic meat. In some stores, the meat is labeled "natural." Since the words "organic" and "natural" have no legal meaning, you should look to see if the meat is certified organic by a state or by an organic-farming association. Failing that, the store ought to provide a description of how the meat animal was raised.

In any event, this is the only meat that deserves first ranking. All other meats rank at level 2 or lower.

Second rank: Choose cuts at either end of the animal

A piece of meat as it comes from the animal still has the solid structure of flesh. It is composed of a tight array of cells that act like water-tight containers. They retain fluids with vitamins, minerals, and, importantly, the 1,001 substances that give cooked meat its characteristic aroma, flavor, and eating enjoyment. Freezing breaks down cell structure. The fluids with the vitamins, minerals, and flavor components escape.

Steaks, roasts, and chops occupy the second rank, providing they are fresh. You should trim visible fat before cooking. Plenty of fat remains, however, some of which you see as streaks (marbling), and much of which you don't see, built into the flesh. The remaining amount of fat varies, but there are three ways you can estimate.

First, look. See how much marbling is present. Second, refer to the USDA grade. The USDA has graded beef since 1927, but the system has nothing to do with nutrition. In their grading system, the more fat, the better. The USDA grades, in ascending order of fat content, are:

Unofficially... Why does frozen meat tastes bland compared to never-frozen meat? Freezing causes a breakdown of cell structure and the loss of key vitamins, minerals, and flavor components.

- Select

- Choice

- Prime

Keep in mind that the USDA grades meat on the basis of fat built into the structure of the meat. So if you want leaner meat nutritionally just as satisfying, choose the choice or select grades.

The third method is to note where on the carcass the cut of beef comes from. Cuts from the middle of the carcass—ribs, loin, sirloin, flank—have more marbling and are more tender. Cuts from the two ends of the carcass include muscles the animal once used to move about—chuck, shank, round—and are tougher but have less fat.

Because of a greater fat content, the middle cuts can be cooked with dry heat, such as grilling or broiling. The end cuts should be braised or stewed. Both methods involve slow cooking. Braising is done in a heavy pot with a lid and a small amount of water. Apart from less fat, end cuts are tougher because they contain more connective tissue, also known as collagen. Slow cooking (the temperature never exceeds the boiling point of water, 212°F) breaks down the collagen, turning it into gelatin; this imparts a tender, juicy feel when the meat is chewed.

Third rank: Hamburger and frozen meats

Hamburger is America's favorite form of beef. In fact, three-quarters of all beef sold in the country is consumed as hamburger. Let's set aside the taste and convenience of hamburger—that's a personal choice—and focus on two matters: nutrition and safety. When the meat is ground, the cell structure is ripped open, allowing the escape of fluids with vitamins and minerals. In addition, the surfaces of all

Bright Idea
When buying hamburger, buy a round steak that you first inspect, then have the meat attendant grind it. This way you know exactly what goes into the hamburger, and you have freshly ground meat.

the little meat bits are exposed to air. The delicate essential fatty acids are rapidly oxidized. Meat is a good source of the omega-3 fatty acids, but they are the first to be destroyed by the air. In short, the nutritional value of hamburger starts decreasing the moment the meat is ground.

Safety is another critical issue with hamburger. An intact piece of meat, such as a steak or roast, resists bacterial invasion. Thus you can cook a steak or roast with a rare center and not have to worry about bacteria, because the interior won't be infected. Hamburger is another story. Having a multitude of surfaces, hamburger is rapidly colonized by bacteria. One study found one-quarter of all hamburger samples taken from supermarkets to be contaminated. To be safe, a hamburger patty must be cooked long enough to eliminate all center pinkness. This is a sign the interior temperature is sufficient to kill the bacteria (about 155°F).

A word about the word *hamburger.* It is a legal term, and ground meat labeled as hamburger must comply with a USDA definition. The term is quite generous. If the starting meat is fairly lean, the USDA allows the maker to add pure fat to bring total fat to 30 percent by weight. In calorie terms, a cooked hamburger patty delivers 1 calorie out of 2 as fat.

Frozen steaks and chops—why do they rank at the third level? As already mentioned, as the meat freezes, ice crystals form inside the cells and cause the cell membranes to deteriorate. The vitamin- and mineral-rich fluids leak out. More damage is caused when the ice crystals thaw. So the freeze-thaw cycle causes nutritional losses compared to the same meat consumed fresh; this drops the meat one quality rank.

Watch Out!
The law allows
the hamburger
maker to grind in
parts of the cow
you might not
normally buy,
such as the
animal's cheeks—
up to 25 percent
of the total
product.

We are talking here, of course, about nutrition. From the standpoint of running a home, meat in the freezer can be handy if guests show up unexpectedly or if you haven't shopped for a while. As always, it's up to you to balance convenience and nutrition.

Remember that, once frozen, meat continues to deteriorate, albeit slowly. The USDA recommends that when you use a separate freezer, store beef cuts no more than 12 months (8 months for pork). The maximum time for frozen hamburger is 4 months. If you use a freezing compartment in your refrigerator, cut the time in half.

Choose a cured ham with a bone

Injecting a saltwater solution (brine) into fresh pork is a curing method that goes back several centuries. Salt pork was a standard dish on wooden sailing ships. Bacteria don't grow in salty water, but the meat tastes horribly salty. Modern curing methods reduce the amount of salt needed by adding a variety of other substances: corn syrup, sugar, nitrite, liquid smoke, preservatives, colors, and chemicals that hold water. The pumped-up ham gains 8 percent in weight. Manufacturers often inject extra water (it's cheaper than pork), in which case the government requires that the label state "extra water added."

Cured ham ranks at level 3 instead of level 2 for a fresh pork roast because of the added chemicals. The chemicals do nothing for your nutrition and burden your body with extra work to get rid of them.

But what's this about the bone? Modern meat processing takes cured ham one step further. Fresh pork is "chunked and formed." The meat is cut into larger pieces, as much as an inch in size. The chunks are tumbled together—"massaged" is the word the industry uses—until the chunks are bruised. The injury causes protein to leach out in a gluey exudate, which coats the chunks. A high-pressure press molds the meaty mass into a ham shape. Like a solid ham, the chunked and formed ham is cured with salt, corn syrup, and numerous curing agents and flavors. As already mentioned, this product can legally be called a ham. As a boneless ham, it is easy to carve, and, in fact, many such hams come pre-sliced.

From the nutritional point of view, the chunking process allows more contact with air, causing destruction of delicate nutrients. In addition, leaching occurs, also removing nutrients. For this reason, the chunked and formed ham drops to the fourth nutitional rank.

The problem for the consumer is that the law allows this restructured ham to be called ham. So how do you know if the cured ham is genuine solid or a chunked ham? Look for the bone. A bone firmly lodged in the ham is a tip-off that the meat is original—third rank.

Fourth rank: Sausages, restructured, and deli meats

Many of the meats enjoyed today, such as sausages, salami, cured ham, and bacon, were invented as a way of preserving meat. Drying the meat, or adding salt or sugar to a meat, prevents spoilage bacteria from absorbing the water they need to grow. Our early ancestors knew nothing about microbes, but they did know that cured meat kept for long periods. The issue at the time was a choice between having cured meat or no meat at all. This is not the issue today, because meats are available year-round. From a cell's-eye view, the cured meats may store

Bright Idea
After you've wrapped your meat for freezer storage, write the date on the package in large letters. Clearly marking dates on packages gives you better control over the contents of your freezer. The recommended maximum storage time of meat in home freezers is 1 year.

well and are enjoyable, but lost nutritional value drops them to fourth rank.

Sausages and wieners: Don't expect much nutrition

Sausages and wieners fall into a class of meats the food industry calls *comminuted*. That word means "pulverized." The meat is ground very fine, much finer than the ground meat of hamburger. The meat is mixed with extra fat, emulsifiers, curing chemicals, coloring agents, spices, flavoring agents, and chemicals that hold water. The mixture is poured into casings. The product may be cooked, such as a wiener, or left raw, such as a pork sausage.

Why do these products fall to the fourth rank? Three reasons:

1. **Low protein quality.** Sausage meat consists of meat trimmings, lips, cheeks, and other scraps that can't be used for anything else. Cows incapable of providing steaks or even hamburger, are ground into sausage meat. These meat sources have a low-protein quality by virtue of a high amount of connective tissue. Connective tissue is an incomplete protein, unable to rebuild body tissues. Sausages, wieners, bologna, and other meats that fall into this category shortchange the consumer when it comes to protein. They particularly fail growing children with their high demand for quality protein.

2. **Fine grinding.** Grinding exposes meat particles to air oxidation. The full spectrum nutrition you obtain from a solid steak or roast plummets as essential fatty acids and sensitive vitamins vanish.

3. **Manufacturing.** The law is lax and producers have an economic incentive to fill the casing

Unofficially...
Pemmican is the earliest cured meat widely used in North America. Native Americans cut buffalo and deer meat into strips, sundried it, and pounded it with crushed blueberries, cranberries, or wild cherries. The berries contain natural antimicrobial agents and, moreover, made the pemmican slightly acid, preventing bacterial growth.

with the cheapest ingredients possible. Cheaper turkey and chicken parts wind up in pork and beef sausages. Water is cheap. Emulsifiers allow the meat to remain solid while holding a huge amount of water. Fat is another cheap ingredient. By law, fresh pork sausages may contain up to 50 percent fat by weight. That translates into 76 percent of the calories after cooking. Fresh beef sausages may contain up to 30 percent fat by weight (50 percent of calories after cooking).

> 66
> People aren't ready to know how their sausages are made.
> —Otto von Bismark, German chancellor in the latter part of the 19th century
> 99

Cooked sausages are ready to eat

While fresh pork and beef sausages must be cooked, a wide range of sausages are precooked by the manufacturer and are ready-to-eat. They may contain up to 10 percent water by weight.

This category includes

- Blood sausage

- Bologna

- Bratwurst

- Braunschweiger

- Hot dogs (wieners)

- Jellied beef loaf

- Knockwurst

- Liverwurst

- Salami

- Thuringer

In addition to these cooked sausages, sausages such as the popular pepperoni and Lebanon bologna are preserved by bacterial fermentation. Fermentation creates lactic acid which retards bacterial growth.

In buying ready-to-eat sausages, remember they are perishable. Check the package date. Unfortunately, there are no national standards for dating. The date can mean: date of manufacture; date to be sold by; date to be used by. Hopefully, the package indicates what the date means and also gives exact instructions on how long the package can be stored.

Flaked and formed steaks

After cutting 10 T-bone steaks out of a beef carcass, what do you do with the rest? From a meat packer's point of view, only a small portion of the meat between tail and head can be carved into expensive steaks. Much of the remaining carcass is ground into cheap hamburger. But meat packers have found a way to upgrade the price of their products—the *flaked and formed* steak. The carcass is mechanically deboned and shredded into cereal-size flakes, which are mixed with chemical binders and flavors, and extruded into laminar sheets. Like a piece of fabric, these sheets are cut into steak shapes, each identical in size. The steaks often come with grill marks printed on them.

This flaking and forming process is so sophisticated that without a microscope it is difficult to tell a genuine steak from a flaked and formed piece. The printed grill marks, though, are a dead giveaway. Restaurant chains, one notch above fast-food outlets, make flaked-and-formed steaks, veal cutlets, pork chops, and chicken breasts the centerpiece of their menus.

This process, incidentally, was developed by the United States Army, which wanted a low-cost, consistent source of meat for its army bases.

Compared to the solid-meat steak and chop, flaked and formed meats fall to the fourth rank for the same reasons that sausage meat occupies fourth rank. With a solid piece of meat you know that it is beef, chicken, or pork. Not so with the flaked and formed meat; other meats may be tucked in. The meat's natural structure is destroyed. Nutritional quality drops with air exposure. Then there are the chemical additives and the processing a solid steak doesn't undergo.

Low-fat meats: A nutritional rip-off

Fat is a four-letter word are far as meat processors are concerned. They have to contend with consumers' wariness of fat, of which meat has plenty. The industry has come up with one response—low-fat meat products. The easiest products to manipulate are the comminuted meats, sausages and deli meats, because meat can be replaced with water. Water is certainly low fat, to say nothing of its cheapness.

The technical trick: How do you add a lot of water and still have a solid sausage, wiener, or sliced luncheon meat? The answer: Add water-absorbing substances, like carageenan, soy protein, sodium polyphosphate, and chemically modified food starch. This mix now needs additional flavoring agents to mask the bitterness of the water-absorbing substances. The net result is a product with less fat, but more water and more additives. If eating less fat is your goal, eat less of the regular product.

Poultry: Chickens and turkeys

Poultry, chicken especially, has become a dominant meat in most American homes. One reason: cost. Chickens grow faster, reaching market weight in a month and a half, compared to about a year and a half for beef. A chicken eats one-sixth of what a beef

Watch Out!
Turkey and chicken meats (cheaper than pork) can be artificially flavored to taste like pork, ham, and sausage. They can even be legally sold as the real thing. An annoyed pork industry screamed foul and sued the turkey producers, but lost the suit. So the pork sausage, instead of starting life grunting "oink oink" may have cackled "gobble gobble."

cattle eats to produce a pound of meat. Chicken and turkey meat is cheap to produce, which is reflected in the price you pay in the supermarket.

Chicken and turkey meat is processed into a variety of products, with varying ranges of nutritional values. If you like chicken and turkey, choose products of higher rank to get superior nutrition. The following table gives a guide to the nutritional value of chicken and turkey products.

TABLE 5.2: A GUIDE TO THE NUTRITIONAL RANKING OF CHICKEN AND TURKEY MEATS

Quality Scale	Meat
1st Rank	Free-range chickens and turkeys, broiled or roasted
2nd Rank	Fresh chicken and turkey, grilled, broiled, or roasted
3rd Rank	Frozen turkey and chicken, whole or parts
4th Rank	Deli-style turkey breast, rolled turkey breast, flaked chicken breasts with grill marks, battered and deep-fried chicken

First rank: Seek free-range birds

Read any article or cookbook in which the writer talks about chickens and turkeys, and the words she or he uses to describe the taste of the cooked meat are "bland," "tasteless," or "dull." Cooks therefore strive to mask the dull meat flavor by using sauces, seasonings, marinades, and the ultimate, deep frying.

The modern poultry factory produces chicken and turkey meat at extraordinary speed and low cost but at a price—a tasteless product. Chicken and turkeys are not normally tasteless, but the manner in which they are raised makes them so. The birds stand on wire mesh, consume antibiotics and other drugs, and eat food scientifically flavored to encourage gorging. High-speed meat hasn't time to develop nuances of flavor.

However, if you give those chickens and turkeys the freedom of open pasture, leisure to grow at a natural rate (half the speed of factory-raised birds), and an opportunity to scratch for tidbits, in the end you have meat with character and taste.

If you look for such birds, gather your wits, because labeling standards are absent. The term *free-range* means the birds have been given some space to move about. They may still be fed high-energy rations and receive all the drugs. You just don't know.

Since 1982, the USDA has allowed the term "all natural." That term applies only to the processing of the meat, not the raising. The additives are not supposed to be artificial, but the meat can come from those drug-dosed, accelerated-growth birds. In short, if you want truly naturally raised birds, forget the labels and trust the vendor to provide you with reliable information on how the birds are raised.

Second rank: Choose fresh, never-frozen chicken

The nutritional value of the chicken starts falling immediately when the bird is killed and dressed. So you want to buy chicken that is fresh. The best instrument to determine freshness is your nose. If the chicken is fresh, you should smell nothing. If you detect the slightest whiff of an odor, the bird has started to decompose.

Commercial broilers achieve an accelerated growth, partly by acquiring fat in a hurry. Unlike beef and pork, where fat is marbled throughout the flesh, chickens lay down most of the fat under the skin. An advantage of buying broilers fresh is that you can discard the skin along with a goodly amount of the fat. To maintain a second rank level, the chicken should be broiled, grilled, or braised—no frying.

Moneysaver
Save money—go directly to the farm. Organic farming associations, which are active in every state, can provide you with a list of farmers who maintain free-range organic flocks.

A word about color. Chicken meat is naturally white, and that is the color people in most parts of the country seem to like. Many folks in the Northeast, on the other hand, like their chicken flesh yellow. The color is induced artificially by feeding the birds marigold petals, a chemical dye, or the yellowish gluten of corn. Color does not influence taste or nutritional value.

Select a fresh turkey

A whole roasted turkey seems to go with the year-end holiday seasons. Since this might be the only time of year you prepare a whole turkey, why not select the best? Buy a fresh bird. A fresh turkey is much more succulent than a frozen one. Not only does the taste of frozen turkey go downhill, so does the nutrition. The turkey industry, however, is geared to producing masses of frozen birds, so order a fresh turkey well in advance of the holiday season.

Turkey meat, like chicken meat, is now packaged in cut-up sizes: whole and half breasts, thighs and drum sticks, and breast cutlets. These turkey parts qualify for a second-rank level only if they come from fresh, never-frozen birds.

Third rank: Frozen birds

The flesh of frozen chicken and turkey, like that of beef and pork, suffers severe degradation when frozen. Fluid leaks out, carrying with it vitamins, minerals, and soluble substances that would have contributed to taste. For this reason, frozen poultry, compared to fresh, never-frozen poultry, drops to third rank.

Supermarkets sell many items—whole turkeys, for instance—obviously frozen. But they also thaw frozen whole chickens, chicken parts, and turkey

Bright Idea
When cooking a stuffed turkey, the stuffing heats up more slowly than the flesh. The USDA, concerned about dangerous bacteria surviving in undercooked stuffing, suggests leaving the stuffing out (you can cook it separately, adding juice from the cooked turkey for flavor). If you do stuff your holiday bird, use a meat thermometer.

parts and display them as if they were fresh. "Freshly thawed" would be the correct phrase. The consumer is left in the dark as to whether the fresh item has never been frozen or is in fact frozen-thawed. The government perpetuates this sleight of hand by allowing frozen-thawed items to be called fresh. The only stipulation is that the freezing temperature not fall below 0. This arbitrary mark seems odd, considering a bird at that temperature has the consistency of granite.

Fourth rank: Restructured chicken and deli turkey

Ever notice the uniform shape and size of those turkey breasts sitting in the deli counter? Can it be possible that they come from turkeys all sized the same? No, but they come from the same mold. What you see in the deli counter is a restructured piece of turkey meat shaped to look like a natural-born turkey breast. This turkey has gone through a chunked-and-formed process.

If you are in the turkey business, probably the greatest invention since the wheel is mechanical deboning. Machines take a fresh turkey carcass and in a flash strip out the bones. The remaining flesh, skin and all, is cut into chunks. Chemical binders, salt, corn syrup, sugar, liquid smoke, nitrite, ascorbic acid (vitamin C), other additives, flavoring agents, and colors are mixed in, and the mass is formed into the breast shape.

The deboned, chunked, and formed turkey meat, called *deli-style,* can also be shaped into ovals, squares, or rounds. The cooked rolls or squares are conveniently sliced. This is the sliced turkey you get in restaurants that serve those low-price turkey dinners.

Watch Out! Supermarkets sell ready-to-eat turkeys roasted to a golden brown. These birds fall into the third rank, because very likely they started out frozen. Moreover, that golden-brown color can be chemically induced, having nothing to do with the way the bird was cooked.

As in the case of chunked and formed hams, the nutritional value of these turkey products suffers because of the extra processing, exposure to air, loss of nutrients, and inclusion of additives.

Deboned chicken meat through the flaking and forming process can be formed into solid-looking breasts (with painted grill marks). All this work is done by machines—cheaper than having human hands carve off breast meat. Thus a solid piece of chicken that would otherwise merit a nutritional rank of two is demoted to nutritional rank of four.

The self-basting turkey may not be buttered

Perhaps because of massive advertising, the self-basting turkey has become increasingly popular. Nevertheless, it ranks at the fourth nutritional level. These birds are injected not with butter but with vegetable oil, often coconut oil, which has a high percentage of saturated fat. Along with the oil, you get emulsifiers, sodium phosphate, color, and artificial flavor. As the turkey cooks, this mixture bubbles to the surface and dribbles down the flesh. *New York Times* food editors, who taste-tested several brands of turkeys, describe the self-baster's taste as "chemical stew."

Battered and fried chicken

Perhaps because of modern chicken's dull taste, the battered and deep-fried chicken is highly popular. The batter compensates for the bird's lack of taste with salt and strong flavoring agents, including MSG and spices. The batter also absorbs the frying oil, in the same way as french fries, which imparts a deep-fried taste and adds to the fat burden. The protein value of the chicken survives. But overall nutrition, compared to chicken meats in higher ranks, is poor value for your money and poor value for your body.

To sum up, remember these seven tips when buying chicken and turkey:

- Buy boneless and skinless breasts.

- Sniff the meat. It should have no smell.

- Save money. Buy a whole chicken and cut it up yourself.

- Buy fresh (never-frozen) turkeys. You may have to order in advance.

- If you buy frozen poultry, avoid packages with free liquid or other signs of seepage.

- Be aware when you buy ready-to-eat chicken or turkey in the supermarket or deli that you have no idea of its history. It could have been abused and stored frozen for a long period. Also, meat deteriorates quickly once cooked. So if you do buy this item, eat as soon as possible.

- Buy "organic" chickens and turkeys, but find out from the vendor what "organic" means.

Eggs are a complete food

Mention eggs and the immediate thought is cholesterol. Eggs contain cholesterol, and this fact gives them a bum rap. Many people have stopped eating eggs altogether. The incessant advertising trumpeting cholesterol-free and low-cholesterol foods has brainwashed the consumer; now everyone wants low-cholesterol foods, and eggs hardly qualify.

Let's look at the claim that eggs are unhealthy. The claim is based on poor reasoning, the idea that a single component could define the food value of the whole egg. This faulty reasoning has been exposed in a study by Frank Hu and colleagues, Harvard School of Public Health, (*Journal American Medical Association*, April 21, 1999). They studied

Moneysaver
Cooking cannot rescue chicken or turkey meat that has a slight odor. All the cooking does is make the flesh safe to eat. If you buy a poultry product that has an odor, save your money and return the item to the store.

Unofficially...
Chickens can
count. A hen is
genetically pro-
grammed to lay a
small number of
eggs at a given
time, then stop.
The hen's inten-
tion is to sit on
the clutch of
eggs and hatch
them. But, as
long as the egg
producer removes
the eggs, the
hen keeps laying,
hoping to reach
the clutch limit.
She, of course,
never does.

117,000 men and women, age 34 to 75, over an 8-year period. Egg consumption among members of this group ranged from one egg a week to two eggs a day. Hu's team found absolutely no correlation between the number of eggs consumed and coronary heart disease. On the basis of this study, Hu concludes that healthy people can eat one egg a day with no problem.

Other studies of real people eating real eggs confirm that eggs eaten in moderate amounts do not affect blood cholesterol levels. If there's a culprit in raising blood cholesterol levels, it's saturated fat, of which eggs have little. Eat a single poached egg, for example, and you get half the saturated fat of eating a 1-ounce bag of potato chips.

Keep in mind, however, that the real test of a heart-healthy diet is not the ups and downs of blood cholesterol but whether or not your heart stays healthy. The Hu study on eggs and heart health speaks to that point.

TABLE 5.3: FATS IN EGG VERSUS POTATO CHIPS

Fat	Poached egg, 2 ounces	Serving of potato chips, 1 ounce
Total grams fat	4.5	10
Saturated fat	1.6	3
Mono- and poly-unsaturated fat*	2.9	7

*The polyunsaturated fats include the trans fats.

The message is simple: If you like eggs, don't be afraid to include them in your dietary regimen. An egg packs everything needed to make a living organism, a chick. Since the chick's nutritional needs match those of humans, an egg is capable of delivering full-spectrum nutrition.

That full-spectrum nutrition is available, however, only in a raw, freshly laid egg. As with other foods, eggs are processed, marketed, and made into a variety of egg-containing products.

The following table provides a guide to the nutritional quality of eggs and egg products.

TABLE 5.4: A GUIDE TO THE NUTRITIONAL RANKING OF EGGS AND EGG PRODUCTS

Quality Scale	Egg or Egg Product
1st Rank	Fresh eggs obtained from free-range ("organic") chickens, omega-3 eggs
2nd Rank	Commercial eggs
3rd Rank	Liquid eggs, dried eggs
4th Rank	Egg substitutes

First rank: Free-range and omega-3 eggs

The organic chicken produces superior eggs. But from a consumer's standpoint, the same issues apply here as we discussed for free-range broilers. With a lack of standard terms—free range may mean no more than walking around inside a shed instead of a cage—you have to probe the supplier to find out how the chickens are managed.

One of the interesting developments in egg production is the omega-3 egg. As mentioned in the previous chapter, omega-3 fatty acid is essential to human well-being but is uncommon in most foods. The more foods you include in your daily diet that contain omega-3 fats, the better.

Chickens don't make omega-3 fatty acids, and whatever omega-3s wind up in the egg reflects the amount in their food. A number of egg producers feed their chickens flax seed, marine oils, and soybean oil, sources of omega-3 fatty acids. The result: The eggs have three times the normal level of

Watch Out!
Watch out for off-center yolks. When an egg is freshly laid, the yolk is centered. As the egg ages, the white breaks down and the yolk moves off center. A membrane encasing the yolk weakens and the yolk flattens. These are all signs of an over-aged egg.

omega-3 fatty acids. Look for such eggs. You find them under different trade names in different parts of the country.

Second rank: Fresh commercial eggs

The fresh commercial egg is the egg that for most people is the easiest to obtain. So let's look at ways to maximize taste and nutrition:

- Refrigerate eggs in their original carton on a shelf, not the door. Opening and shutting the door shakes up the yolk and may cause cracking. Keep no longer than 4 to 5 weeks after pack date.

- If you wish, remove the rare blood spot you see with the tip of a knife. In fact, such a spot signals a fresh egg. The spots disappear with time.

- Fertile eggs aren't necessarily more nutritious. The fact that a rooster has chased the hen, however, is a sign they have room to do the chasing.

- The greenish-gray color you occasionally see around the yolk of a hard-boiled egg is nothing dangerous. It is iron sulfide, formed when iron in the yolk comes in contact with sulfur in the white.

- Brown and white eggs have no nutritional difference. The color is due to the genetics. Some breeds of hen lay a brown pigment in the shell.

- Eat eggs raw? The greatest fear is salmonella infection, but such infections are rare. The rate of contamination of eggs is extremely low, less than 1 egg in 10,000. The more likely source of contamination lies in the handling, that is, in the egg-producing facility or in the home kitchen (see Chapter 13 on food safety). To be safe, lightly cook eggs for 3½ minutes at 150°F. You don't need a thermometer. Cook until the white is opaque and set but not hard, and the yolk has begun to set but not runny.

Third rank: Frozen omelet mixes

The frozen omelet mix you buy in the supermarket has its convenience. It's simple to thaw and pour onto a griddle. You pay a price, however, in loss of nutritional value compared to making an omelet from fresh-cracked eggs. The industrial processing and pasteurization degrade the more delicate vitamins.

Fourth rank: Egg substitutes

Seeing a profit in the cholesterol fright, food companies started making cholesterol-free eggs. The egg's cholesterol is located in the yolk, so to make such an egg it is a simple matter to get rid of the yolk. From a cell's-eye view, however, the cholesterol-free egg doesn't make sense. In throwing out the yolk, you throw out the egg's nutritional value. The white of the egg is pure protein. Every other nutrient the egg possesses is dissolved in the yolk.

The egg substitute uses egg white, but instead of the nutrient-rich yolk, the substitute gives you nonfat milk, tofu, hydrogenated vegetable oil, emulsifiers, stabilizers, antioxidants, gums, artificial color, and added vitamins and minerals. Not the sort of mix that could produce a chick.

Finally, another word about eggs and cholesterol. Consider the total nutrition an egg offers, which is all-around, superior. The fact that eggs contain cholesterol is immaterial. For a small percentage of people, whom doctors can easily identify, eggs do increase the level of cholesterol in their blood. But for most people, as a 1999 study published in the *New England Journal of Medicine* found, eating two eggs a day has no effect on blood cholesterol.

The results of this study point out the folly of making blanket recommendations for the entire population because of a problem that may affect a few.

From sea to plate

Fish offer the pleasure of eating along with a treasure of nutrient values. Rich in protein, vitamins, and minerals, seafood (unlike land-based animals) offers an abundance of essential fatty acids, especially those hard-to-get omega-3s. This is the theory, anyway. But the practical challenge of moving fish from sea to plate with most of that nutritional treasure reasonably intact is formidable.

Problems begin the moment the fish is caught. Commercial fishermen use gill nets, which have a mesh like a volleyball net. The net, however, is made of plastic filament, invisible in the water. The fish swims into the net and the head penetrates the mesh, but the body is too big to pass through. The fish can't back out because its gills are caught. It struggles and drowns. At this point, the flesh is already bruised and starting to deteriorate.

In another type of netting, trawlers drag a net along the ocean bottom, as long as three hours per run. Fish caught early in the run are long dead and banged about before being brought to the surface. The more a fish is jostled, the mushier it becomes, and mushiness indicates nutritional degradation.

The least damaging way of catching a fish is the old-fashioned hook and line. Cod, skate, tuna, and

Bright Idea
Want to savor really fresh fish? Short of catching your own, go to a top restaurant. Such restaurants have special connections and get fresh fish from sea to your dinner plate much faster than supermarkets or fish stores. But of course, you have to be prepared to pay top price.

some salmon are caught this way. You may see the term "line caught" in the fish market.

Catching a fish is just the start of the race against rotting. Icing slows destruction, but the fish has to be moved fast to consumers. Salmon and cod, if not bruised and iced immediately, last 8 days. Mackerel and herring last even less time, 5 days. In general, the colder the water the fish swims in, the faster it deteriorates.

Given the time required for the fish boat's travel, warehousing, wholesaling, and transportation, by the time you see the fish in the fish market, there's not much quality time left.

In any event, truly fresh, wild fish occupies first rank in the guide to the nutritional quality of seafood.

TABLE 5.5: A GUIDE TO THE NUTRITIONAL RANKING OF SEAFOOD

Quality Scale	Seafood
1st Rank	Wild fish, fresh, broiled, grilled, baked; live lobsters, boiled or steamed
2nd Rank	Farmed fish, fresh
3rd Rank	Frozen fish, shrimp, and crab
4th Rank	Fish sticks, fake crab, canned fish

Second rank: Farmed fish, big business

If you order salmon in a restaurant, the fish likely never saw the open ocean. It probably grew up in a pen anchored in a narrow inlet along the North American coast or a Norwegian fjord. Chefs love farmed salmon because they are all the same size—this makes it easy to portion the fillets. Best of all, the fish are guaranteed fresh.

No waiting for the fish boat to arrive in port! Farmed salmon are caught, processed, and chilled one day and have arrived in the restaurant or fish market the next day. The idea of eating a noble fish that has been factory-raised appalls many people. For this reason, few restaurants advertise the source of their fish, and fish markets don't always put a sign next to the fish. You can tell, however, because the code word for farmed salmon is "Atlantic."

Wild Atlantic salmon have been fished almost to extinction. The species lives on, however, because it adapts to the close confines of the sea pens. Pacific salmon like sockeye, coho, and chinook don't survive the confined space.

Fish farming is a rapidly growing enterprise. Half the salmon now sold is farmed. Farming keeps up with demand as the world's sea life declines. Fishing fleets with their super-efficient fish-locating gear literally vacuum the oceans of fish. But the diversity of wild sea life that presently shows up in fish stores will shrink. Few wild species like Pacific salmon can be successfully raised in pens. The following table lists species currently farmed.

TABLE 5.6: FISH SPECIES THAT ARE FARMED

Fin fish	Crustaceans and Shellfish
Arctic char	Clams
Atlantic salmon	Crayfish
Catfish	Mussels
Red fish	Oysters
Striped bass	Shrimp
Sturgeon	
Trout	

From the consumer's point of view, farmed fish can be moved faster to market than wild fish and thus are likely to be fresher. Some species, such as trout and shrimp, are generally frozen, so freshness is not an issue.

The downside of farmed fish is that, like the crowded cattle feed lots, the fish are packed into a confined space. They eat a concentrated diet that makes them grow almost twice as fast as a wild fish. They are prone to disease and thus receive antibiotics and other drugs. Shrimp and salmon are given a synthetic dye to color their flesh pink.

Many people say the taste of farmed fish is inferior to that of their wild cousins. A fish that eats a variety of wild food and develops its muscles is bound to be tastier than a pen-raised fish. But again, in making choices, you have to balance freshness with whether or not the fish came from a pen.

Third rank: Frozen fish may be called fresh

Given the realities of moving a highly perishable product to market, much of the fish as it comes off the boat is frozen. The fish is kept frozen as it moves through the distribution system until it is thawed for display at the retail fish market. This fish is labeled "fresh." Surprisingly, that's legal. As with the "fresh" chickens, as long as the temperature of the frozen fish doesn't fall below 0°, the government allows the thawed fish to be called fresh.

When you approach the fish counter, you're on your own. You don't know exactly how long the fish has been in transport, how much abuse the fish has taken, or if it has been frozen.

Use your eye and sense of smell. No scientific instrument beats human senses. Fresh fish should have absolutely no odor—at most a fresh, ocean smell. Here are other tips when buying fish:

- The eye of a whole fish should be clear, bright, and bulging. If cloudy, the fish is spoiling.

- The skin should have a vivid color, with no blemishes, tears, or exudate.

- Fillets should have moist, solid flesh with a translucent sheen. Watch for dryness. Rub your hand across the fillet. If particles rub off, the fish is old.

- Check the display. Fish should be well-iced; it's best if the fish species are kept in individual, iced pans.

- Ask the clerk to put your purchase in a plastic bag together with a couple of scoops of ice.

Fourth rank: Fake crab, fish sticks, and canned fish

A reminder: The quality scale refers only to nutritional level, not enjoyment. Canned tuna has to be one of the most popular sandwich fillings, and canned salmon is delightful in a salad. The canned fish provide quality protein, omega-3 fats, vitamins, and minerals. But compared to the fresh tuna or salmon, the total nutrition has dropped significantly.

Fake crab, shrimp, and lobster, otherwise known as surimi, are also popular and much cheaper than the real sea creatures. Fake crustaceans begin life as pollack, a relatively cheap fish. The process is similar to the making of a flaked and formed steak. Frozen pollack is flaked, mixed with binders, stabilizers, and a huge dose of salt, and massaged into a crablike texture, which is baked in flat sheets. The sheets are cut into strips and rolled into the shape (more or less) of a shrimp, crab leg, or lobster tail. The final touch: a red dye is streaked on the surface. About all that can be said for the nutritional value of the fakes is that they provide some protein.

Finally, there are fish sticks and other deep-fried fish. Since the taste of these products comes from the batter and the soaked-in frying oil, you have no idea what fish you are eating, or indeed if it is fish.

The versatile textured vegetable protein (TVP) can be manipulated into a fishlike texture and infused with artificial fish flavor. If you ate this vegetable fish embedded in a deep-fried batter or bread crumbs, you would swear it was real fish. Commonly, the TVP fish is mixed in with the genuine fish so that the word "fish" can appear on the label.

In any event, battered and deep-fried fish sticks deliver fat calories, mostly from the frying oil, which consist of 30 to 60 percent trans fats. Compared to the riches of fish in higher ranks, these items are nutritionally impoverished.

Fish contain omega-3 fats

As pointed out earlier, the average American diet supplies a shamefully low amount of the essential omega-3 fatty acids. So a rich source such as fish is welcome. But the omega-3s are only part of the bountiful nutrition fish supplies.

Take for example the link between these essential fats and heart disease. A study of 8,000 Canadian Inuit (Eskimo) found they had one-quarter the heart disease of Canadians as a whole. Could it be the omega-3 fatty acids of the Arctic fish they eat? Other studies suggest that indeed, while the omega-3s help, supple arteries and a strong heart come from eating the total nutrition of fish.

Balancing safety with nutrition

Finally, a word about undesirable things in fish—toxic chemicals. Unfortunately, the world's waterways and oceans are also the world's garbage dump. Pesticides, agricultural runoff, and industrial wastes such as mercury, PCBs, and dioxin funnel into the waterways, where they enter the aquatic food chain.

Watch Out!
Are you swayed by the name of a fish? Apparently, a lot of people are. The slimhead, a fish in New Zealand waters, didn't sell. Enterprising fishermen changed its name to orange roughy. It became a bestseller. The Patagonian toothfish didn't sell either, until fishermen renamed it Chilean sea bass.

Carol Browner, administrator of the Environmental Protection Agency (EPA), has stated that 40 percent of the nation's rivers, lakes, and streams are not suitable for swimming or fishing. Federal and state governments issue fish advisories warning pregnant and nursing women not to eat any fish caught in these waters. Adults should not eat more than one fish meal a week and, in some areas, once a month.

Ocean fish can be just as contaminated. The situation poses an unfortunate dilemma. Fish deliver super nutrition. They also deliver toxic chemicals, but you don't know how much. There is no easy answer. Toxic chemicals accumulate in the fishes' fat, so one solution is to trim visible fat or choose relatively low-fat fish. A table in Appendix D lists species of fish arranged according to their habitat and fat content. Generally, freshwater fish are the most contaminated; nearshore fish, less contaminated, and offshore fish the least contaminated.

Since the fishing industry is unlikely to label fish with their chemical contaminants, you will never know to what degree a fish is contaminated. Your best approach is to follow the general government guideline—one fish meal a week.

Just the facts

- Meat from free-range cattle, hogs, and poultry deliver better nutrition and better taste. The definition of free-range and natural, however, is elastic. Get a description from the vendor of how the animals are raised.

- To get the best nutrition (and taste) from red meat (beef, pork, and lamb) and poultry, buy the meat fresh and grill, broil, or bake it.

- The largest-selling meat item is hamburger, but it deteriorates rapidly. Your best bet is to buy round steak and ask the butcher to grind it for you.

- Deli-style turkey breasts, hams, and luncheon meats are restructured meats. The original meat is chunked and reformed into a breast, a round, or a square. Nutritional value ranks low compared to the intact, solid meat.

- Fresh fish is best. Given a choice between a farmed fish and a wild fish of equal freshness, take the wild. It has better taste—and better nutrition.

GET THE SCOOP ON...
Lactose intolerance ▪ The differences between
nonfat and low-fat milk ▪ Processed cheese and
cheese foods ▪ Fat and cholesterol in cheese ▪
Artificial whitening of skim milk

Dairy: Milk, Cheese, Ice Cream, and Yogurts

Most Europeans visiting the United States are amazed to see adults drinking fluid milk. They think of milk as food for infants and toddlers, not for anyone older. To some extent, nature agrees. The majority of adults on the planet have difficulty digesting fluid milk, or to be more precise, digesting the milk sugar, lactose. They lack the enzyme, lactase, that breaks down lactose in the intestines, allowing the sugar to be absorbed. If not broken down, lactose passes into the lower bowel, causing bloating and intestinal distress. About 70 percent of African-American adults, for example, are lactose intolerant, while only about 10 percent of white Americans are intolerant.

An inability to handle fluid milk among our forebears, however, sparked an inventive urge. Because fresh milk is available year-round and also portable (the cow), peoples in different parts of the world solved the lactose problem by creating milk products that eliminated all or most of the lactose: butter, cheese, cottage cheese, yogurt, and ice cream.

These dairy products can be made by simple methods. In fact, if you want, you can make them in your own kitchen. Milk products spoil quickly. Thus, when milk and its products passed from being a cottage industry to being a commercial enterprise, production methods changed. Simple home methods for making cheeses and yogurts were adapted to mass marketing.

Yogurt, for example, is smoothed out and given a fuller body with the plant gum, carrageenan. Sugars, flavoring agents, preservatives, and other additives are introduced. The dressed-up yogurt may be more appealing and, importantly from the commercial point of view, have longer shelf life than plain yogurt. But nutritional values have deteriorated.

In this chapter, we look at traditional dairy products in their modern guises and identify the range of nutritional changes. With this insight you will be able to go into the supermarket or restaurant and make smarter choices.

Fluid milk: Homogenized, low-fat, and skim

Few people seem willing to contend with non-homogenized milk in which milk fat (cream) separates. The cream, being lighter than the water of milk, rises to the surface. Moreover, once separated, the cream cannot be mixed back into the milk. To avoid these problems and make milk more convenient to use, dairies homogenize it.

Homogenization changes the nature of the fat. The fat globules in the milk as it comes from the cow are relatively large and enveloped in the same type of membrane that envelops cells. The globules tend to aggregate and rise. Homogenization shatters the large fat globules, creating tiny fat particles that bind with proteins. Unable to aggregate, the fat particles distribute evenly throughout the milk.

Pasteurization

Heat treatment (pasteurization) of milk kills disease-causing microorganisms—if the milk is contaminated. Few states are willing to trust dairy farmers to produce uncontaminated milk and thus ban the sale of raw milk to the public. Nevertheless, in only a few areas of the country is certified (government-inspected) raw milk sold. So for most people, the option to buy raw milk is unavailable. All milk sold in stores is pasteurized. *Pasteurization* is named after the French scientist Louis Pasteur, who in the 19th century discovered microbes and realized they could be killed by heat.

Milk, however, is a delicate substance. Heat destroys some of the heat-sensitive vitamins and proteins, thus nutritional value falls. The trick in pasteurizing milk, therefore, is to heat it sufficiently to kill dangerous microorganisms, but not so much that the milk develops a "boiled milk" flavor. Dairies use one of two methods. They hold the milk at 144°F (62°C) for 30 minutes. In a much faster method, they heat the milk for 15 seconds at 160°F (71°C). The higher temperature borders on scorching the milk.

Milk that has gone through homogenization starts to spoil immediately. Therefore, dairies combine homogenization and pasteurization in one continuous production line. Pasteurization, in addition to killing disease-causing microbes, has an advantage of extending shelf life. The process also

Unofficially...
It's unclear how homogenization affects milk's nutritional value, but the character of the milk changes. Homogenized milk has a blander taste compared to the nonhomogenized product.

kills spoilage microbes and destroys normal enzymes that split the milk fat. If the enzymes attack the fat, they create an unpleasant odor and taste.

Proteins, the curds and whey of milk

Milk contains a variety of proteins. Some, like casein, are intended to nourish the calf. Others, like the lactoglobulins, fight disease (at least diseases that might infect a calf). From the viewpoint of a human consumer, all proteins are part of fluid milk's nourishment. Nevertheless, when dairies make cheeses and yogurts, milk proteins fall into two distinct classes, the traditional curds and whey of Miss Muffet fame.

Cheese is made by adding *rennet,* an enzyme obtained from a calf's stomach, to the milk. Rennet causes casein to coagulate into curds. The lacto-globulins remain dissolved in the fluid along with the lactose—the whey.

Casein also gives yogurt its semi-solid character. Casein coagulates when the lactobacilli convert some of the lactose to lactic acid, turning the milk acid. In making yogurt nothing is discarded, so you get the full spectrum of milk proteins. With cheese, conversely, you eat only part of the milk protein, the casein.

> **"**
> With organic methods, fertility is built up with the use of manures, compost, and cover crops which improve nutrient balance and microbial life. Research has shown that crops grown in such soils are more disease and pest resistant.
> —The Northeast Organic Farming Association of Vermont
> **"**

Fluid milks

You might feel that in terms of nutritional quality, among fluid milks, differences in nutritional quality are slight. Milk is milk and the big concern is over how to avoid milk fat. Well, not exactly. The fat issue is indeed important, but apart from fat, nutritional differences do exist. The following Table 6.1 gives a guide to the nutritional ranking of fluid milks.

TABLE 6.1: A GUIDE TO THE NUTRITIONAL RANKING OF FLUID MILKS

Quality Scale	Fluid Milk
1st Rank	Milk from organically raised cows
2nd Rank	Pasteurized, nonhomogenized, 2%, 1%, and nonfat milks
3rd Rank	Pasteurized and homogenized milks
4th Rank	Ultra-pasteurized, canned, or condensed milks

We'll now explain the rankings for the fluid milks. We start where it all begins—with the cow.

The super-efficient, hormone-treated milk cow

Raising milk cows, like raising beef cattle, has become a high-tech, no-room-for-error production. The milk cow has been bred specifically for producing milk. Unlike the bulky, muscular beef cow, the milk cow is large-framed, bony, and drags a huge udder. The goal: convert feed as cheaply as possible into milk.

To that end, the nutrition of the feed is scientifically balanced. When a cow enters the stall to be milked, a sensor reads an identity tag clipped in her ear. A computer analyzes the cow's recent production record and feed consumption and triggers a feed dispenser. A bolus of mixed grains, whose composition has been tweaked to match the cow's inner physiology of the day, drops in front of her nose. The cow munches while being milked.

The cow's grain-based food, unnatural for a ruminant, pumps up her physiology and pumps out the milk. A stressed physiology, however, is susceptible to infection, and cows have to be treated with a variety of antibiotics and other drugs. There is always a worry that drug residues will pass into the milk supply. Although a cow normally lives 15 to 20 years, the high-production cow burns out after 2 or 3 years of intense milking. Her scrawny frame goes directly to the hamburger factory.

The bovine growth hormone: Good for the consumer?

Unofficially... The United States is the only country that has approved the use of the synthetic bovine growth hormone, rBGH, in dairy herds. Australia and New Zealand have banned it, and the countries of the European Union have declared a moratorium on its use.

There's nothing new about factory-style milk production. Dairy farms have operated this way for decades. But that all changed in 1993, when the FDA approved the use of the bovine growth hormone (BGH). The hormone also goes under the name bovine somatotropin hormone (BST), and sometimes you see the term written *rBGH*. The "r" refers to the fact that the hormone is genetically engineered.

Animals, humans included, secrete a growth hormone, which causes the young to grow to adult size. Even in adulthood the hormone is important in maintaining tissue tone. Factory-produced rBGH is similar but not identical to the natural hormone the cow secretes. From the point of view of milk production, the hormone works wonders. Injected into a cow, rBGH boosts milk production by 10 to 15 percent. Thus, a cow producing 40 quarts a day could produce an extra 4 to 6 quarts. But extra production comes at a cost, and herein lies a storm of controversy.

The Canadian government in 1999 refused to approve the use of rBGH, citing as one reason for refusal the FDA's research on the safety of rBGH. Canadian government scientists say the research the FDA used to validate rBGH's safety is deeply flawed. Moreover, in looking over dairy herds in the United States that use rBGH, the Canadian scientists were stunned to find:

- The cows have a 25 percent greater risk of udder infections.
- Fertility has gone down 18 percent.
- Lameness has shot up 50 percent.

The Canadian government cites these facts as evidence that the cow's physiology, already stressed by its high production, is stressed even more. The FDA in response says that the composition and wholesomeness of milk from rBGH cows is the same as milk from non-rBGH cows.

But another issue looms. The addition of rBGH causes cows to secrete extraordinary amounts of a normal milk protein, called insulin dependent growth factor 1 (IGF-1). This is a milk protein humans don't need, and the larger amount in milk from rBGH cows may be a health problem.

Two ongoing Harvard studies, the physician's health study and the nurse's health study, found a link between IGF-1 and an increased risk of breast and prostate cancer. How serious the risk is remains to be seen, but critics of rBGH, like Marion Nestle, director of the Department of Nutrition and Food Studies at New York University, have called for more testing (*New York Times,* Jan. 19, 1999). The American Medical Association has weighed in with the comment that the science on the effects of oral ingestion of IGF-1 is incomplete. In short, we don't know enough about the safety of drinking milk produced in cows injected with rBGH.

How does this controversy affect consumers of dairy products, and what can you do about it? As of 1998, 30 percent of the United States's 9 million dairy cows were in herds that use rBGH. Since milk comes into a commercial dairy from different farms and is mixed together, you have to assume that all

Watch Out!
A word of caution about the word "organic." As mentioned in previous chapters, the word has no legal definition, so you have to trust the information the producer puts on the carton's label. Also look for the phrase "certified by," followed by the name of an organic farming association or state certification agency.

the milk in your local grocery contains a portion produced in rBGH cows. You won't know for sure, because the government doesn't require milk from rBGH cows to be labeled as such.

On the other hand, dairies that sell milk from cows that are not injected with the hormone can state that information on the label. So in terms of overall nutritional quality, organically produced, hormone-free milk occupies first rank on the quality scale of fluid milks.

Why organic? A concern over rBGH, drug use, and pesticides used in commercial farming causes many consumers to seek organic milk. Farmers have obliged, and in most areas of the country you can find organically produced milk and milk products. At one time you could find them only in natural food stores, but mainstream supermarkets now sell organic milk products.

Fluid milk comes with four degrees of fat

At one time most fluid milk sold was homogenized whole milk (3.5 percent fat). Then the concern over fat and, especially saturated fat, seized the public. The dairy industry started producing milks with four levels of fat: whole, 2 percent, 1 percent, and skim.

The names describing the reduced-fat milks vary. The FDA permits the following names:

- 2 percent—reduced-fat or less-fat

- 1 percent—low-fat

- skim—fat-free, no-fat, nonfat

If the terms confuse, just look for the percentage of fat in the milk.

Don't be misled by the fact that low-fat milks are referred to as containing only 1 percent and 2 percent fat. That amount doesn't sound like much, but the percentage refers to the milk's total weight, which is mostly water (87 percent). A more informative way of stating fat content is to state the amount of fat as a percentage of total calories. This gives a better idea of the amount of food value you get from fat. The following table shows the percentages of calories derived from fat.

TABLE 6.2: PERCENTAGE OF FAT CALORIES IN FLUID MILK

Milk	Fat calories as percent of total calories
Homogenized whole milk (3.5% fat)	48
Less-fat, 2%	35
Low-fat, 1%	23
Nonfat (0.4%)	4

You see from this table that even 1-percent milk gives you one-fifth of its calories as fat. Two percent milk on a caloric basis is one-third fat. This is something to keep in mind, if you are trying to reduce fat calories.

Fluid milk has additives

Fluid milk falls under government standards which strictly regulate what can and what cannot be put into milk. One item permitted in milk—one you'd never know about—is the metal oxide, titanium dioxide. Companies are not required to indicate its presence on the label. Titanium dioxide has a dense whiteness to it, and for this reason paint manufacturers use it in white paint. Nonfat milk has a thin, bluish look to it, so dairies may add titanium dioxide

Watch Out! Countries of the European Union, concerned over both deception and safety, have banned the use of titanium dioxide in milk.

to give the milk a whiter look. The metal is also used in butter, ice cream, and cheese.

Fluid milk is fortified with something more than a cosmetic touch-up. Vitamins A and D occur naturally in milk, but as they are dissolved in the fat of the milk, they are lost when cream is removed. But with vitamin A and D fortification, low-fat and nonfat milks now have ample amounts. With respect to vitamin D, you sometimes see the term D_3. This is the active form of the vitamin.

Vitamin fortification for some people has been a benefit. Health authorities credit the vitamin D fortification of milk with eliminating rickets, a disease that affects growing children. Bones require vitamin D to accumulate calcium. If not enough of the vitamin is present, calcium circulates in the blood unused. Without the calcium deposits, the long bones of the legs weaken and are unable to support the child's weight. As a result, the bones bow out, leading to the classic bow legs of rickets.

This disease was once a major public health issue for children living in northern sections of the country. Kept indoors and swaddled in clothes during long winters, they never received the sun to produce sufficient vitamin D in the skin. And diets often did not provide the necessary amounts of the vitamin. But the introduction of vitamin D has solved the problem.

Keep your milk fresh

Because milk is a highly perishable product, here are three tips for preserving the milk's freshness:

- Milk dating lacks any standard. From personal experience, I'd say the milk goes sour about the time of the printed date. So at best, select milk with the farthest-ahead date. Since supermarkets invariably put the newest cartons at the rear of the shelf, rummage around to find the best date.

- Light is an enemy. Light induces rapid destruction of milk fats, creating unpleasant tastes. Since nonfat milk contains some fat, it too is vulnerable. Light also causes loss of some vitamins, particularly riboflavin. Therefore, keep the milk away from light sources.

- The milk you buy is sterile. To keep the milk fresh as long as possible, try to maintain that sterility. Pour out the milk you need and close the top. Also, never pour back into the container unused milk. It will contaminate the container and cause the milk to spoil much more rapidly.

All fluid milks have roughly the same amount of protein and lactose. Eight ounces of milk (1 cup) contains 12 grams of lactose, 8 grams of protein, and roughly 300 milligrams of calcium. To put those numbers in perspective, a 6-year-old child drinking 8 ounces of milk gets one-quarter of his or her protein requirement for the day and about one-third of the calcium.

The amount of fat in different milks varies, of course, but fat composiztion remains the same. Of the total fat, about two-thirds is saturated fat. The remaining third is mostly monounsaturated with a small amount (about 3 percent) polyunsaturated. The following table summarizes the basic components of fluid milks.

TABLE 6.3: COMPOSITION OF FLUID MILKS

Milk, 1 cup (8 ounces)	Calories	Protein grams	Total fat	Saturated fat	Calcium milligrams
Nonfat	86	8.4	0.4	0.3	302
Low-fat, 1%	102	8.0	2.6	1.6	300
Less-fat, 2%	121	8.1	4.7	2.9	297
Whole milk	150	8.0	8.0	4.9	288
Buttermilk	99	8.1	2.2	1.3	285
Chocolate milk, 2% fat	179	8.0	5.0	3.1	284

(Source: Bowes and Church's Food Values of Portions Commonly Used, 17th ed. Revised by Jean A. T. Pennington. Copyright © 1998 Lippincott-Raven Publishers.)

The lower-ranked products: chocolate milk, ultra pasteurized, and condensed

Chocolate milk ranks at the third level because it has additives and a quantity of added sugar to make it sweet. It retains the protein, fat, and vitamins of the corresponding regular milk.

Ultra-pasteurized milk, as the name implies, has been subjected to intense heat (280°F/138°C, far above the boiling point of water). The idea is to ensure that all spoilage microorganisms are killed and also that fat-splitting enzymes are totally destroyed. But a process severe enough to wreak this damage among microorganisms also damages proteins and other delicate milk components. Nutritional value falls and, moreover, the milk has a cooked flavor to it. Ultra-pasteurized milk may be convenient, but you pay a nutritional price.

Condensed (or evaporated) milk is manufactured by evaporating about half the water. The concentrate is sterilized at high heat, a process similar to the canning of vegetables. The heat causes lactose to partly caramelize, which accounts for the characteristic taste. Sweetened condensed milk has a large amount of sugar added, which has the value of preventing microbes from growing. Thus, sweetened condensed milk need not be sterilized.

Powdered milk takes evaporation to the extreme, all the water being removed. It is generally made from low-fat or nonfat milk, because any fat retained in the powder would soon go rancid. Powdered milk mixed with water as a drink is hardly appealing, so it winds up in baked goods. Powdered milk is also added to low-fat milk under the term "nonfat dry milk solids." The intention is to increase the protein content of the milk and thicken it. The dry milk solids are composed of proteins, lactose, and minerals.

The condensed and dry milks rank at the fourth level by virtue of the heat treatment, with subsequent deterioration of nutritional quality.

Milk chocolate, a medicine?

People eat chocolate because they like it, not because it has medicinal value. Yet chocolate contains substances, called *polyphenols,* that are potent antioxidants, excellent protectors of our bodies. How? We come back to this fundamental problem of human life. We live in a bath of oxygen. While our bodies need oxygen to burn foodstuffs for energy, oxygen at all times threatens to react with vital structures of the body much as iron exposed to the oxygen of air rusts. Not that we are likely to rust! More precisely, cell components are damaged. Cells, whether muscle cells or heart cells, function less efficiently. Oxygen can cause premature aging, greater risk of heart disease and cancer, and loss of skin tone.

Bright Idea
Adding milk to chocolate does two things. It modifies the cocoa butter, giving it a creamy texture, and it cuts the natural bitter taste of cocoa.

The body protects itself from the harmful effects of oxygen by antioxidants it produces itself and by antioxidants received in the diet. The dietary antioxidants are critical. In Chapter 2, "Smart Nutrition in Your Basic Food Categories," we noted the strong antioxidant properties of phytochemicals in fruits and vegetables. The polyphenols are a specific class of phytochemicals, which also occur in red wine. The wine industry promotes the drinking of red wine—a glass a day suffices—as a way of staving off heart disease. While wine makers obviously have a vested interest in increasing wine consumption, there is some truth to their claim for the protective value of red wine. Red wine drinkers have fewer heart attacks, and the polyphenols have been pinpointed as the reason.

Why specifically do polyphenols come to the aid of the heart? Several classes of lipoproteins (particles comprising a mixture of fat and protein) circulate in the blood. Oxygen attacks one class, known as the low density lipoproteins (LDL), causing them to deposit as artery-clogging plaques. Polyphenols help to stop this from happening.

Where does milk chocolate come in? Say you don't drink alcohol or don't care for red wine, but you like chocolate. You get the same heart-protecting benefit of a 5-ounce glass of red wine by eating a 1½-ounce chunk of milk chocolate.

So if you like chocolate, dismiss any guilt feelings about eating it, unless of course you overindulge. Milk chocolate is only one variant of chocolate making, but the most popular. To make milk chocolate, manufacturers use either fresh milk, evaporated milk, sweetened and condensed milk, or nonfat milk solids. The label should tell you which milk product is used.

Milk chocolate outsells all other forms of chocolate by a five-to-one margin. The composition of milk chocolate and other chocolates is shown in the following table. You can see from this table that chocolates consist of a sugar/fat combination with the cocoa taste thrown in. We humans have a particular affinity for that sugar/fat combination, which of course is the basis of ice cream, confectionery, cakes, cookies, and other dessert foods.

TABLE 6.4: COMPOSITION OF CHOCOLATE PRODUCTS*

Chocolate	Cocoa Paste	Cocoa Butter	Sugar	Milk
Plain	✔	✔	✔	
Milk	✔	✔	✔	✔
White		✔	✔	✔

*Cocoa paste is the part of the cocoa bean containing the colors, flavors, and aroma. In the dried form it is cocoa powder.

Cocoa butter is the mix of fats found exclusively in the cocoa bean.

The proportion of each chocolate component varies with the product and manufacturer.

Cocoa butter, the fat of the cocoa bean, is largely responsible for the dense caloric value of chocolate. If you eat an ounce and a half of a milk chocolate, you add 225 calories to your diet. Cocoa butter is mostly saturated fat, but a fat with an unique property: It melts in your mouth. Cocoa butter is solid at room temperature, but at a temperature slightly below body temperature, it melts. It's this quality that gives chocolate confections their unparalleled popularity.

Ice cream: Four ways to make smart choices

If you ate four ice cream cones in the past week, you are a typical consumer. That's the average ice cream consumption, 52 weeks a year, for every adult and

Moneysaver
So-called white chocolate is milk chocolate without cocoa. Because the heart-protecting polyphenols are located in the cocoa, white chocolate lacks the excuse (if you need one) for eating chocolate. So if you want real chocolate, save your money and buy the dark stuff.

child in the country. Although ice cream seems typically American, it was not invented here. Ice cream goes back to the time of the ancient Romans and was popular in Europe in the 1700s. It took American ingenuity in the mid–19th century, however, to invent a paddle ice cream maker and begin the commercial exploitation of this delightful dessert.

Hitherto, ice cream had been made by simply cooling a mixture of cream, milk, sugar, and other ingredients, such as fruit. Ice cream made this way was coarse and crystalline. The paddle solved that problem by keeping ingredients evenly mixed while they froze, giving the product a velvety, smooth texture.

The basic process for making ice cream may be straightforward, but ice cream makers select from a stunning variety of ingredients and employ a variety of manufacturing shortcuts. The result: Ice cream quality varies. There are four things about commercial ice creams you ought to know to help you make smarter choices:

- The basics of ice-cream making

- The differences between ice cream, sherbets, and frozen yogurt

- Why low-fat ice cream is not low-calorie

- Why the fresher the ice cream, the better

Know the basics of ice cream making

Ice cream is basically a frozen foam. Freeze a cream mix and you get an unappealing lump—eating it would be like sucking on a solid block of ice. Manufacturers, therefore, whip air into the cream mixture as it freezes, creating a foam. A small amount of air, about 15 percent by volume, produces a creamy ice cream that melts into the taste buds of your tongue. As it melts, it gives that pleasant cooling sensation.

Super-premium ice creams contain anywhere from 10 to 20 percent air. Since ice cream is sold by the pint or gallon and not by weight, cheaper ice cream has much more air whipped, as much as 50 percent total. Buy a half gallon of bargain ice cream for three dollars, and you buy a quart of air.

You can estimate the amount of whipped-in air by looking at the label and the number of grams per serving. An ice-cream serving is standardized at ½ cup. Here is the difference in weight between super-premium and premium ice creams:

- Super premium, 100 to 110 grams
- Premium, 60 to 70 grams

The taste and feel of ice cream as it glides through your mouth depend on creams, and lots of it. This fact is inescapable. Start putting in more air and reducing the amount of cream, and the feel can be maintained only through added emulsifiers and stabilizers. The downside of the added chemicals is that they may impart a sticky feeling and sometimes a chemical aftertaste.

Ice cream, sherbets, and frozen yogurt

Fruit sherbets are manufactured in a way similar to ice cream. They have less cream than ice cream and are thus thought of as low-cal desserts. But because of the acidity of the fruit in a sherbet, a whopping amount of sugar and corn syrup is added. As a result, a sherbet delivers about the same number of calories as premium ice cream, about 135 calories per ½-cup serving. A nutritional breakdown of ice cream, sherbet, and low-fat frozen yogurt follows.

Watch Out!
Don't serve ice cream too cold. If the ice cream is overly cold, it doesn't melt smoothly in the mouth. Serve regular ice cream at about 10°F and soft ice cream at 22°F.

TABLE 6.5: NUTRITIONAL COMPOSITION OF VANILLA ICE CREAM, SHERBET, AND LOW-FAT FROZEN YOGURT (PER ½ CUP)

	Premium Vanilla Ice Cream	Sherbet	Low-fat Frozen Yogurt
Calories	135	127	124
Total fat (grams)	7.3	1.7	5
Saturated fat (grams)	4.5	1	2.9
Total sugars (grams)	16	27	22
Cholesterol (milligrams)	29	4	18
Protein (grams)	2.3	1.2	9

(*Source:* Bowes and Church's Food Values of Portions Commonly Used, *17th ed. Revised by Jean A.T. Pennington. Copyright © 1998, Lippincott-Raven Publishers.*)

In terms of calories, there is no real difference between ice cream, sherbet, and low-fat frozen yogurt. Composition, however, differs. With ice cream, you have more fat and less sugar, and with the other two you have less fat and more sugar. This is not to mention the added stabilizers, such as carrageenan, guar gum, and methylcellulose, and emulsifiers such as lecithin, phosphates, and polyoxethylene derivatives of fatty acids. In general, sherbets have greater quantities of additives to keep the cream, fruit, corn syrup, and sugar from separating. The number and amounts of additives vary with individual manufacturers, so read the labels.

Ice cream, sherbets, and frozen yogurts are blank canvases. Imaginative cooks can paint them with an infinite variety of flavors and added items, like crumbled cookies, exotic spices mixtures, nuts, fruit chunks, alcoholic liquors—practically anything that freezes. Since we are talking about dessert foods, this book makes no attempt to assess nutritional values. Enjoy what you like, but do so in moderation.

Why low-fat ice cream is not low-cal

If your taste runs to super-premium ice creams, you are definitely consuming more fat than with the less-expensive ice creams. Four ounces of one brand of super-premium ice cream gives you 18 grams of total fat, as much fat as an 8-ounce porterhouse streak.

The high fat content and high calories of super-premium ice creams drive many ice-cream lovers to low-fat versions. But don't think you're winning on the calorie score. Take out the cream and you have to add something else to get a semblance of the typical ice cream mouth sensation. That something else is the corn syrup and sugar, plus stabilizers and emulsifiers to make the ice cream hold together. As a result, low-fat ice creams provide about the same number of calories as their high-fat counterparts. A smarter choice is to stick with the regular ice cream you like but eat smaller portions. Order a cone with one scoop instead of two or three scoops.

The fresher the ice cream, the better

Ice cream doesn't keep well. Its subtle flavors dissipate, and the texture becomes more crystalline and maybe even gritty. Unfortunately for the consumer, ice cream is not dated. You don't know how long the ice cream has been warehoused before being sent to your local supermarket. There are two solutions:

- Patronize mom-and-pop ice cream outlets. In most areas, you can find enterprising individuals who make their own ice cream on the premises. You can count on it being fresh.

> 66
>
> No one is saying these reduced-fat ice creams are low calories.
> —Betty Campbell, FDA's office of food labeling
>
> 99

Moneysaver
When shopping
for ice cream,
beware of car-
tons in the
store's freezer
covered with
frost. Those car-
tons have sat
there a long
time. Don't
bother buying
them.

- Make your own ice cream. The task is greatly simplified with home ice-cream makers. These machines range from the old-fashioned, hand-cranked machines to fully electric, self-refrigerated machines. You know exactly what goes into the mixture, and you have absolutely fresh ice cream.

Know your cheese

Most cheeses are made from cow's milk, but many varieties are also made from goat's and sheep's milk. Basic cheese making is similar for all cheeses. Here are the six steps for making the most popular of all cheeses, cheddar:

1. Milk is warmed to about 70°F (21°C) and a bacterial culture is added that creates lactic acid, causing the milk to coagulate (curdling).

2. The temperature is then raised to 80°F (27°C) and rennet is added to complete the curdling. The curds consist of a mixture of the protein, casein, and milk fat.

3. The mixture of curds and fluid (whey) is heated to about 104°F (40°C); this cures and hardens the curds.

4. The whey is drained off. The curds, now about the size of baby carrots, are "cheddared" by being pressed together into a solid mass. The cheese begins to gain a fibrous texture and a tangy taste.

5. This mass is broken into small cubes, salt (1.5 to 2.0 percent by weight) is added, and the cubes are pressed into molds.

6. The molded cheese is put in temperature-controlled storerooms and cured at 55 to 60°F.

The longer it cures, the more flavor the cheese develops and the tangier it becomes. Mild cheddar is aged about 6 months, medium about 12 months, and sharp, 18 to 24 months.

The natural color of the cheese is a pale yellow. The bright yellow-orange color you see in many cheddars is due to annatto, the ground seeds of the annatto plant, a tropical evergreen shrub. To get the pure white color of some cheddars, the milk is bleached with benzoyl peroxide (this won't be mentioned on the label) or by canceling the color with a blue dye.

Variations on the basic cheese-making process include:

- Different bacterial cultures, each of which imparts a distinctive taste.

- Curing at a higher or lower temperature, which changes texture and taste.

- Varying the firmness at which the curds are compressed.

- Addition of spices and herbs.

The net result is an infinite variety of cheeses, as individual as the different cheese makers. Going into a specialty cheese shop or the gourmet cheese section of your local supermarket, you can be overwhelmed by the sheer number of different cheeses. To simplify choosing, cheeses can be grouped into broad categories depending on a special feature of manufacturing or the cheese's hardness. The harder the cheese, the less water it contains. The following table lists the nutritional composition of representative cheeses from different categories.

Bright Idea
Remember to remove a cheese from the refrigerator an hour or two before you plan to eat it. You can only savor a cheese's full flavor when it is at room temperature.

TABLE 6.6: NUTRITIONAL COMPOSITION OF REPRESENTATIVE CHEESES, BASED ON A 1-OUNCE SERVING

Cheese	Calories	Protein (g)/ percent of calories	Total fat (g)/ percent of calories	Calcium (milli-grams)
Blue (semi-soft)	100	6.1/25%	8.2/75%	150
Camembert (soft)	85	5.6/27%	6.9/73%	110
Cheddar (hard)	114	7.1/25%	9.4/75%	204
Gouda (semi-soft)	101	7.1/29%	7.8/71%	198
Mozzarella (fresh)	80	5.5/23%	6.1/71%	147
Parmesan (extra hard)	111	10.1/38%	7.3/62%	336
American (pro-cessed) cheese	106	6.3/24%	8.9/76%	174

(*Source:* Bowes and Church's Food Values of Portions Commonly Used, *17th ed. Revised by Jean A.T. Pennington. Copyright © 1998, Lippincott-Raven Publishers.*)

Cheese is basically a mixture of the milk's protein and fat. A cheese's calories, therefore, are split between the two. As you see from the preceding table, regardless of the type of cheese, the majority of calories come from fat. As already mentioned, three-quarters of the fat is saturated. Enjoy your cheese, but do it in moderation, and think twice before you order that triple cheeseburger.

What follows now is a brief description of the major cheese categories.

■ **Extra-hard cheese (30 percent water).**
Originally developed in the Parma region of Italy, these hard cheeses are suitable for grating. Parmesan—or to give it its Italian name, Parmigiano—is the best known. Romano cheeses are closely related but tend to be sharper. Pecorino Romano is made from sheep's

milk. The Italian grana cheeses and the Swiss Sbrinz and Sapsago also fit into this group.

- **Hard cheese (30 to 40 percent water).** At least in the United States, cheddar is the queen of this group. Colby and provolone are similar to cheddar but with a milder flavor. The English cheeses—Cheshire, Gloucester, Lancashire, Derby, and Caerphilly—are members of the cheddar family.

- **Swiss-style cheeses (35 to 40 percent water)** are also hard. Emmentaler is the best known. Close relatives are: Appenzell, Gruyere, and Formaggio. The big holes in the cheese develop during curing as the bacterial culture releases gas (carbon dioxide).

- **Semi-soft cheese (40 to 50 percent water).** This group includes a large variety of mild, stable, all-purpose cheeses. They tend to be unpronounced in flavor and aroma, but are firm and easily sliced, making excellent sandwich cheeses. The group includes Edam, Fontina, Gouda, Havarti, and Monterey Jack.

- **Soft cheese (50 to 75 percent water).** Soft cheeses, like Camembert and Brie, are also known as surface-ripened because they are ripened by a Penicillium mold that grows on their surface. Enzymes produced by the mold penetrate the surface of the cheese and give it a characteristic flavor. When you cut into one of these cheeses at its peak, the paste bulges out from the rind. Other surface-ripened cheeses are Bel Paese of Italy, Port du Salut of France, and the all-time king of smelly cheeses, Limburger.

Unofficially...
Because of chemical additives, *restricted cheese* remains solid to 350°F (176°C), whereas an ordinary cheese at this temperature would turn into a smoking puddle. The food industry loves restricted cheese, because it doesn't run during cooking and create a messy entree. They use it in precooked frozen dinners containing a cheese sauce.

- **Blue cheese (40 to 45 percent water).** This group also includes Danablu from Denmark, Gorgonzola from Italy, Roquefort from France, and Stilton from England. During the curing phase, the cheese is pierced with dozens of small channels and inoculated with a Penicillium mold. The mold grows through the interior of the cheese, giving it the characteristic blue-vein look.

- **Mozzarella,** an unripened cheese (55 percent water), starts out like a cheddar. But the curd is not pressed; Instead, it is heated in hot water and stretched and molded into irregular, stringy, spherical shapes. Mozzarella is not cured and is eaten fresh.

- **Pasteurized processed cheese (American cheese) (40 percent water).** The starting cheese is a mixture of cheeses, principally cheddar but also cheeses from a diverse roster, including, surprisingly, Limburger. The cheese mixture is ground into fine particles and heated sufficiently (pasteurized) to kill all ripening bacteria and enzymes. The ground cheese is mixed with chemical plasticizing agents and emulsifiers and rolled into bricks or sheets, which are cut into sandwich-size slices. The character and flavor of the original cheeses vanish, replaced with a bland flavor and soft texture.

  Because the cheese is pasteurized, all ripening stops and the cheese retains the same taste and texture no matter how long it is stored. In fact, the cheese is popular for this very reason. It has consistent flavor and keeps well.

Bright Idea
Find a quality yogurt by reading the label. Look for few added ingredients and the presence of live microorganisms. Here's an example, the ingredient list of one top yogurt brand: Grade A pasteurized certified organic milk, certified organic maple syrup, pure vanilla, living yogurt cultures: *L. acidophilus*, *L. bulgaricus*, *S. thermophilus*.

- **Pasteurized processed cheese foods and spreads.** Pasteurized processed cheese food is 51 percent processed cheese. The rest is milk, cream, whey, or powdered milk, which gives a softer texture and milder taste. This type of cheese is often mixed with vegetables or meats. Pasteurized processed cheese spreads have less fat and more moisture (47 to 60 percent), which enables them to be spread with a knife. They cannot be labeled as cheese, and are sold under the manufacturer's trade name.

- **Cream cheese.** Cream—milk with a butterfat content of 10 to 12 percent—is inoculated with lactic acid bacteria, causing the curds to separate. The curds are salted and worked into a smooth paste with the help of emulsifiers and gums like guar gum and carrageenan. Cream cheese has high moisture (55 percent) and high fat (33 percent) content. It does not keep well and should be consumed fresh. A similar cheese with less fat is called Neufchatel.

- **Imitation cheese.** Food chemists have been remarkably successful in creating from a mixture of hydrogenated vegetable oil, modified food starch, casein, and a variety of chemical stabilizers and emulsifiers a product that has a cheeselike texture. Flavor chemists have re-created a palette of cheese flavors, each distinct for a specific cheese. Between the artificially textured product and the artificial cheese flavors, manufacturers create imitation cheeses as different as provolone, cheddar, and mozzarella. Such cheeses essentially replace the milk fat of real cheese with hydrogenated vegetable oil, which delivers the undesirable trans fatty acids.

You'll not likely meet such cheeses in the cheese section of your market. You will find them, however, as part of precooked frozen pizzas, dinners, or other prepared food products containing a cheese. It is sometimes difficult to figure out if a cheese-containing frozen dinner has the imitation product, because the maker will put in some real cheese so it can be named on the label.

Imitation cheeses also show up in restaurants where cheese is part of the dish, like pizza. Restaurants are not required to disclose ingredients—perhaps for good reason. Would you order a pizza if the pizza parlor posted a sign saying "Our pizzas are made with imitation mozzarella"?

■ **Cottage and Ricotta cheeses.** These cheeses are consumed fresh. Cottage cheese is made from skim milk by adding a small amount of rennet and inoculating it with a lactic acid bacteria. The bacteria produce lactic acid, which causes the protein to coagulate. The curd is separated from the whey, water-washed to remove the acid, and salted. The curds may be left as such and sold as dry-curd cottage cheese. Most cottage cheese is creamed with added cream, giving a fat content from 1 to 4 percent. Ricotta cheese is produced in a similar manner from whey and is therefore referred to as a whey cheese.

Look for cottage cheese with the shortest list of additives

Quality cottage cheese doesn't need emulsifiers and stabilizers to make it smooth and appealing. Some cottage cheeses contain a long list of gums and emulsifiers, added to smooth the rough edges and also to extend shelf life. The additives contribute nothing to the nutritional value of the cheese and burden your body with the work of separating them from genuine nutrients. The following table lists the ingredients of two brands of cottage cheeses, one with few additives, one with many.

TABLE 6.7: INGREDIENTS OF TWO BRANDS OF LOW-FAT (1%) COTTAGE CHEESE

Brand A	Brand B
Cultured, pasteurized, grade-A skim milk	Cultured, pasteurized skim milk
Milk	Whey protein concentrate
Salt	Whey
Vitamin A palmitate	Cream
	Salt
	Potassium sorbate (preservative)
	Color
	Guar gum
	Vitamin A palmitate
	Enzyme

Read the labels of the cottage cheeses in your supermarket and select the one with the least number of additives.

Look to the total nutritional value of milk and milk products

Dairy products, of all the major food classes, attract the most controversy. Its severest critics say milk is for calves only—humans should not touch it. Proponents, on the other hand, often zero in on a single component, like calcium, and say you should drink milk for that one benefit. But such claims take a narrow view of dairy products. Here's a cell's-eye view of the pros and cons of three controversial topics.

Moneysaver
Butter comes in two forms, salted and unsalted. Save your money—buy the unsalted. Why? Salt masks undesirable flavors, so unsalted butter has to be of higher quality to stand on its own.

1. **Milk and heart disease.** The leading theory is that saturated fat raises the level of blood cholesterol and, thus, the risk of heart disease. No question, whole milk, butter, and cheese have lots of fat, two-thirds of which is saturated fat. On the other hand, milk contains substances that seem to lower blood cholesterol. In addition, the calcium and magnesium of milk help keep blood pressure down. And then there's evidence that peoples of countries like the Netherlands eat a diet rich in dairy products yet live long lives. They also eat more vegetables.

   The question from the cell's-eye view is not whether dairy products raise blood cholesterol, but whether your total diet raises blood cholesterol or, in the larger sense, whether or not your total diet contributes to long-lived health. You need to see dairy products in the context of your total diet. For most Americans there is good reason to reduce total fat, because they eat more calories than they need. Drink the lower-fat milks and eat cheese, ice cream, and butter in moderation as part of an overall balanced diet. In later chapters we revisit this concept of a balanced diet.

2. **Milk, calcium, and osteoporosis.** The dairy industry makes a big point of the rich calcium level in milk, suggesting that you will never get enough calcium unless you drink fluid milk. But other foods contain calcium. Asians eating a traditional diet get most of their calcium from green vegetables and rarely consume milk or milk products. Compared to Americans, they have a low rate of osteoporosis. Moreover, there is evidence that the

calcium of milk is not all that well absorbed, perhaps because of the high protein level of milk.

In any case, don't consider milk as having to be your main source of dietary calcium. Eat those vegetables.

3. **Milk and allergies.** Genuine milk allergies are due to milk proteins. For people who have such an allergy, the recourse is to avoid milk. Lactose intolerance, on the other hand, is generally not absolute. Most lactose-intolerant individuals can drink a glass or two of milk— better at mealtime—without discomfort. And don't forget those dairy products that don't contain lactose: cheeses and yogurts.

Just the facts

- Highest-quality milk and milk products come from cows that are organically raised.

- Low-fat milks offer the same nutritional benefits as whole milk without all those fat calories.

- Ice cream depends on cream for its smoothness. Fat-reduced ice creams replace the cream with emulsifiers, stabilizers, and sugar, but calories aren't reduced. Stick with creamy ice cream and just eat less.

- Enjoy cheeses made the old-fashioned way, from curdled milk. Beware of the imitation cheeses often found in precooked frozen meals and inexpensive restaurant pizzas and other cheese dishes.

Special Features of Smart Nutrition

PART III

GET THE SCOOP ON...
Spotting the hidden degree of food processing
in a product ▪ Reading the Daily Values ▪ Why
the focus on fat is misleading ▪ When the label
says "natural"

Reading Between the Lines of Nutrition Labels

Chapter 7

What's gone wrong with the FDA's nutrition labeling system? Introduced as a result of the 1990 Nutritional Labeling and Education Act, the new labels on food products were supposed to turn everyone into informed food shoppers. But the FDA hasn't kept up with the times. Trends in eating habits and technical advances in food manufacturing have overtaken the FDA's 1990 labels. The standard label you see on food products provides some of the needed information, but not enough to make sound decisions. You are not being informed as well as you may think you are.

Here are three key pieces of information the FDA omits from a nutrition label.

1. **How the food product is processed.** Manufacturing can be harsh, bringing down the product's total nutritional value. From a cell's-eye

view, it's total nutrition that counts. Suppose, for example, the label on a package describes cheese as part of the product. Is it genuine cheese, cheese food, imitation cheese, or a mixture? The label is silent on this issue, yet the nutrition of the product varies greatly depending on which type of cheese is used.

2. **Critical nutrients.** The label ought to tell you if a food product contains crucial nutrients that are relatively scarce in the general food supply, such as the omega-3 fatty acids. This information is absent.

3. **Lack of a balanced view of the food's nutrition.** The nutrition label spotlights the negative—food components you should be wary of, such as total fat, saturated fat, and cholesterol. The negative focus encourages consumers to choose foods on the simplistic basis of avoiding fat. It would make more sense to give a balanced view of the total nutrition the food offers.

All, however, is not lost. While the nutrition label doesn't explicitly tell you anything about manufacturing and omega-3 fatty acids, you can glean this information reading the labels in a way the FDA never intended. This chapter gives you an unofficial guide to interpreting nutrition labels—reading between the lines, so to speak. It isn't hard. You'll learn how to spot key words and phrases on the label that clue you in to a product's total nutritional value.

Changing eating habits

Before getting into the details of the nutrition label, we need to put nutrition labeling into the larger context of people's lifestyles. A broader question is: How does the nutrition information help people lead healthier lives?

Consider the following scenario. It's 4 p.m. Carol B. has no idea what she's going to prepare for dinner this evening. The kids are in the pool, but she's thinking about how she can get one child to dance class and another to soccer practice. The ballet school and soccer field are located on opposite sides of town. The thought of dinner hasn't even crossed her mind.

Carol's meal planning—or lack of it—is not unusual. The American Meat Institute found that 60 percent of adults surveyed have no idea what they're going to prepare for dinner. People don't want to think about food until they feel hungry or the supper hour has arrived.

When folks finally enter the kitchen, they want to exit fast. They allot no more than half an hour to preparing and cooking a meal. They won't use any ingredient or follow any recipe if they can't get food on the table within 30 minutes of entering the kitchen. *Scratch* cooking used to mean starting with vegetables that needed washing, meat that needed trimming, and a sauce and dessert that needed preparing. Today scratch cooking means assembling bagged lettuce and other prepared meal ingredients.

Avoidance of kitchen time is one of several trends sweeping the country. There's a food revolution going on, and we are all part of it. The revolution changes the way we eat, the way manufacturers produce foods, and the way we use nutrition information.

Consider the following signs of the revolution in eating habits.

■ Both adults in two-adult families work and thus have less free time to plan and make a meal.

- Food is readily accessible at all times of the day. Convenience stores selling snacks are found everywhere. Your local garage has turned into a food center. Fast-food restaurants stay open from dawn to midnight. Supermarkets offer sandwiches and complete meals.

- Half the meals people eat in their homes are prepared outside the home. You pick up a hot, take-out meal on the way home from work, or microwave a frozen dinner purchased earlier at a supermarket, to say nothing about pizza delivery to the door. As we discuss elsewhere, the food industry calls such meals *home meal replacements* or HMRs.

- There has been an explosion in the variety and availability of finger foods. Tear open a package or box, and out comes something to eat, no worry about dealing with cutlery and plate.

- A revolution in food technology has swept the food industry, making HMRs, finger foods, fast foods, frozen meals, and other technical innovations possible.

66
Despite major educational programs, Americans still consume a diet that is skewed towards fat and is low in nutrient-dense foods.
—Fran Katz, Editor, *Food Technology*
99

There are two revolutions going on—one social, one technical. The social revolution can be summarized as a switch from eating three set meals a day to grazing. People react to hunger, not time of day. They wait until hungry, then seek something to satisfy that hunger. The universal availability of ready-to-eat foods makes it easy to graze.

Chris B., a young man we counseled, was a part of this revolution in eating habits. He had grown up in a family that believed in the traditional three meals. But when he got to college, he became an ardent grazer. He ate only when he felt hungry, and then he would just go to the nearest vending machine. He passed his college years relying on machines for daily nourishment. And he eventually paid a price: He ended up taking two rolls of antacid tablets a day to keep his stomach quiet.

Chris's story is hardly unusual. It is against this backdrop of changing eating styles and types of food people buy that we have to think about the information conveyed by nutrition labels. What information would have helped Chris make antacid-free choices and still eat out of a vending machine? Or, what information does Carol B. need when she stocks her refrigerator or freezer so she can have nutritious choices waiting there at suppertime?

The answer is an updated way of interpreting the information printed on a nutrition label. We're stuck, so to speak, with the label as it stands. So let's see what we can learn from it.

The official nutrition label consists of three parts.

1. Nutrition Facts

2. Ingredient List

3. Nutritional Claims

Nutrition Facts

The Nutrition Facts on all packages conforms to a government-mandated format. The format is the same on all packages. So we use as an example the Nutrition Facts for a common product, *Chicken Nuggets: Breaded Nugget Shaped Chicken Patties.* The label is reproduced on the following page. We'll start at the top of the panel and work down.

What is a serving?

The first listing is the serving size for the product. A serving is supposed to represent the amount of food a person would normally eat at one time. The FDA provides manufacturers with guidelines. Thus, a

Chicken Nuggets
Nutrition Label.

Chicken Nuggets
Breaded Nugget Shaped Chicken Patties

Nutrition Facts
Serving Size 6 Nuggets (96g)
Servings Per Container about 3

Amount Per Serving	
Calories 300	Calories from Fat 180

	% Daily Value
Total Fat 20g	31%
Saturated Fat 5g	25%
Cholesterol 30mg	10%
Sodium 670 mg	28%
Total Carbohydrate 19g	6%
Dietary Fiber less than 1g	0%
Sugars 2g	
Protein 10g	

Vitamin A 0%	Vitamin C 2%
Calcium 0%	Iron 5%

* Percent Daily Values are based on a 2,000 calorie diet. Your daily values may be higher or lower depending on your calorie needs.

		Calories	2,000	2,500
Total Fat	Less than		65g	80g
Sat Fat	Less than		20g	25g
Cholesterol	Less than		300mg	300mg
Sodium	Less than		2,400mg	2,400mg
Total Carbohydrate			300g	375g
Dietary Fiber			25g	30g

Calories per gram
Fat 9 • Carbohydrate 4 • Protein 4

Ingredients: Boneless chicken, water, wheat flour, TVP [textured vegetable protein], bleached wheat flour. Contains 2% or less of the following, corn flour, modified food starch, dried whey, partially hydrogenated soybean oil, hydrolyzed soy and corn protein with hydrogenated soybean oil, sodium tripolyphosphate, glucose, flavorings, sugar, autolyzed yeast extract, Guar gum, leavening (sodium acid pyrophosphate, sodium bicarbonate, monocalcium phosphate), oleoresin paprika. Fried in partially hydrogenated vegetable oil.

Watch Out!
The listed serving size of some foods can be ridiculously small, to give the impression that the product is low in fat. The serving size of some muffins, for example, is given as half a muffin. If you normally eat a whole muffin, do a quick doubling of the fat grams to see how many grams the product actually gives you.

serving size is relatively uniform among competing products.

For meat products, the standard serving is about 3 ounces. For Chicken Nuggets, the 96 grams works out to six nuggets. Most people, when they eat, eyeball the quantity. If you put one serving of Chicken Nuggets (six) on a plate, they cover an area about the size of your palm. Whether that represents a serving to you depends on what else is for dinner, your body size, and how hungry you are. In any event, on a hunger scale between a small child and a hungry man, the 3 ounces meat serving is about midway.

Other products have different serving sizes. A serving of bread is defined as 50 grams (2 ounces), or two slices. In some cases, smaller packages, like cans of soft drink, are considered to be a single serving. Whatever the serving size, the actual amount is given in grams and, for some items, in cup size. Thus you can figure out what a serving means in terms of your own preferred quantity.

Why metric? Foods are sold by the ounces and pounds, but nutrition facts are given in the metric system. This can be confusing. Here is a quick conversion guide:

1 ounce = 28 grams

2.2 pounds (2 pounds, 3 ounces) = 1 kilogram

1 tablespoon = 15 grams (of salt)

1 teaspoon = 5 grams (of salt)

How many calories per serving?

Under "calories per serving," you see two values. For one serving of Chicken Nuggets, the values are: total calories, 300; calories from fat, 180.

If the amount of fat you eat concerns you, these two values enable you to calculate the percentage of fat calories in the food. For a serving of Chicken Nuggets, 180 divided by 300 equals 60 percent. By comparison, a skinned chicken breast or leg delivers only 50 percent of its calories from fat.

Some might argue that the amount of fat calories in a single item isn't so critical; it's the amount of fat in the total meal that is important. Low-fat items on the dinner plate balance out the high fat of chicken nuggets. That is true, but when the percent of calories in a meat product creeps over the 50 percent mark, the nutritional quality of the meat sinks. The more fat in the cut, the less vitamins and minerals the meat delivers. These nutrients are located in the protein portion of the meat

Daily Value? What's this?

Before going any further, we need to talk about *Daily Values*. When FDA officials designed the nutrition label, they asked: What is the amount of particular nutrients a person should consume to maintain good health? These values are the Daily Values, but

Bright Idea
Meat products are not required to carry nutrition labels. Supermarkets, however, are supposed to display the nutrition information on posters in their meat sections. Read the posters, and choose cuts that don't exceed 50 percent total fat.

Timesaver
Give your child a
balanced meal
you prepare
yourself instead
of a pre-
packaged 56-
additive meal.
You'll save time
in the long run
by avoiding trips
with the child to
the doctor's
office.

they are hardly set in stone. They are intended as reference points to help people gain a perspective on overall dietary needs.

Look at the panel to the right of Nutrition Facts. This panel, appearing on all nutrition labels, lists Percent Daily Values based on persons consuming 2,000 and 2,500 calories per day. For example, the Daily Values for fat is 65 grams for the 2,000 calorie diet and 80 grams for the 2,500 calorie diet.

How many calories do you burn in a day? If your caloric expenditure differs from the reference 2,000- and 2,500-calorie diets, you need to adjust the numbers for total fat and saturated fat calories. Table 7.1 provides a guide to help you. (The Daily Values for cholesterol and sodium don't change with number of calories).

TABLE 7.1: DAILY VALUES FOR TOTAL FAT AND SATURATED FAT AT DIFFERENT CALORIE LEVELS

Individual	Calories	Daily Value Total Fat, grams	Daily Value Saturated Fat, grams
Kindergarten child	1,300	42	13
Average-size woman, limited activity	1,600	53	18
Average-size woman, active	2,000	65	20
Average-size man, active	2,600	80	25
Teen-age boy, active	3,000	100	27

The FDA calculates the Daily Values for total fat as 30 percent of total calories, and for saturated fat as 10 percent of total calories. More details on how FDA arrives at the Daily Values are given in Appendix D.

Nutrients the FDA considers important to your health

The third section below Nutrition Facts, starting with "Total Fat," is what the FDA calls "nutrients considered important to health." In designing the nutrition label, the FDA faced the dilemma of either overloading consumers with data or not giving enough. The FDA struck a middle road, selecting a few key nutrients it deems important to health. Significantly, the FDA chose to list not nutrients you must *have*, but nutrients you should *limit*:

- Total fat

- Saturated fat

- Cholesterol

- Sodium

Limit your total fat

Total fat is the top-listed item. A serving of Chicken Nuggets provides the eater with 20 grams. Based on the 2,000-calorie reference diet, the 20 grams works out to 31 percent of Daily Value. Individuals wary of over-consuming fat will find 20 grams high for a food that is one part of one meal. Doesn't leave much room for eating other fat-containing foods over the rest of the day.

Saturated fat is listed as 5 grams, 25 percent of Daily Value. Why does the FDA list this particular breakdown of total fat? Saturated fat is thought of as the bad member among classes of fats, often called an artery clogger. It provides no nutritive value, except calories. Because of the negatives, the FDA requires manufacturers to include this amount on the label.

Now we come to a great void in information about fat. In Chicken Nuggets, one serving contains 5 grams of saturated fat. What about the other $20 - 5 = 15$ grams? What's this 15 grams? The FDA doesn't require the manufacturer to let you know the identity of this mystery fat. Suffice to say, the 15 grams of fat falls into the categories of three types of fats:

Unofficially...
The FDA is considering requiring labeling for trans fats. In the meantime, you can use the nutrition label to calculate trans fats by taking the total fat grams and subtracting saturated, monounsaturated, and polyunsaturated fat.

- Monounsaturated fat
- Polyunsaturated fat
- *Trans* fat

While listing total fat and unsaturated fat is mandatory, the law gives manufacturers the option to list or not list polyunsaturated and monounsaturated fats. You see these two items listed on the labels of some products. Manufacturers can also list stearic acid if they choose. Stearic acid is the main saturated fat of beef. The FDA *forbids* manufacturers from ever listing *trans* fats. In our example here, Chicken Nuggets doesn't list any of these fats, which is the prerogative of the manufacturer.

Can we fill this 15-gram void? There are two pieces of information that would help evaluate the nutritional worth of chicken nuggets:

- The amount of essential fatty acids, especially the omega-3 fatty acids
- The amount of trans fat

Since the FDA doesn't require a listing of essential fatty acids or trans fat, can we figure them out? The trick in estimating the amounts of these two types of fats is to look at the ingredients. Chicken muscle contains small amounts of essential fatty acids, including the omega-3s, so we can assume Chicken Nuggets supplies some. How much is a guess, so let's leave it at "a little."

Estimating the amount of trans fat is easier. Chicken Nuggets consist of chicken pieces wrapped in a flour and oil batter, which are deep fried in vegetable oil. The chicken meat doesn't contain trans fat, but the oils do. You get this information from reading the ingredient list and spotting the code word for oils with trans fat—hydrogenation. There are, in fact, two sources.

- Partially hydrogenated soybean oil used in the batter

- Hydrogenated vegetable oil used in frying Chicken Nuggets

Partially hydrogenated oils contain a substantial percentage of trans fat, up to 40 percent (see Chapter 4). Thus, we can reasonably estimate that for Chicken Nuggets a few grams of that mystery 15 grams is trans fat, a fat linked with increased risk of heart disease.

Not a satisfactory way of arriving at answers. But until the FDA mandates fuller disclosure of the fat breakdown, we have to make such estimates. In any event, by reading between the lines we have figured out that Chicken Nuggets contains trans fat, perhaps quite a bit. Given a choice between plain chicken with no trans fat and Chicken Nuggets with trans fat, the better choice is the plain chicken.

Cholesterol—what's it doing here?

As pointed out in Chapter 1, cholesterol is not a nutrient. You don't need even 1 milligram in your diet. It is listed here because health authorities believe you shouldn't eat too much of it. Three hundred milligrams (less than one-eighth of a teaspoon) represents the maximum (Daily Value) the FDA believes you should eat in a day. The 30 milligrams in Chicken Nuggets is low relative to total fat for a meat product, 10 percent of Daily Value. The reason is that the major source of fat in Chicken Nuggets is the vegetable oils, which don't contain cholesterol.

Sodium is a measure of salt

Health authorities insisted that sodium be included in the mandatory list of substances in a food product. Why? Sodium chloride, or common table salt, is

Moneysaver
Buying battered, deep-fried chicken is an expensive way to buy chicken. Buy instead skinless breast or leg. You'll save money and, from a cell's-eye view, save your body from diminished nutrition.

the major contributor of sodium. Health authorities believe that too much salt in the diet increases the risk of high blood pressure. Why don't they just say "salt" on the label instead of listing sodium? Other substances that might be in the food product, such as monosodium glutamate (MSG) and baking soda (sodium bicarbonate), also contribute sodium, but not much compared to table salt.

It is hard to visualize what milligrams of sodium mean in real life. Chicken Nuggets contains 670 milligrams per serving, which translates into 1.8 grams of salt, $1/16$ of an ounce, or $1/3$ of a teaspoon.

The salt in Chicken Nuggets comes from the batter, and one serving supplies almost one-third (28 percent) of Daily Value—another reason for selecting plain chicken over the battered chicken.

Total carbohydrate includes starch and sugars

The items listed so far are substances you should try to *limit*. We finally arrive at an item, carbohydrate, your body needs in quantity. As mentioned in Chapter 1, carbohydrates includes starch, a complex carbohydrate, and sugars, simple carbohydrates.

The label also states the amount of sugar, so you can figure out the amount of complex carbohydrate, or starch, simply by subtracting. Chicken Nuggets contains only 2 grams of sugar, so this product contains $19 - 2 = 17$ grams of starch. The starch in Chicken Nuggets comes from the wheat flour that goes into the batter. The meat itself doesn't provide carbohydrate.

Dietary fiber keeps you regular

Although not a nutrient in the strictest sense, fiber eases the passage of food through your intestinal system. So fiber in food is beneficial. The law requires the manufacturer to list total fiber. As an option, if the manufacturer wishes, the amount of fiber is divided into soluble and insoluble. Chicken Nuggets don't include those two options, but you will see the fiber breakdown listed on other products.

Sugars: Too many?

Note that the word "sugars" is plural. When you look at the ingredient list of a product you see one or more of the following:

- Sugar
- Raw sugar
- Brown sugar
- Dextrose
- Fructose
- Glucose
- Lactose
- Maltose
- Sucrose
- Fruit juice concentrate
- Molasses
- Honey
- Maple syrup
- Corn sweetener
- Corn syrup
- Corn syrup solids
- High fructose corn syrup

Every one of these items is a sugar. Because ingredients of a product are listed in descending order of quantity, manufacturers of highly sugared products add different sugars so that each product individually falls farther down the ingredient list. Otherwise, sugar would be the first-named item, a tip-off of extreme sweetness.

Watch Out!
Remember, only fruits, grains, and vegetables contain fiber. In any other foods, it has to be added artificially.

Unofficially...
Some products may list sugar alcohols (it's the manufacturer's option), which are added as substitute sweeteners. Unlike the sugars mentioned here, sugar alcohols don't provoke an insulin response. These substances are xylitol, mannitol, and sorbitol.

This point is not an issue for Chicken Nuggets, because it contains only 2 grams of sugar, about two-thirds of a teaspoon. From a cell's-eye view, the body handles carbohydrates much better when they arrive in the stomach as a complex (starch), not as an added sugar.

Protein

Protein on the product label is simply listed as number of grams. As a guide, the National Research Council of the National Academy of Sciences has established reference daily intakes of protein (RDIs), listed in Table 7.2.

TABLE 7.2: THE REFERENCE DAILY INTAKE (RDI) OF PROTEIN

Individual	RDI in grams
Infant (under 12 months)	25
Child (under 4 years)	28
Adults and children over 4	65

Note, the protein RDIs are simply guides, not hard-and-fast values. The number depends on who does the calculating. The FDA calculates the Daily Value for protein as 10 percent of calories. For a woman eating 2,000 calories per day, that works out to 50 grams of protein per day. Sufficient protein in the diet is not an issue for people who eat meat and dairy products. It may be an issue for strict vegetarians, a point we take up in Chapter 9.

Why only two vitamins and two minerals?

Your body requires a long list of vitamins and minerals (see Table 1.1). Government officials, however, decided that only two vitamins, vitamin A and vitamin C, and two minerals, calcium and iron, would be most likely lacking in the average diet. A person should make special effort to ensure their daily intake is adequate.

If the product is fortified with added vitamins, like many breakfast cereals, the vitamins so added will also appear in this section of the label.

When reading the data listed under Nutrition Facts, make a mental note to do the following:

- Adjust the percentage Daily Value up or down to fit your size and level of activity.

- Check to see if the label lists grams of mono-unsaturated or polyunsaturated fat. If it doesn't, seek a comparable product that does.

- Check the sugar grams. If high, question whether you should eat this product. Keep in mind that excess sugar can be converted to fat.

The table of Daily Values

The second panel of the nutrition label contains a table of the Daily Values for two diets, 2,000 and 2,500 calories a day. This information appears on the nutrition labels of all products. It is put there so you'll know how Daily Values are calculated and can adjust the values to fit your own caloric intake (check Table 7.1).

You also see at the bottom of this table a section called *calories per gram:*

- 1 gram of fat = 9 calories
- 1 gram of carbohydrate = 4 grams
- 1 gram of protein = 4 calories.

Knowing the weight in grams, these conversion figures allow you to calculate the number of calories. For instance, the 10 grams of protein in one serving of Chicken Nuggets delivers $10 \times 4 = 40$ calories. This little table also reminds you that 1 gram of fat delivers more than twice the number of calories as a gram of protein or carbohydrate.

Bright Idea
Exercise common sense in deciding whether or not the amounts of vitamins and minerals in a particular food product are important. Meat products, for example, contain almost no vitamin A and C. That doesn't mean the meat you're thinking of buying is low-quality—it just means you have to look elsewhere to get those nutrients.

What is the unofficial message in the Ingredient List?

We turn now to the ingredient panel of the product label. This panel lists the ingredients the assembler of the food puts in the product. It doesn't include chemicals and other items that went into the manufacture of the ingredients. For example, bread flour is treated with potassium bromate. The bread maker who used the flour as an ingredient, however, lists only "flour" on the package label. Nevertheless, we can learn a great deal about the product from the ingredient list—perhaps more than the manufacturer intended.

When reading an ingredient list, keep these three points in mind.

1. Ingredients are listed in descending order of quantity.

2. Look for a small number of ingredients (listed below) that are red warning flags of an inferior product.

3. Don't worry about deciphering the significance of every last ingredient. Try instead to get an overall impression.

What is this mystery meal?

Earlier, we talked about the revolution in food processing. In addition to freezing and canning, processes that have been around for a long time, food manufacturers now upgrade their products. Upgrading means that the food item costs more—it has nothing to do with nutritional worth. In general, as financial value goes up the nutritional value goes down. Chicken Nuggets are a case in point. They go from plain chicken to a battered chicken product. Whereas plain chicken can rank at a quality level of 1 or 2, however, Chicken Nuggets ranks at level 4.

Bright Idea
When reading the ingredients list of a product, see if you can spot the actual food ingredients as opposed to the additives. If you find it difficult, reconsider your choice.

One way to upgrade price is to manufacture complete meals. You find them in the frozen food section of the supermarket. In learning how to read between the lines of the ingredient list, we take a frozen dinner as the example.

First, a little guessing game. Table 7.3 lists the ingredients of a four-course frozen dinner. Can you guess what's in the meal from this list? Normally, ingredients are listed on the label in descending order by weight. Table 7.3 rearranges the list for all four courses alphabetically.

TABLE 7.3: INGREDIENT LIST OF A FROZEN MYSTERY MEAL, ARRANGED ALPHABETICALLY

Anatto coloring
Artificial vanilla flavor
Autolyzed yeast extract
Beta carotene
Breader wheat
Carnauba wax
Cellulose gum lecithin
Cheddar cheese
Cheddar cheese blend
Cheese culture
Chicken
Citric acid
Cocoa powder
Confectioners glaze
Corn
Corn (yellow) flour
Corn oil
Cornstarch
Cream
Dextrin
Disodium guanylate
Disodium inosinate

TABLE 7.3: INGREDIENT LIST OF A FROZEN MYSTERY MEAL, ARRANGED ALPHABETICALLY (CONT.)

Disodium phosphate dihydrate

Durum semolina

Egg white solids

Enzymes

FD & C Blue #1

FD & C Red #3

FD & C Red #40

FD & C Yellow #5

FD & C Yellow #6

Folic acid

Garlic powder

Glycerin

Guar gum

Hydrolyzed corn, soy and wheat gluten

Iron

Macaroni, cooked

Lactic acid

Modified food starch

Monocalcium phosphate

Natural vanilla flavor

Niacin

Nonfat milk

Nonfat dry milk powder

Oleoresin paprika

Partially hydrogenated cottonseed oil

Partially hydrogenated soybean oil

Potassium carbonate

Riboflavin

Salt

Sodium acid pyrophosphate

Sodium bicarbonate (baking powder)

Sodium caseinate (milk protein)

Sodium tripolyphosphate

Soy protein isolate

Soybean oil

Spices

Thiamin mononitrate

| Torula and brewers yeast protein |
| Wheat starch |
| Whey |

A four-course, frozen meal

When you first look at the items in Table 7.3, you may rightly wonder if this is a book on nutrition or a book on chemistry. Have no fear—we aren't getting into a chemistry lesson. But we are going to see if we can make some sense out of this list.

The mystery list is, in fact, a list of ingredients in a child's frozen dinner, consisting of four courses:

- Breaded chicken balls

- Corn niblets

- Macaroni and cheese

- Chocolate pudding

The dinner has already been factory-cooked and needs only thawing and heating—about 5 minutes in the microwave.

Suppose you cooked the same meal from scratch in your kitchen. All you would need are the main ingredients: chicken plus bread crumbs, corn, macaroni, cheddar cheese, salt, and for the pudding, starch, milk, sugar, and cocoa. That's nine ingredients. The frozen meal lists 65. Why does the manufacturer need an additional 56 ingredients, and would you find them in your kitchen cupboards?

Manufacturing meals by the ton puts huge stresses on food ingredients—that is, the ingredients that are supposed to provide the nourishment. These stresses are much more destructive than what happens in home cooking. The chicken, corn, and macaroni lose the delicate array of substances that make up the food's aroma and taste. Texture collapses. Original colors fade.

As we note elsewhere, the meal at this point would be pale, bland, and unappetizing, impossible to sell. The manufacturer thus adds flavors, flavor boosters, and artificial colors to make the meal look attractive and taste good. The taste, however, will not be the taste of freshly cooked chicken, corn, and macaroni. It is generally much more intense, to mask off-flavors.

Texturing chemicals are added to restore texture, to give the food good *mouthfeel*, as they say in the food industry. Finally, the meal has to withstand freezing, lengthy storage, eventual thawing, and microwaving, and ultimately has to appeal to the eater. It takes 56 additives to do the job.

The consumer gets convenience, a meal in five minutes. But from a cell's-eye view, the meal is weighted with nutritionally unnecessary baggage. Let's have a look at some of this baggage.

Not all vitamins are restored

Industrial cooking and processing destroys vitamins and leaches out minerals. The manufacturer in this case has added back some of the losses:

- Beta carotene (Provitamin A)
- Folic acid
- Iron
- Niacin
- Riboflavin
- Thiamin mononitrate

Nevertheless, addition of these vitamins and the one mineral, iron, does not make up for the full spectrum of vitamin and mineral loss. To be fair, when you cook a meal at home, the food loses some of its vitamin and mineral content, too. But when a meal is cooked on a family scale and consumed

Watch Out!
Many chemical additives to foods are legally exempt from inclusion on the ingredients list.

immediately, losses are far less than the losses resulting from factory-scale manufacturing.

Additives enhance taste

We add salt and pepper and, often, spices to flavor
our foods. As you well know from personal experience, these additions rarely work when the food
lacks flavor to begin with. The mass cooking of
foods is a powerful enemy of the delicate components that give foods their characteristic taste, but
food manufacturers have still found ways to produce
flavor. Look at the ingredients in the frozen meal,
added to pep up weak flavor:

- Autolyzed yeast extract

- Hydrolyzed corn, soy, and wheat gluten

- Disodium guanylate

- Disodium inosinate

- Garlic powder

- Natural vanilla flavor

- Spices (unspecified on the ingredients list)

The first two items on this list are powerful taste
boosters—they contain monosodium glutamate or
MSG. MSG has a bad connotation in some peoples
minds. Manufacturers use these listed substances,
therefore, so they can legally avoid putting MSG on
the label.

The second two items, disodium guanylate and
disodium inosinate, are also taste boosters, like
MSG. They are purines, not easily digested.
Although purines are natural components of meat
and plants, the average diet contains relatively small
amounts, insufficient to cause any difficulty. There
was a time, however, when rich people, in particular,
ate high quantities of the flesh of game animals and

Unofficially...
Andy Rooney, in
a TV essay, won-
dered about the
food additives
you see listed on
product labels.
When you look
through the *Joy
of Cooking* and
other cookbooks,
you never see
these additives
mentioned.
"Why," Rooney
asked, "aren't
they used in
home cooking?"
(*60 Minutes*,
January 24,
1999.)

birds, food sources rich in purines. They paid the price with gout, which became known as the disease of the rich and famous. Whatever the source, purines in excess can lead to this painful and threatening disease.

Artificial colors: Who needs them?

This particular food product contains an interesting palette of artificial dyes, made from coal tar.

- FD&C Blue #1 (brilliant blue)
- FD&C Red #3 (erythrosine)
- FD&C Red #40 (allura red)
- FD&C Yellow #5 (tartrazine)
- FD&C Yellow #6 (sunset yellow)

With a set of primary colors, the manufacturer paints any hue or color desired to replace the faded colors of the main foods. In fact, the dyes give colors nature never dreamed of. Since the frozen meal is intended for children, the vivid, kindergarten colors are likely designed to appeal to that age group.

FD&C refers to the Food, Drug and Cosmetic Act under which the government approves these dyes for use in foods. While the five dyes impart primary colors, they raise severe questions about safety. Take Red #3, for example. As long ago as 1979, scientists at the National Institute of Health, Bethesda, MD, claimed this dye, also known as *erythrosine*, interfered with nerve impulses in the brain. Three years later, tests conducted by the food industry showed that ingestion of the dye caused tumors in rats, and in 1983, the FDA officially declared this dye a carcinogen (cancer-causing).

This declaration should have been enough to have the dye banned. But because of its intense red color, cherry growers and the makers of canned fruit cocktail said they couldn't get along without it. The politicking delayed action for several years. The dye was finally outlawed in 1990—sort of.

FDA banned FD&C Red #3 in all drugs and cosmetics applied externally. The FDA, however, permitted use of this coal tar dye in drugs taken internally and in foods. It's a curious decision. If it's unsafe to be applied to your skin, why is it safe to be eaten? In making its decision, the FDA claimed that "any human risk posed by FD&C Red #3 is extremely small."

The other four coal-tar dyes, although permitted in foods in the United States and Canada, have been banned in European countries. Blue #1 and Red #40 are banned in countries of the European community; Yellow #5 and #6 are banned in Scandinavian countries. Scientists and health officials in these countries believe the health risks posed by these artificial dyes are not worth the pretty colors.

Are natural flavors really natural?

You see on the list of ingredients (Table 7.3) the item "natural vanilla flavor." What does *natural flavor* mean?

Consider, first, what taste means to you as a biological creature. Your taste buds are your first line of defense against being poisoned. Within 50 milliseconds of a food entering the mouth, the taste buds signal the brain how the food tastes—plenty of time to spit the food out if the signal spells danger. This rapid response is nature's protection against swallowing toxic food.

At least that was the idea in the days before food protection laws and food labels. People relied on their taste buds to sense dangerous foods and, of

Watch Out!
Some herbal teas contain "natural flavors." When you brew the dried leaves, stems, or flowers, you think you're getting a totally natural brew. You also get a brew of microbial chemicals.

course, to savor the pleasures of safe and tasty foods. But taste buds are easily fooled.

The natural flavor of a food, say a raspberry, consists of a thousand or more chemical substances. These substances, some volatile, some soluble in the berry's juices, some clinging to the berry's seeds, mingle and caress the taste buds. Put a raspberry in your mouth and you experience the characteristic raspberry taste with all its vibrating overtones.

So if you buy a raspberry sorbet and see on the label *natural flavor,* you might assume the sorbet is flavored with an extract of raspberries carrying those thousand and one natural flavor substances. Wrong. Labeling laws allow the manufacturer to flavor the sorbet with a chemical mix that has never been near a farm, let alone a raspberry.

One way to produce a so-called natural flavor is to use bacteria and yeasts. Special strains of these hard-working microbes produce a variety of chemical substances, including some of the same substances that give a fruit or vegetable its characteristic flavor. Chemical companies grow the specific microbes in three-story vats. They then extract the flavor chemicals and distill and bottle them. One company, for example, sells 45 of these pure chemicals.

Pure flavor chemicals are like keys on a piano. Play different combination of keys and you create different tunes. A flavor specialist, by selecting the right combination of a few of the pure substances, creates a flavor characteristic of raspberry. Another combination gives a peach flavor, and so on.

The upshot: A pure chemical mix flavors the "raspberry" sorbet. The carton carries a picture of a cluster of raspberries and the label, with the full backing of the law, carries the words, "natural flavor."

The artificial—oops, I mean natural—chemical mix in fact carries only the dominant flavor note of raspberry. The mix lacks the hundreds of other flavor components a real raspberry conveys to your taste buds. The "natural" flavor, because it lacks those subtle overtones, is more intense. Do people care?

The *New York Times* (Jan. 3, 1996) carried a story entitled "Do Artificial Flavors Spoil Us for the Taste of Real Food?" The article noted that few people have eaten real raspberries. They lack any reference to the real thing. Consequently, they get used to the intense flavor of the artificial, and they come to expect that intensity.

The artificial natural-flavor mix is not necessarily dangerous. It is more a matter of deception. People have an expectation that natural means *natural*.

Not all natural flavors are artificial

Not all "natural" flavors are synthetic mixtures of pure chemicals. Some manufacturers extract the flavor essence from the fruit or vegetable. This genuine essence carries the thousand or so substances that make up a vegetable or fruit flavor. Unfortunately, because of the labeling law, consumers can't tell if the flavor added to the food product comes from a microbe or from the fruit or vegetable itself.

You'll also see the words *artificial flavors* on nutrition labels. In this case, the flavors have been synthesized in a chemical factory and bear no resemblance to any flavor substance in the plant or animal world.

Avoid products that contain modified food starch

The ingredient list includes substances that have already undergone extensive chemical modification, but that fact is hidden in some innocuous

Moneysaver
Modified food starch is a cheap filler for food products. If you see it listed on the label, save your money for a better product that doesn't contain the chemically treated substance.

phrase. Consider, for example, modified food starch (an ingredient in the mystery meal, Table 7.3). Starch undergoes coarse chemical treatment, which changes its benign nature. It's no longer anything found in the natural world. The treatment does not aid digestion or improve nutritional value. Chemical treatment is done solely to prevent the starch from breaking down during the high heat of industrial food processing. You, the consumer, receive no benefit.

Already in 1970, the Food and Agriculture Organization (FAO) and World Health Organization (WHO) raised their voices, concerned about the health hazards from consuming this product. Nevertheless, it is still permitted in foods. You would never guess from the friendly phrase, *modified starch*, the severe chemistry the starch undergoes, or the health concerns associated with it.

Watch Out!
Reading an ingredient label can be tortuous. To construct Table 7.3, the author had to read the ingredient list on the package with a magnifying glass. Moreover, the list was printed against a dark blue background, making it doubly hard to read. Manufacturers aren't doing us a service when their disclosures are so expertly hidden!

Beware of products with a lengthy list of ingredients

In fairness to the manufacture of the frozen meal (Table 7.3), every item on the ingredients list is legally approved by the FDA. But from a cell's-eye perspective, would your body approve? We don't really know for sure, because of insufficient safety testing of chemicals approved as food additives.

What testing is done is unrealistic, done in a way that often has little or no bearing on how you eat. When you eat a food product, you ingest everything in the food, including every last one of those chemical additives. If you eat the mystery meal, listed in Table 7.3, you ingest some 56 additives. The FDA has never tested the effect on the human body of eating all 56 additives at one time.

Whether the food product contains 56 additives or 3, the FDA never tests the combination. Food additives are tested for safety one at a time, as if each were the only additive in a food. The FDA gives a green light on this basis.

Do toxic effects of several additives acting in concert in your body or your child's body exceed a safety threshold? Does the combination trigger an unhealthy event in the body? We can't be sure. But when choosing food, particularly for children, beware of products whose list of ingredients and additives is lengthy.

Watch for these five red warning flags

When shopping in the supermarket, scan the ingredient list of food products for the following red warning flags:

1. The ingredient list is long.
2. The ingredient list is hard to read.
3. You see any of the FD&C artificial dyes.
4. You see hydrogenated or partially hydrogenated oil
5. You see multiple sugars, such as sugar and corn syrup.

If you see any of these red warning flags, put the product down and look for a comparable product without the flags.

Health claims: Are they valid?

You often see some health claim blazoned across the package or in advertisements for the product. This

Unofficially...
Although restaurant menus are exempt from nutrition labeling, if a restaurant makes a nutrient or health claim on the menu, sign, or poster, the food must meet FDA criteria for that claim.

fairly new advertising phenomenon results from the food industry's desire to capitalize on consumer interest in food and health. The industry lobbied the government hard to allow this doubtful practice. Nevertheless, a manufacturer can't just make any claim it wants. The FDA reviews the claims, allowing only those that it deems reasonably "factual and truthful." The intent is to show a connection between some nutrient in the food or the food itself with a reduction in the likelihood of a disease or health-related condition.

The problem is that the claim can get wildly out of hand. Take the example of oat bran, which is a soluble fiber. The FDA allows the claim, "fruits, vegetables, and grain products that contain fiber, particularly soluble fiber, may reduce the risk of heart disease."

In the manufacturer's hands, that phrase *soluble fiber* takes on unwarranted significance. It's true that oat bran when consumed as part of oats may be beneficial. But when the bran is extracted and added to a muffin loaded with sugar and fat, that's a different nutritional context. You lose the other beneficial feature of oats that contribute to the reduction of heart-disease risk. Yet the muffin maker would have you believe that this nutritional dessert, because it contains a bit of oat bran, is the way to avoid heart disease.

While the connections between a food item and health are not always unreasonable by themselves, the way manufacturers use the claims to promote products is questionable. Smart eaters disregard all health claims on food packages as nothing more than advertising gimmicks. (The 10 health claims the FDA allows are listed in Appendix D.)

Reading the nutrition label: A wrap-up

Reading a nutrition label is like looking at a painting. While you may examine some of the painting's details, your enjoyment comes from the total view, your overall impression. This chapter has given specifics and clues on interpreting label information. The trick in reading between the lines is to take an overview. Combine data in the Nutrition Facts panel with what you see in the Ingredient List to get an overall impression.

Based on that impression select those food products that give you the best nutritional value. Keep in mind that nutritional value goes beyond vitamins, minerals, and protein. That value includes an absence of items in the food, like unneeded additives that pose a drag on your body.

Finally, a comment on that part of the food universe that doesn't carry any labeling whatsoever. The FDA exempts the following foods from carrying a nutrition label:

- Fresh fruits and vegetables

- Meats

- Fish

- Baked goods from the corner bakery

- Items scooped out of a bulk bin

- Food ordered in restaurants, fast-food outlets, cafeterias, and from street vendors

- Food from vending machines

(For fresh fruits and vegetables, meats, and fish, the nutrition information may be posted at point of sale.)

As this list suggests, of the total food consumed in this country, a sizable fraction doesn't carry any nutrition labels. The food revolution in people's eating habits and food manufacturing technology has swept far ahead of government attempts to let consumers know how foods affect their health and daily nutrition. People are moving more and more to ordering their food from restaurants, delis, and takeouts.

Some information is better than no information at all, of course. For the packaged goods that carry nutrition labels, however, you have to be aware of the label's shortcomings. And for the universe of unlabeled foods, you are on your own.

Well, not really. This book is here with behind-the-scenes information to help you make smarter choices, whether the food is labeled or unlabeled.

Just the facts

- American eating habits have turned upside down. There is more grazing and eating finger foods, and less sitting down for meals.

- If you know how to read them correctly, ingredient lists of food products reveal hidden information about nutritional losses during processing. In general, beware of long labels.

- Nutrition labels emphasize fat information. Nutritional quality goes beyond fat content. You risk making poor choices if the amount of fat is the only criterion for choice.

■ Specific health claims for food products are
generally taken out of context. Beware of such
claims. Food is food, not a drug.

To Supplement or Not to Supplement Is No Longer the Question

C an 175 million Americans be wrong? That's the number of people who supplement their diet with vitamins, minerals, herbs, or phytochemicals. What drives this broad acceptance of dietary supplementation? Is it because people don't trust the food supply to deliver needed vitamins, or is it something more?

Indeed, it is something more. At one time people who took vitamin pills were considered cranks. Medical and nutrition authorities discouraged the practice, saying American foods gave all the necessary dietary components. But the authorities have changed their minds, now saying dietary supplements have an important role in maintaining good health.

Basically, medical thinking has shifted away from the idea that the only purpose of vitamins and minerals is to prevent deficiency diseases. Medical authorities believe vitamins and minerals in larger amounts help ward off chronic diseases. Thinking has gone from short term to long term.

Consider vitamin C, for instance. Vitamin C was identified as the vitamin that prevents scurvy, a deficiency disease in which a person's connective tissue disintegrates. The body literally falls apart. If an evil genie removed all vitamin C from your food, your body would use up residual stores and you'd eventually collapse in a little pool like the Wicked Witch of the West. That's the short term, and nutrition scientists figured that 30 to 60 milligrams a day of vitamin C is all you need to prevent scurvy.

New research, however, shows that vitamin C does more than prevent scurvy. It has long-term benefits. Vitamin C helps keep your heart in tone and reduces the chances any of your cells will turn cancerous. We are talking about 500 to 1,000 milligrams a day, a whopping dose compared to the anti-scurvy amount. You'd have to eat 17 fresh Valencia oranges to get 1,000 milligrams of vitamin C. You should still eat an orange or two every day, but vitamin C supplementation has become a practical way to help build long-term health.

The vitamin C example illustrates the basic switch in thinking from short-term to long-term health, and it is in this light that we examine the whole issue of dietary supplementation. In fact, the concept of dietary supplements has taken on new meaning. While vitamins and minerals are traditional supplements, new types and new ways of supplementation greet you in the marketplace. This chapter takes up the following:

- **Vitamin and mineral supplements.**

- **Nutraceuticals.** These are plant substances—phytochemicals, for example—that, unlike vitamins and minerals, are not needed to stay alive. In the long term, nutraceuticals may help prevent disease and promote health.

▪ **Functional foods.** These are processed foods fortified with vitamins, minerals, herbs, or nutraceuticals. The manufacturer, because of the fortification, may make certain claims about the food's health-promoting benefit.

Beware: Supplements cannot rescue a poor diet

Before we get into the specifics of dietary supplements, we have to get one thing quite clear. Supplements cannot rescue a low level or inadequate diet. Supplements are not intended to replace food. Remember, the word is "supplement."

There are two reasons why supplements cannot replace food:

▪ We don't know everything about human nourishment. Foods supply substances of which we are only dimly aware that still contribute to overall vitality. Supplement manufacturers can only put things in pills that are known. We know about vitamin C, so that can be put in a pill. We know about lycopene, a phytochemical from tomatoes that is supposed to help fend off cancer. So lycopene goes into a pill. But manufacturers can't bottle things they don't know about.

▪ Natural foods supply the total spectrum of vitamins, minerals, phytochemicals, fiber, and so forth in a balanced way. Balance is critical for absorption of the these substances from the gut. Too much of one mineral or vitamin can interfere with the absorption of another. Too much phosphorus, for example, depresses calcium absorption. Supplementation can be overdone, a critical point we take up in more detail in a moment.

A word of caution: Before you start thinking about supplements, think about a balanced diet. The USDA Food Pyramid in Chapter 1 is a good place to start, but as mentioned earlier, it is only one of many ways of achieving nutritional balance in your daily foods. In any event, keys to a balanced diet include the following:

- Above all, choose upper-level foods—that is, foods that rank at level 1 or 2 in the guides given in Part II.

- Make fruits and vegetables, plus whole grains, your base.

- Eat relatively smaller amounts of meat, poultry, and dairy products. If you are vegetarian, make sure you eat other sources of protein every day.

- As in the USDA pyramid, eat only tiny amounts of sweets, if any.

Having said that, we have to recognize that a well-balanced diet is elusive, and greatly depends on your lifestyle and available foods. Say, for example, you live in the northern tier of the country: long winters, short growing season. When fresh vegetables and fruits are available locally, your family's level of nutrition goes up. During winter, you rely on produce trucked from a continent away, and quality level goes down a notch. The answer is to do the best you can, recognizing that, although it will not be perfect, your best attempt at a balanced diet underpins any supplementation program.

Understanding labels on supplement bottles

Supplements are regulated under the 1994 Dietary Supplement Health and Education Act. The act's intent is to make information about dietary supplements widely available to consumers. Here are things you should know.

- A supplement manufacturer does not require FDA approval before selling a product to the public. Thus, supplements are regulated differently from drugs. A drug manufacturer has to prove a new drug's efficacy and safety before the FDA approves its sale.

- The FDA does not analyze the contents of a supplement pill. The manufacturer is responsible for ensuring that the ingredient list is accurate (as is true of drugs).

- The ingredients of the supplement pill or capsule must be listed on the label. The list also includes binders and fillers used in making the product.

- A dietary supplement cannot make any claim as a new treatment, diagnosis, or cure for a specific disease or condition. If it does, then the product is no longer considered a dietary supplement and would be regulated as a drug. The product, however, can make general health claims: It can say "enhances memory" but not "cures schizophrenia." If the manufacturer makes a claim not approved by the FDA, then a disclaimer must be put on the label saying the FDA has not evaluated the claim.

The upshot of all this is that, when you buy a dietary supplement, forget government guarantees.

> **"**
> In the guise of oversight of the nutrient supplement industry, the Congress managed to create a law (the 1994 Dietary Supplement Health and Education Act) that essentially exempts most nutrient supplements from meaningful regulation.
> —Mark S. Meskin, California State Polytechnic University, Pomona
> **"**

The FDA does not guarantee efficacy, safety, or accuracy of labeled ingredients, though it does have the power to remove misleading, misbranded, or dangerous products from the market. You have to trust the manufacturer.

Vitamins and minerals

While everyone can benefit from taking vitamin and mineral supplements, there are subgroups for which supplementation becomes imperative.

- **Anyone over age 60.** As people get older they eat less. But the body's need for vitamins and minerals doesn't diminish. In fact, need goes up because absorption from the gut becomes less efficient as people age.

- **Pregnant women.** Pregnancy places unusual stresses on the body. Vitamin and mineral supplementation on top of an excellent diet help ensure that mother and baby do well. Special attention should be given to folic acid, a delicate vitamin, easily destroyed during food processing and heating (cooking).

- **People who are dieting.** Dieters eat less and, just as for older folk, their bodies' need for vitamins and minerals does not diminish.

- **Heavy drinkers.** Since these individuals drink a large portion of their daily calories, the amount of real food in their diet is small. They need supplements.

- **Stressed individuals.** A body under stress consumes vitamins and minerals more rapidly. Therefore, such individuals need to take in more.

To repeat, everyone can benefit from dietary supplements. But individuals in the above categories, if

Watch Out!
Smokers beware. Tobacco smoke soaks up vitamins, particularly vitamin C. A smoker has to take two-and-a-half times the amount of this vitamin as a nonsmoker to achieve the same benefit. Nonsmokers living with smokers are also at risk—secondhand smoke drains a person's vitamin C.

they aren't taking vitamin and mineral supplements, place their long-term health at risk.

What are the acronyms RDA, USRDA, RDI, and DV?

We can talk of the benefits of taking vitamin and mineral supplements, but the burning question is: How much? How much is enough and, just as important, how much is too much? To answer these questions, we need a baseline, a minimum value that one ought to ingest for each vitamin and mineral.

The Food and Nutrition Board of the National Research Council established such a target, called the *Recommended Dietary Allowance (RDA)*. The RDAs are levels of vitamins and minerals considered adequate to meet the nutritional needs of healthy adults. The United States RDAs (USRDAs) are based on the RDAs and used specifically for the labeling of products. You often see "USRDA" on bottles of vitamin and mineral supplements. Trust the government, however, to make things unduly complicated. They use yet a third baseline, the Reference Daily Intake (or RDI). To top off bureaucratic confusion, they've created a fourth baseline, the Daily Value or DV. It's the percent DV you generally see on the label. This is the same Daily Value used on the nutrition labels of food products and described in Chapter 7. From a consumer's point of view, RDAs, USRDAs, RDIs, and DVs are sufficiently similar. Don't worry which term is used on the supplement label.

For instance, you may see a listing such as the following:

Vitamin A, 10,000 IU (International Units),
200 percent DV

This means that one vitamin pill contains twice the Daily Value established for vitamin A, which is 5,000 IU.

What to look for in a multivitamin

You can become bleary-eyed reading the lists of vitamins and minerals on the dozens of supplement brands. How do you know that the amount of each vitamin and mineral listed is right for you? Fortunately, there is a fair amount of latitude in optimal amounts. Nevertheless, you should have some sense of proportion, because you get vitamins and minerals in your daily food as well as in any supplement.

The Daily Value baseline is a good place to start. The following lists of vitamins and mineral supplements are a general recommendation. You should consult a qualified health professional for recommendations covering your specific case.

Bright Idea
Take vitamin E capsules with meals. The vitamin needs fat in the food to be absorbed.

1. **Antioxidant vitamins.** If you don't take any other vitamin and mineral supplements, take at least these two vitamins. They help protect your cells against the ravages of oxygen, which can lead to cancer and accelerated aging. A comment on vitamin E. The natural form extracted from vegetable oils is better absorbed than the synthetic form. It is actually a mixture of eight related compounds. Whether natural or synthetic, look for the name d-alpha-tocopherol. This is the principal form of vitamin E.

   - Vitamin E. Consume at least 200 to 800 IU a day.

   - Vitamin C. Consume 200 to 500 milligrams a day. Some authorities suggest larger amounts, 1,000 to 3,000 milligrams a day. Whatever amount you select, divide it into three or four doses over the day. Vitamin C is rapidly excreted in the urine.

2. **The B vitamins.** These are water-soluble vitamins easily destroyed or leached out during food processing and cooking. They could be lacking in a general diet. Look for 200 percent of DV of the following B vitamins:

- Thiamin (B_1)
- Riboflavin (B_2)
- Niacin (B_3)
- Pyridoxine (B_6)
- Vitamin B_{12}
- Folic acid

3. **Supplements equal to Daily Value.** Take supplements on a daily basis containing 100 percent of the Daily Values of these vitamins and minerals.

- Vitamin A (Some of the vitamin may come from beta-carotene.)
- Chromium
- Copper
- Iron
- Magnesium
- Selenium
- Zinc

4. **Supplementation unnecessary.** Some vitamin and minerals are present in adequate amounts in a general diet and thus supplementation is not important:

- Biotin
- Iodine
- Pantothenic acid
- Phosphorus

Bright Idea
Here's a tip.
Don't look for all
the vitamins and
minerals in one
pill—it would
have to be huge.
Buy vitamin E
and C as separate pills or capsules.

- Potassium
- Vitamin K

Is more better?

Since you buy vitamin and mineral supplements over the counter, you are legally free to take as much as you wish. But a word of caution. Too much of some of them can be dangerous. Besides, you might waste money. Here are suggested limits:

- **The B vitamins.** Up to 200 percent of Daily Value is okay, and many are safe at higher levels.

- **Vitamin A.** This vitamin can be toxic at high levels, but the toxic level is highly variable among individuals. To be on the safe side, limit the daily supplement to 15,000 IU.

   Vitamin A capsules may also contain or consist solely of beta-carotene, which in the body is converted to vitamin A. beta-carotene is more benign, and you don't have to limit it as much as you do the pure vitamin A. Taking 25,000 IU as beta-carotene a day is okay. To put that amount in perspective, one large carrot gives you 10,000 IU of beta-carotene.

- **Vitamin D.** This vitamin can be toxic at high levels. For most people, a daily supplement of 1,000 IU (250 percent of DV) should have no adverse effect.

- **Iron.** Don't go overboard with this mineral. If you have a medical problem, like iron-deficient anemia, consult a healthcare professional. Otherwise don't go over the suggested 100 percent of Daily Value, which is 18 milligrams.

   For healthy people, only 10 to 15 percent of iron ingested is absorbed. The gut has a

Watch Out!
Keep all vitamin and other supplement pills out of reach of kids. An overdose can be dangerous to a small child.

protective system that regulates the amount of iron absorbed. If the body needs more, then more is absorbed. In certain individuals, however, this regulation has gone awry. They absorb as much as 75 percent of the iron they ingest. Their internal organs fill up with iron, developing a disease known as hemochromatosis. Even for those without a hereditary predisposition to this disease, an overdose of several iron pills can make adults very sick and could kill a toddler.

Should you take a calcium supplement?

Calcium is another mineral you need, but don't need in excess. Since your food, depending on what you eat, supplies calcium, you need to take that into consideration when deciding whether or not to take a calcium supplement. The total amount an adult needs is about 1,000 milligrams a day. Older people, women over age 50 and men over age 65, need 1,200 to 1,500 milligrams.

There's more to a bone than calcium. Magnesium is another mineral that works closely with calcium. If you take a calcium supplement, choose one that contains both minerals, preferably one with a 2:1 ratio of calcium to magnesium (some authorities prefer 1:1, 1:2, or 3:2). You can also find supplements that combine calcium, magnesium, and vitamin D (calcium needs the vitamin to enter bones).

Make sure you get enough folic acid

Medical researchers report that women who have inadequate levels of folic acid are more likely to have a baby with the birth defect spina bifida (open spine). They say ingesting 400 micrograms of folic acid a day is sufficient to prevent this birth defect.

Unofficially...
The calcium panel for the National Academy of Sciences says not to rely on supplements to get adequate calcium. The panel recommends eating foods rich in calcium, such as dairy products, fish, green leafy vegetables, tofu, and almonds.

The good news is that if you consume the requisite five servings of vegetables and two to four servings of fruit, you stand an excellent chance of getting 400 micrograms. Supplements may also be helpful in this case—these studies showed a benefit from supplements as well as food.

For women who don't eat sufficient fresh fruits and vegetables, health authorities now recommend a folic acid supplement (the vitamin is a form of folate).

There is another reason for getting adequate amounts of folic acid—your heart. Folic acid has a beneficial effect on one's arteries. Studies at Tufts University Human Nutrition Research Center on Aging (Boston, MA) showed that men with low levels of folic acid had more deterioration of the arteries leading to the brain (a prelude to stroke).

The study, incidentally, shows there's more to preventing heart attacks and stroke than worrying solely about cholesterol and saturated fat in one's diet.

Take the antioxidants, vitamins C and E

As mentioned in the previous chapter, our bodies are subject to a slow burn, a gradual breakdown of key body tissues due to oxidation. Consider the problem from a cell's-eye view. Cells are full of oxygen, delivered by the blood. Cells need the oxygen to oxidize sugars and fat for energy, the energy that keeps us alive. Oxygen at the same time bounces around the inside of the cell, a spray of cannon balls battering vital cell components. What stops the oxygen from doing its dirty work? An assortment of *antioxidants:* substances the cell makes and substances from the diet. Dietary antioxidants are crucial. Without them, the cell's own defenses are overwhelmed, and serious tissue damage results.

There are two ways to ensure your body is not enveloped in the slow burn. First, take vitamins C and E as supplements. They are both potent anti-oxidants. Second, eat fruits, vegetables, and whole grains. They are rich in a group of yellowish plant pigments known as *carotenoids*. Some 500 carotenoids have been identified, including beta-carotene. Beta-carotene is available in capsules and is advertised as an antioxidant. Don't make the mistake of relying on a beta-carotene supplement to beef up antioxidant action. While a beta-carotene supplement has value because it is converted to vitamin A, its role as an antioxidant is less secure. The reason is that carotenoids work as a team, and thus the only way to reap the benefit of their antioxidant strength is to eat the plant foods. The carotenoids are produced only in plants. Because cattle and chickens eat plant food, relatively small amounts of the yellowish carotenes occur in egg yolks, cheese, butter, and milk with fat.

The health benefits of antioxidants are manifold. People who take vitamins C and E supplements in addition to eating fruits and vegetables benefit in the following ways:

- They have a reduced risk of heart attacks and strokes
- They have decreased risk of cancer
- They have less chance of suffering from cataracts

FAQs concerning vitamin and mineral supplements

Here are 10 questions frequently asked concerning vitamin and mineral supplements.

1. **Question:** Does the government guarantee the potency of the vitamins in the pills I buy?

Watch Out!
The Federal Trade Commission (FTC) controls the advertising of dietary supplements in the media, including the Internet. Unlike product labels, an ad can claim the product prevents a disease if the manufacturer backs up the claim with scientific studies. But policing thousands of Web sites selling supplements is proving difficult. Many make exaggerated and unsupported claims of health benefits.

Answer: Only if the ingredients are labeled USP (U.S. Pharmacopeia). In that case the vitamins must conform to a rigid standard. Most vitamin manufacturers don't run the necessary tests and therefore don't label their products as USP. Thus, as a consumer you have to take the manufacturer's word the vitamins are up to strength.

2. **Question:** Should vitamin E capsules be kept in a refrigerator?

   Answer: No. The soft-gel capsule keeps the vitamin safe from exposure to air. But keep the capsules bottled and cool or the gelatin will soften.

3. **Question:** Regarding vitamin E, what is the difference between d- and d,l-alpha tocopherol?

   Answer: Tocopherol is the chemical name for vitamin E. The natural form is d-alpha tocopherol. The d,l-alpha tocopherol is a synthetic product that has half the potency of the natural d- form. Some vitamin E supplements contain beta-, gamma-, and delta-tocopherols. These related tocopherols have some vitamin E activity, but much less than the alpha form. Sometimes you see the word "acetate"—for example, d-alpha tocopherol acetate. Acetate doesn't change potency. Ignore the word.

4. **Question:** What is the difference between niacin and niacinamide (vitamin B_3)?

   Answer: Both are active forms of the vitamin. If you take a niacin supplement you may get a flush—your face and upper body get hot. It's momentary, however, and soon goes away. (Note that taking niacin with food can reduce

Moneysaver
Avoid paying premium prices for vitamin and mineral supplements labeled with fancy names such as Morning Vitamins, Evening Vitamins, Women's Supplements, Men's Supplements, Stress, Vitamin Mixture, Silver Supplements, and Vision Vitamins. Read the labels. Buy plain vitamin and mineral supplements.

the severity of the flush.) Niacinamide doesn't cause the flush.

5. **Question:** I see amino acids sold as supplements. Are they worth the money?

   Answer: Not necessarily. Although research suggests that specific amino acids, such as glutamine and aginine, are beneficial, amino acid supplements are often sold in quantities too small to achieve a benefit. Amino acids are components of proteins, and for them to work their best, I recommend that you eat them as protein from food.

6. **Question:** I'm confused by a calcium supplement. It lists 500 milligrams of calcium phosphate, yet there are only 200 milligrams of calcium.

   Answer: Calcium phosphate, as the name suggests, consist of two parts, the phosphate and the calcium. This supplement lists the weight of the calcium phosphate (500 milligrams), which gives you 200 milligrams of calcium. Bones also need the phosphate, but since phosphate is readily available in the diet from other foods, this mineral is not one you need worry about. In fact, too much phosphorus can deplete calcium in bone.

7. **Question:** What is retinoic acid and how does it relate to vitamin A?

   Answer: Retinoic acid is a chemical name for vitamin A. Beta-carotene is converted to retinoic acid in the body.

8. **Question:** Are there restrictions on the amount of a vitamin or mineral a manufacturer can put in one pill?

Answer: No. The decision as to how much to put in the pill is made by the manufacturer and does not require FDA review (except for folic acid and iron).

9. **Question:** Where can I get information about a specific dietary supplement?

    Answer: You have to contact the manufacturer. The government does not maintain a database on the contents of dietary supplements.

10. **Question:** Who ensures the safety of dietary supplements?

    Answer: Don't look to the government. The FDA does not require products to be reviewed and evaluated before they reach the market, nor do they routinely and proactively test most of the products to ensure safety and reliability. They can, of course, remove products that show evidence of being dangerous.

Unofficially...
People might buy two or three cars or a second home, but they won't buy more food than they can eat. A food company can only increase the sales of one product at the expense of another competing product. Companies are always looking for novel ways to enhance the perceived value of their products and gain a marketing advantage. Adding nutraceuticals is one way.

Nutraceuticals: Foods in a bottle?

Nutraceuticals are substances extracted from a natural source and either put into a supplement or added to a food product. Unlike vitamins and minerals, we don't need nutraceuticals to stay alive, but when they are added to the diet they may confer some benefit.

To illustrate the concept behind nutraceuticals, take broccoli, a member of the cruciferous plant family. Broccoli is well known and appreciated as a vegetable that thwarts the cancer process. Broccoli contains a phytochemical, sulphoraphane, believed to be central to broccoli's anticancer properties.

The nutraceutical industry looked at the sulphoraphane connection and said, "Aha! Let's bottle the chemical and market it." They can either extract it from broccoli or synthesize it. Either way, it can be marketed as the natural phytochemical from broccoli that fights cancer.

For many folk, swallowing a pill is easier than eating broccoli. But wait a minute. Can we be sure that the protective essence of broccoli now resides in the pill? No. The broccoli's sulphoraphane is one of dozens of other phytochemicals, vitamins, minerals, and plant hormones that work in close harmony against cancer. There is no guarantee that sulphoraphane in a pill offers anything like the same potency as a serving of broccoli. In fact, without extensive clinical trials we don't know whether or not it has any potency at all.

Research on the health benefits of phytochemicals is still very much in its infancy. It is premature to expect that the complex phytochemical mixture in broccoli can be captured in a pill. The moral of this story: Eat your broccoli. You don't like broccoli? Eat other members of the cruciferous family: kale, cabbage, cauliflower, collard greens, or brussels sprouts.

Are phytochemicals the new wonder drugs?

The leaves, roots, stems, and fruits of plants contain tens of thousands of substances, which we call phytochemicals. Plants don't make these often-complex substances just for the fun of it. They are present for definite purposes. Phytochemicals include colorants, which give the infinite spectrum of hues and colors in the plant world. They color blueberries blue and tomatoes red. Other phytochemicals drive away insects, and still others flavor fruits so animals will eat them and thus distribute the seeds. Phytochemicals give each plant and fruit a distinct character.

Bright Idea
Phytochemicals, as the name implies, are plant chemicals. There are no comparable substances in animal foods. Thus, to take advantage of the health benefits, you have to include plant foods in your daily diet or find supplements.

As fruit and vegetable consumers, we appreciate the flavors and colors that make these foods attractive and tasty. Beyond that, we now find the phytochemicals in our everyday fruits and vegetables enhance a person's health, warding off degenerative disease, such as heart disease, cancer, arthritis, and cataracts. To say the least, these substances are powerful components of our overall nutrition.

Some 4,000 phytochemicals have been identified, a tiny fraction of what's in the plant world. Of these, only about 150 have been extensively studied. In short, while we know in general about phytochemicals and the fact that they enhance health, we know relatively little about the details of how they work or which combinations of phytochemicals are needed to attain a specific health goal. So, while in individual cases there are studies to give us a sense of their effects, in the big picture we're only just beginning to identify phytochemicals and learn their effects on humans.

Nevertheless, a new research thrust has taken shape that has sparked a new industry. Its goal: Identify specific phytochemicals in plants that have a specific health benefit, put the chemicals in pills, and promote the pills as having the same benefit as the plant. These new supplements are called *nutraceuticals.*

For the record, the following table presents a list of foods known to have long-term health benefits and some of the phytochemicals they contain.

TABLE 8.1: FOODS, PHYTOCHEMICALS, AND POSSIBLE HEALTH BENEFITS

Food	Phytochemicals	Possible Benefits
Berries: blueberries, blackberries, boysenberries, cranberries, raspberries, strawberries	Flavonoids (they belong to the larger class of polyphenols), ellagic acid	Antioxidants, prevent cancer and heart disease. Also rich in soluble fiber.
Citrus Fruits: grapefruit, lemons, limes, oranges	Flavanones, coumarins, carotenoids (includes beta-carotene), flavonoids, limonoids	Prevent cancer. Carotenoids and flavonoids are antioxidants.
Cruciferous Vegetables: broccoli, brussels sprouts, cabbage, cauliflower, kale	Carotenoids, isothiocyanates, sulphoraphane, indoles	Prevent cancer. Sulphoraphane believed to be the most active agent.
Flax Seeds	Lignans and the omega-3 and omega-6 fatty acids	Lignans may have an anticancer effect.
Garlic Family: chives, garlic, leeks, onions, scallions, shallots	Allylic sulfides, flavonoids	Prevent cancer and may benefit the heart.
Grains, Whole	Saponins, phytic acid, phtoestrogens, terpenoids	Prevent cancer. Phytic acid may help reduce risk of heart disease.
Green Tea	Flavonoids, polyphenols	Prevent cancer.
Legumes: beans, lentils, peas	Isoflavonoids, phytic acid, phytosterols, saponins	Prevent cancer. Protect against heart disease.
Nuts: almonds, brazil, cashews, walnuts	Ellagic acid, saponins	Benefit the heart.
Red Grapes	Flavonols, polyphenols, anthocyanins	Prevent cancer and benefit the heart.
Spices: cumin, ginger, oregano, rosemary, sage, thyme	Carnasol, phenols, curcumin, gingerols	Antioxidants.
Soybeans	Isoflavonoids (daidzein and genistein); lignans, phytosterols, saponins	Isoflavonoids and lignans are converted to estrogen-like substances.
Tomatoes	Ellagic acid, carotenoids, such as lycopene	Prevent cancer.
Yellowish Fruits and Vegetables and Leafy Vegetables: apricots, carrots, corn, mangoes, pumpkin, spinach, sweet peppers, sweet potatoes	Carotenoids, lutein, zeaxanthin	Prevent cancer. Strengthen immune system.

Bright Idea
Although fresh raw tomatoes have many nutritional advantages over canned tomatoes, the canned tomato has one advantage. The lycopene—and presumably the other carotenoids—becomes five times more available on cooking. Maybe there is something to those Mediterranean tomato sauces.

In reading this table, keep in mind the state of the science. Science has indeed identified some of the phytochemicals associated with health benefits listed in the third column. But, in fact, the benefits you see in the third column stem from eating the fruits and vegetables you see in the first column. The identified phytochemicals may play a part in winning the benefits, but only a part. Importantly, there is no clinical evidence that putting any of these phytochemicals in a bottle will give you the expected benefit.

A case in point is lycopene, a member of the carotenoid family. A study of 1,379 European men found that those eating foods rich in lycopene halved the risk of a heart attack compared to men who ate few such foods. You might jump to the conclusion that lycopene prevents heat attacks. But the head of the research team conducting the study, Lenore Kohlmeir, professor of epidemiology and nutrition at the University of North Carolina, Chapel Hill, said they weren't sure that lycopene is the protective agent. It could be another phytochemical that travels with lycopene. According to a report in the *New York Times*, she noted that you can't assume that a pill with lycopene offers the same benefit as ingesting lycopene through food.

Turning food into a pill goes beyond the edge of science. Look at it this way. You are 40 years old. Your doctor says to you: I'll give you two choices:

- Eat a balanced diet with the fruits and vegetables listed in the preceding table, and I guarantee you'll have a low risk of heart disease and cancer, and other wonderful health benefits, for the rest of your life.

- Swallow all these pills containing a tiny selection of phytochemicals for the rest of your life.

They are said to fight against cancer and heart disease, but we have no idea if they will work in a pill. Are you willing to take the chance?

What choice would you make? Take the second choice and you will be nothing but a human guinea pig. Luckily, in life you probably won't be forced to make such an either/or choice. Be sure to eat a balanced diet, but if you want to augment it with phytochemicals that are well-researched, by all means do so.

Beware of claims too good to be true

Nutraceuticals, like vitamins and minerals, are classed as neither food nor drug, meaning they are hardly regulated at all. As noted earlier, the FDA controls a little of what's printed on the product label—the manufacturer can make no claim that implies treatment or cure of a specific disease. Other than that, the manufacturer has freedom to stake out a claim about health.

Take the case of cranberry juice. Folk wisdom has it that the juice protects against urinary infections. A 1994 study at Harvard University Medical School put this folk wisdom to the test. The researchers gave a group of elderly women 10 ounces of sweetened cranberry juice a day. Compared to an equal group of non–cranberry juice drinkers, the juice-drinking women cut their amount of urinary tract infections by 40 percent.

Enter a nutraceutical product consisting of a dried cranberry extract in a pill. The label on the bottle claims, "research indicates cranberry fruit may help maintain a healthy urinary tract by preventing the adhesion of bacteria (*E. coli*) to the bladder."

The statement on the label is correct, assuming they are citing the Harvard study. But to suggest the contents of the cranberry pill will produce the same

> **"**
> Vivid and fanciful descriptions imply that use of a product will improve performance or ameliorate or boost a condition. Gone is the line between what science has documented a product or ingredient can do and what description suggests it will do.
> —Joyce A. Nettleton, D.Sc., R.D., director, Science Communications, Institute of Food Technologists
> **"**

result as drinking cranberry juice is not well-founded. Two reasons: Scientists don't know what the active ingredient in the cranberry juice is, and they don't know if it would survive the heating and other rigors of processing into a pill. In short, eat cranberries or drink the whole juice, and forget the pills.

If you think that bottle labeling pushes the envelope of truth, consider advertising claims for nutraceuticals. Product advertising in magazines, newspapers, and TV and radio come under the jurisdiction of the Federal Trade Commission (FTC). Unlike the FDA prohibition against claims of cure or treatment, the FTC allows such claims. While the FTC insists that the claim be backed up by research, the quality of such research can vary widely. And while the manufacturers are forbidden to make misleading claims, they, like the proponents of many products, have an economic interest in emphasizing claims favorable to the product, discarding unfavorable results.

Ginkgo biloba is a good example. It was long advertised as improving memory and concentration and enhancing mental focus. Recent studies such as those in the *Journal of the American Medical Association* have supported these claims, while others have not. Even if studies should ultimately support the claims for gingko biloba, however, the problem is that people widely assume its abilities even before the scientific evidence is well-established. The lesson? Don't believe everything you hear from a friend or see on a label. Do a little research on your own, and in the meantime, use food—not supplements—as the basis for your good diet.

Unofficially...
The distinction between foods, supplements, and drugs is becoming ever more blurred. We seem to be moving back to a Wild West era when hucksters advertised snake oil as a cure for every imaginable ailment. This is all the more unfortunate because many *good* products are out there. They deserve your attention but are drowned out in the shrill cries of unproven claims.

Foods fortified with vitamins and minerals

Fortified foods, such as breakfast cereals fortified with added vitamins and minerals, have long been on the market. Since there is merit in taking vitamin and mineral supplements, is there merit in getting extra vitamins and minerals in food? The question goes deeper. Do health claims riding on the added vitamins or minerals make sense? Do you buy the food for whatever nutrition or enjoyment it provides, or do you buy it for the fact that it gives you vitamins or minerals? Is it a food or a supplement? Can it be both? Consider the case of young girls, calcium, and bones.

Can added calcium up the value of juice drinks?

Many teenage girls have two strikes against their skeletons. They are physically inactive, and they eat nutritionally low-level foods—"junk foods." Bone structure is set for life at this age, and a flimsy, underdeveloped skeleton primes the individual for osteoporosis later in life.

Researchers at Pennsylvania State University wanted to see if they could improve bone strength in that age group. They gave a group of girls a supplement of calcium citrate-malate. Sure enough, over 18 months, the bones of girls receiving the supplement grew more dense compared to a group of girls not receiving extra calcium.

This research on calcium caught the fancy of juice drink companies, and they started adding calcium citrate to juice drinks—10 percent juice, 90 percent sugar water. Having added the calcium, the companies promote the sweetened water drink as a source of calcium. They highlight the fact that calcium is good for your bones. The implication is that drinking this product strengthens bones.

Here's the rub. We don't know if calcium mixed with a dollop of sugar, water, and a little juice offers the same benefit as taking a calcium supplement. Calcium in a juice drink is not the same as calcium in a supplement, and it may not be absorbed as well or present in a useful amount. The FDA does not require the juice drink company to do separate clinical trials to prove that calcium in the drink works (and in this case, there is reason to doubt that it would work—sugar may well interfere with the absorption).

The smart thing to do is to take a calcium supplement if you feel that it is necessary, and not rely on a food product to provide you with the correct amount.

Get your vitamins and minerals from food or a pill?

There are two schools of thought on the nutritional merits of fortifying processed foods with vitamins and minerals. One school is appalled by the idea. They say adding vitamin and minerals to nutritionally limited foods discourages people from getting their essential nutrients the old-fashioned way— fruits, vegetables, and whole grains. People will say, "Why bother? My breakfast cereal provides me with all the vitamins and minerals I need."

Proponents of fortification say, "That's life. Ninety percent of the population doesn't eat the recommended number of fruits and vegetable servings. We've been telling people for years to eat their vegetables. People just don't listen." So, they claim, the only way to get essential nutrients into the population is to fortify foods people like to eat.

> **66**
> Although fortification makes many food products even more nutritionally sound, foods such as candy and sugary fruit drinks with only 10 percent real juice should not be fortified because they have little or no nutritional value from the outset. It can be a gimmick.
> —Paul A. Lachance, director of the Nutraceuticals Institute, Rutgers University
> **99**

The argument over the merits of fortifying foods with vitamins and minerals is less one of nutrition than of social engineering. Proponents of fortification see large numbers of people who eat junky diets and refuse to change their habits. It is these people that proponents would reach with fortification, hoping to make some improvement in their nutrition.

Be that as it may, this approach to vitamins and mineral supplementation is not smart nutrition. When you eat extra vitamins and minerals in a food, you lose control over the dosage. The manufacturer controls what vitamins and minerals you get and how much. A vitamin and mineral supplement, on the other hand, lets you decide exactly how much is suitable for you. You can adjust the amounts for your age and for the lifestyle you lead.

Avoid iron overdose: Avoid fortified breakfast cereals

One problem with depending on processed foods to supply vitamins and minerals is the possibility of overdose. As already described, too much can be a bad thing. One hundred grams (about 4 ounces) of Total, a fortified breakfast cereal, delivers 60 milligrams of iron, three times the Daily Value of 18 milligrams. Perhaps you wouldn't eat 100 grams—that's a large bowlful—but still that's a lot of iron in one food, far beyond the amount in a natural food. A comparable whole-grain, unfortified cereal delivers only 3 milligrams of iron per 100-gram portion.

A premenopausal woman may handle the amount of iron in the fortified breakfast cereal well, but that amount pushes the envelope for a postmenopausal woman or for a man.

To be sure, statistically speaking, the likelihood of overdose on other vitamins and minerals is a great deal less than that of iron, in part because these nutrients are usually not present in fortified foods to such a relatively high degree as iron. The issue here, however, is not whether a ready-to-eat breakfast cereal fortified with vitamins and minerals is desirable or undesirable. It may, in fact, be of value for some people. The issue is smart nutrition. Smart nutrition is all about eating a good, high-level diet. When you do this you are already getting a full spectrum of vitamins and minerals your body uses.

Supplementing your diet with more vitamins and minerals is not to be taken lightly. Ingesting too much of certain nutrients can decrease absorption of others. From your body's perspective, each vitamin and mineral is like the link of a chain. You need every link. The fact that some links are super-strong does not compensate for weak links. That's where the chain breaks down.

The recommended amounts of vitamins and minerals presented at the beginning of the chapter represent what I regard as a safe and reasonable level of supplementation. You should remember, of course, that other authorities have differing views of the exact levels that are "safe" and "reasonable." Many holistic health advocates, for example, advocate significantly higher levels than those I've indicated here. The bottom line is control and information. Keep control over the supplements you put in your body. And stay informed about the latest research, which can often change our best estimates of what are the optimal nutritional levels for one's diet.

Remember these tips:

- Eat unfortified foods for the nourishment and the enjoyment they provide, not as supplements.

- Take supplements in pills or capsules. You know exactly what is in the pill and how much you take.

- The word is "supplement"—that is, supplement to a high-level, basic diet.

Herbs: Medicine or food?

How does this drink strike you? One orange-mango soft drink contains three herbs: St. John's wort, ginkgo biloba, and gotu kola. The drink carries the promise "to promote calm and focused thought." St. John's wort has been called the herbal Prozac, and ginkgo biloba has been reputed to sharpen memory. But will herbs work with healthy people and at the doses in the fruit drink? The medical literature suggests that for many herbs, the amount present in most of these drinks is too low to be effective. In such cases, FDA regulation against misleading health claims would be welcome, but unfortunately the agency often takes no action.

This drink is part of a new surge in the food industry. Food companies, seeing an expanding market for functional foods, have expanded beyond vitamins and minerals and now add herbal supplements to products. As a consumer, beware.

Nothing against herbs. They have a long and honorable tradition of being used as medicines and for easing the vicissitudes of life. But, except as seasoning, should they be put in foods? Herbs, like drugs, are two-edged swords. If an herbal

Watch Out!
St. John's wort is usually prescribed in doses of 300 milligrams per day (or even three times per day) to achieve a desired affect. One brand of juice drink advertises it contains this herb, but amounts are low. You'd have to drink 15 bottles a day to get a therapeutic dose.

Unofficially...
Varo Tyler, an expert on herbs and professor emeritus of pharmacognosy (drugs from natural sources), Purdue University, says herbs used as nutrition-boosters should be taken as supplements, not as part of food. That way you keep track of how much you ingest.

supplement is potent enough to have a positive therapeutic effect, then it's conceivable that, like drugs that are usually beneficial, it could have an adverse effect in highly sensitive people. Who wants to be made ill from drinking what they thought would be a refreshing fruit drink?

The next time you see a food product with added herbs, remember these facts:

- Foods are foods and herbs are herbs, and they should not be mixed.

- Companies who mix food and herbs do not have to prove that their products deliver the advertised benefits, though legally, the claims are not supposed to be misleading.

- Some herbs have potent therapeutic powers (both negative and positive) and should be treated as such. Take herbs separately and under guidance of a health professional trained in use of herbs.

Just the facts

- Vitamin and mineral supplements alone cannot rescue a substandard diet. Your first priority is upgrading your diet and then thinking about supplements.

- Vitamin and mineral supplements play a role in one's daily nutrition that goes beyond preventing deficiency disease. Over the long term, they help ward off heart disease and cancer and pump up the immune system.

- Nutraceuticals are natural substances, like phytochemicals, that can be bottled or added to foods. In so doing, the substance is removed from its natural context. Unlike with drugs, the FDA does not require the manufacturer to prove that the nutraceutical on its own provides a health benefit, though it does require the product claims not to be false or misleading.

- Fortified foods are regular food products with added vitamins and minerals. Smart nutrition says that, if you supplement, do it with pills, not foods. With pills you know exactly what vitamins and minerals you get, and how much of each.

- Herbs have a centuries-old tradition of use in helping people. Adding herbs to food, however, is a different matter. The FDA does not require manufacturers of foods with added herbs to prove that the food with the herb rewards the consumer with any health benefit.

GET THE SCOOP ON...
Health benefits of a vegetarian diet ▪ Lacto-ovo
vegetarians ▪ Vegans ▪ The Mediterranean diet
and heart disease ▪ Vegetable sources of
protein ▪ Getting sufficient vitamin B_{12}

Vegetarianism: Should You Move Towards a Plant-Based Diet?

Chapter 9

If you look at all the different diets peoples of the world follow and pick the healthiest, you find a common thread. The healthiest diets are loaded with fruits, vegetables, and whole grains, and are short on meat and diary products. Many Americans are catching on to this fact. The USDA estimates that 20 million adults practice some form of vegetarianism and, of those, 12 million are strict vegetarians. The National Restaurant Association reports that one diner out of three seeks a restaurant that offers meatless dishes. When asked why, these folks cite healthier food as the reason.

But health benefits don't flow automatically by merely avoiding meat and dairy products. You can be a vegetarian and still eat a low-level diet with a lot of highly processed foods. Such diets cancel the benefits of going vegetarian. This chapter shows you how to avoid such blunders. It gives you the know-how for choosing nonanimal foods that keeps your diet perking at a high level. The chapter is intended for those who are committed vegetarians as well as those seeking to reduce the quantity of meat and dairy products in their diet.

The term *vegetarian* covers a broad range of eating styles, from those who eat meat occasionally to strict vegetarians—those who eat no animal products whatsoever, not even honey. For the purposes of our discussion, however, we can divide vegetarians into two main groups:

- **Lacto-ovo** vegetarians eat plant foods plus dairy products and eggs

- **Vegans** are strict vegetarians, eating only foods from plant sources

The chapter addresses both types of vegetarians as well as such issues as whether or not vegetarians get sufficient protein, vitamin B$_{12}$, and calcium.

Are vegetarians healthier?

The answer to the question "Are vegetarians healthier?" is an unequivocal yes. The reason is that these individuals eat a much higher proportion of fruits, vegetables, legumes, nuts, and grains. From a cell's-eye view, plant foods give the human body the wide spectrum of nutrients that make the difference between so-so health and long-term vitality.

Here's how vegetarians fare with six major health issues.

Heart disease

Vegetarians enjoy a vastly lower risk of heart disease, especially if they become vegetarians early in life. However, it is never too late to start. Why is a vegetarian diet more heart friendly? Four main reasons:

- Cholesterol and saturated fat, the two bugaboos of individuals eating meat and dairy

Moneysaver
A healthier body means less illness, lower medical and drug costs, and lower out-of-pocket healthcare expenses. Consider vegetarianism as one route to better health.

CHAPTER 9 ■ VEGETARIANISM: SHOULD YOU MOVE
TOWARDS A PLANT-BASED DIET?

247

foods, are not problems. Cholesterol doesn't exist in the plant kingdom, and with rare exceptions plant foods do not have significant levels of saturated fats.

- Vegetarians on average have substantially lower blood cholesterol than meat eaters. The soluble fiber of plant foods sweeps cholesterol out of the intestinal tract, one way the body can rid itself of excess cholesterol.

- Phytochemicals (antioxidants), which exist by the thousands in plant foods, prevent oxygen from damaging heart and brain arteries.

- Adequate folic acid, which plant foods have in abundance, is essential to maintaining heart health.

Cancer

A New Zealand study of 11,000 adults compared death rates between vegetarians and meat eaters. The vegetarians experienced a 20 percent lower rate in deaths from any cause as compared to meat eaters. But the biggest drop was in death due to cancer. Vegetarians experience a 40 percent lower death rate than the meat eaters. Other studies find that the more meat—especially beef and pork—a person eats, the greater the risk of colon cancer. For every vegetarian male who contracts colon cancer, four red-meat eaters (five meals a week) get the disease. Heavy red-meat eaters are also twice as likely to develop prostate cancer as vegetarians are.

Stroke

The brain also enjoys the same benefits the human heart gets from a vegetarian diet. Plaques (fatty deposits) that build up inside coronary arteries and block blood flow are the cause of heart attacks. The same plaques also build up in the arteries leading to

Unofficially...
Fifteen percent of college students are vegetarians. College cafeterias catering to this group provide one or more meatless dishes at every meal.

the brain, blocking the flow of blood. This is the paralyzing cause of a stroke. A study over 20 years of 832 middle-age men found that, for every three servings of fruits and vegetables they ate a day, their risk of stroke dropped 20 percent.

Bone density

Vegetarian women over age 55 were found to have a higher bone density than meat-eating women. The higher bone density means less chance of developing osteoporosis. This finding coincides with the observation that Asian women who are traditionally vegetarian rarely experience osteoporosis.

Diverticulitis

This disease results when pouches (diverticuli) form in the walls of the colon and become inflamed. People who have a low level of fruits, vegetables, and whole grains in their diet often have compact, rough stools. The bowel has to strain to force these lumps through. The severe mechanical stresses on the colon's walls over the years cause the pouches to form. Individuals experience constipation, flatulence, or diarrhea. The vegetarian diet, by contrast, helps avoid this condition.

Weight

It's hard to become fat on a well-ordered vegetarian diet. Such diets are nutrient-dense and calorie-light. For every calorie a vegetarian diet delivers, the consumer is rewarded with a high level spectrum of vitamins and minerals. Why?

> 66
> A man of my spiritual intensity does not eat corpses.
> —George Bernard Shaw
> 99

- Fruits and vegetables, by their nature, are rich in vitamins and minerals.

- Fruits and vegetables are bulky. They contain a lot of water and fiber.

CHAPTER 9 ▪ VEGETARIANISM: SHOULD YOU MOVE
TOWARDS A PLANT-BASED DIET?

249

Thus, you have the advantage of filling foods, rich in needed nutrients yet not providing an overwhelming number of calories.

Overall, as a group, vegetarians are a thinner and healthier group than average Americans. In addition to the six health issues, vegetarians who develop adult-onset diabetes are less likely to die from the disease than meat-eating diabetics. Vegetarians are also less likely to suffer elevated blood pressure, and this fact is independent of sodium intake. From a cell's-eye view, a vegetarian's body biochemistry functions at a higher degree of efficiency. Immune defenses are more robust, and the natural processes of aging are slowed.

Having said that, we should repeat: To gain these benefits, you need to eat a well-balanced diet of upper-level foods, ones that rank first and second on the quality scale.

In addition to our central concern, good nutrition, there is another factor—the health of the environment. Vegetarians like to point out that animals consume vast quantities of grain. Beef cattle consume, for example, 14 pounds of grain for every pound of hamburger they yield. The intensive growing of crops for animals burdens the environment. Excess fertilizer and pesticides contaminate groundwater. Land erodes. Animal manure pollutes land and waterways. All this could be reduced by lessening the consumption of meats and animal products.

> 66
> Vegetarianism is harmless enough, though it is apt to fill a man with wind and self-righteousness.
> —Sir Robert Hutchinson, early-20th-century London physician
> 99

Lacto-ovo vegetarians

Lacto-ovo vegetarians eat eggs and dairy products, although some eat eggs but not dairy, while others eat dairy but not eggs. In any event, the main focus of the diet is plant foods.

Let's take a specific example of such a diet. Cynthia F., a woman in her mid-30s, is a lacto-ovo vegetarian. At 5'7" and 130 pounds, she is a fit, active woman. Her diet over a week varies, but the listing of 1 day's foods is typical for her diet.

TABLE 9.1: LACTO-OVO VEGETARIAN— TYPICAL ONE-DAY'S DIET OF CYNTHIA F.

Food	Calories	Protein, grams	Fat, grams	Carbohydrate, grams
Breakfast				
Cooked oatmeal (³/₄ cup), garnished with ²/₃ T of ground flaxseed, ¹/₂ T of honey, and ¹/₂ cup skim milk. 1 orange.	330	16.6	7	50
Lunch				
Egg salad sandwich on whole-wheat bread. Green salad: lettuce with 2 T of walnuts and 1 chopped apple, 2 T fresh lemon juice.	500	14.2	23	58
Dinner				
Vegetable lasagna. 1 cup bulgur wheat pilaf with 1 cup of mixed vegetables. Fruit smoothie: 1 cup of strawberries, sliced banana, 1 cup fresh apple cider.	745	32	9.6	141
Snacks				
3 T of hummus and crackers, 1¹/₂ T of mixed nuts.	260	3.75	24	7.5
Totals	1,835	66.5	63.6	256.5

The number of calories and number of grams of protein, fat, and carbohydrate are calculated from USDA databases. T = tablespoon.

Cynthia's total energy intake of about 1,900 calories is right for her size and level of activity. Her diet

CHAPTER 9 ■ VEGETARIANISM: SHOULD YOU MOVE
TOWARDS A PLANT-BASED DIET?

251

is well balanced, giving her a full spectrum of vitamins and minerals. Four points deserve special comment.

Unofficially...
Many vegetarians would be best described as "almost" vegetarian, or meat avoiders. They eat seafood, dairy products, and eggs. And on social occasions when meat is served, they eat it.

1. **Protein.** Cynthia's protein intake of 66.5 grams is well above the RDA level of 44 grams. It's important to get protein from a variety of foods. In her case, beans, nuts, cheese, and milk are major contributors.

2. **Fat.** Her total fat intake is in the range of the 60-gram limit recommended in the USDA guidelines and represents 30 percent of total calories. But of this total fat, only about 15 grams is saturated fat, chiefly from the cheese, egg, and butter. The rest is the healthful mono- and polyunsaturated fats. The latter includes a good helping of the omega-3 fats. Her fat balance is excellent.

3. **Vitamin B$_{12}$.** Neither plants nor animals make this vitamin; only specialized bacteria do. Food animals, obtaining the vitamin from their diet, pass it on to human consumers. Cynthia gets about 1.5 microgram (one millionth of a gram) from the eggs in her luncheon sandwich and the cheese snack. This amount is half the RDA of three micrograms a day. Vitamin B$_{12}$, however, is stored in the liver, and daily fluctuations in the diet are not serious. Cynthia does not eat cheese or eggs every day and so takes a vitamin B$_{12}$ supplement.

4. **Calcium.** Cynthia's menu for this day gives her about 750 milligrams of calcium, less than the recommended 1,200 milligrams. She can make up the difference with a calcium supplement.

In short, Cynthia's diet is an excellent example of a lacto-ovo vegetarian, emphasizing plant foods with relatively small amounts of dairy and egg. She likes cheese, and on days when cheese does not appear in main meals, she will have an ounce or so of cheddar cheese on crackers as a snack. On this particular day, the vegetable lasagna contained cheese.

Importantly, her choice of plant foods is varied, not weighting any single plant group.

If you are a lacto-ovo vegetarian, here are tips to ensure that you get the most out of this style of eating:

- Eat upper-level foods—that is, foods that rank at levels 1 and 2 in the guides presented in Chapters 2 to 6. In practice, this means selecting fresh fruits, vegetables, and whole grains, and shunning processed foods.

- Include legumes in at least one meal during the day. They maintain protein balance.

- Emphasize plant foods in your daily menu. Don't make the mistake of merely substituting dairy products and eggs for meat.

- Eat as wide a variety of fruits and vegetables as you can find in your region. Each fruit and vegetable offers a slightly different spectrum of food values.

- Make sure every day your menu includes raw fruits and raw vegetables (for example, salads).

Vegans

The vegan diet is true vegetarian—only plant foods. People following a vegan regimen must pay careful attention to the foods they select and how the foods are prepared. Compared to meat-eating individuals,

Watch Out!
Vegetarians have many reasons for not eating meat—some nutritious, some political, some practical or moral. For Linda McCartney, the late wife of Paul McCartney, the moment of truth came when she saw lambs gamboling in a field. "Wait a minute," she said. "We love those sheep. They are such gentle creatures, so why are we eating them?"

CHAPTER 9 ▪ VEGETARIANISM: SHOULD YOU MOVE
TOWARDS A PLANT-BASED DIET?

253

vegans risk making serious nutrition mistakes. The most serious mistake is to eat most of one's calories from one group, for example, the grain group or fruit group. Nevertheless, vegans as a group enjoy the health benefits already mentioned, plus a vigorous, busy-bee energy level.

The vegan diet draws solely from the four basic plant groups:

- **Vegetables:** all classes. Mix root vegetables (like carrots, parsnips, and turnips) with above-ground vegetables (like broccoli, chard, and tomatoes). Shoot for at least five different vegetables (excluding salad greens) every day. Include a large salad of green leafy vegetables every day. Finally, potatoes, because of their high starch content, count in the grain group.

- **Fruits:** Take advantage of the large selection of local and imported fruits. Eat fruits raw. Vary the way you eat fruit by making smoothies or a mixed fruit medley.

- **Grains:** Breads, pasta, rice, polenta, bulgur, and other grains. Make sure grains and grain products are whole. Potatoes fit into this group. Forget french fries.

- **Legumes and nuts:** Beans, peas, lentils, peanuts, and other nuts.

People not familiar with a vegan diet might ask how one constructs a well-rounded diet out of these groups. Consider a vegan, Jennifer S. She stands 5'5" and weighs 125 pounds. Like Cynthia, she eats a varied diet, choosing a different selection of foods each day. The following table is a 1-day's menu which is typical of how she eats.

TABLE 9.2: VEGAN—TYPICAL 1-DAY'S DIET OF JENNIFER S.

Food	Calories	Protein, grams	Fat, grams	Carbo-hydrate, grams
Breakfast				
Buckwheat pancakes, pat of margarine (no hydrogenated fat), 1 T maple syrup. Fresh mango.	413	7.7	4.2	90
Lunch				
Pea soup, 1 cup. Green salad: lettuce, tomato, bell pepper, 1 T olive oil. Whole-wheat roll, pat of margarine.	466	17.3	19.3	61
Dinner				
Bean-rice casserole (1 cup of cooked dried pinto beans, ⁴/₅ cup of cooked brown rice, ¹/₄ cup of tomato juice). Steamed vegetables: 1 small beet, 1 medium carrot, both chopped, and 1 stalk of broccoli, and 1 section of a cauliflower, 1 T of margarine. Fresh fruit medley (equivalent to 2 pieces of fruit).	760	28.6	7.5	144
Snacks				
Crackers with 6 T of hummus.	220	5.7	10.2	28
Totals	1,859	59.3	41.2	323

The number of calories and number of grams of protein, fat, and carbohydrate are calculated from USDA databases. T = tablespoon.

Jennifer's menu uses items from all four, plant-based groups. Within each group, choice is endless. Her menu represents her particular choice for one day. Note the following points:

CHAPTER 9 ▪ VEGETARIANISM: SHOULD YOU MOVE
TOWARDS A PLANT-BASED DIET?

255

- **Protein.** Her intake of 59.3 grams is well above the RDA of 44 grams for women.

- **Fat.** Jennifer's fat intake at 41.2 grams works out to 19.5 percent of total calories. Practically none of that fat is saturated. It's all mono- and polyunsaturated fat with an excellent ratio of the two essential fats, omega-3 and omega-6.

- **Vitamin D.** Plants do not make this vitamin. Unless a person has sun exposure from time to time (it doesn't take much—casual exposure on face and hands suffices), a vegan should supplement.

- **Vitamin B$_{12}$.** This vitamin is absent from a vegan diet, and supplementation is the only way to get adequate amounts.

- **Calcium.** The recommended DV of 1,200 milligrams for calcium does not seem to apply to vegans. Remember, only a portion of the calcium one eats is absorbed. Calcium absorption may be better in vegans due to the high level of vitamin C in fruits and vegetables. Also, because vegans eat less protein than meat eaters, their urine is less acidic, which may help avoid calcium excretion. Whatever the exact reasons, vegans, as already noted, rarely suffer from osteoporosis, an indicator of calcium imbalance.

- **Iron.** One often hears that, although plant foods contain plenty of iron, it is poorly available to human consumers. The iron in meat is in the form of heme, which comes from hemoglobin, the blood protein that ferries oxygen. Heme iron, indeed, is better absorbed than

Moneysaver
Buy nuts in bulk. Store what you don't need in the freezer. You save enormously with bulk prices.

iron in plant foods. It's easy, however, to get carried away in arguments over how much is absorbed. The bottom line is function. Are vegans more likely to suffer from iron-deficient anemia than meat eaters? No. Studies show that the percentage of vegan women suffering iron-deficient anemia is no greater than women in the general population.

To sum up, a good vegan regimen does not present any nutritional problems. The diet provides a full spectrum of vitamins and minerals, with the exception of vitamins D and B_{12}. The diet provides plenty of protein and fuel for daily activities without risk of a fat-generating surplus. The key to a good vegan diet is variety. The general experience of vegans is that they thrive best when they don't over-emphasize any single plant group, maintaining a balance among all four groups.

Finally, nonvegetarians may think of vegan foods as dull and unappealing. On the contrary, they can be just as exciting as dishes containing meats. Several excellent cookbooks devoted to vegetarian cooking are listed in Appendix B.

Protein: Do vegetarians get enough?

For a person thinking of switching to a vegetarian diet, the first question is: Will I get enough protein? Protein is commonly associated with meat and dairy products. Plant foods are thought of as weak in protein. Moreover, plant proteins are said to be of low quality. You often see the term "incomplete" derisively applied to plant proteins. Weak? Incomplete? Let's bury these two myths.

Are plant proteins incomplete?

As mentioned in Chapter 1, "The Basics of Smart Nutrition," humans are unable to make 9 of the 20 amino acids considered essential, and therefore must get them in the proteins they eat. "Incomplete" suggests that a plant protein does not supply these 9 essential amino acids.

Nonsense. Plant proteins supply all 20 amino acids, including the 9 essential ones. The amounts of different essential amino acids vary in different plant sources. But for a vegetarian eating a variety of plant-based foods, the different plant proteins over the day complement each other. The result: The spectrum of essential amino acids evens out. A vegetarian gets all 20 amino acids in an optimum balance.

Does a vegetarian diet provide enough protein?

An individual entertaining the idea of becoming a vegetarian often worries about getting enough protein, but this is not an issue. Consider the protein in the daily diet of Jennifer S., the vegan. Her day's intake was 59.3 grams of mixed plant proteins. The Food and Nutrition Board of the National Academy of Sciences has set the RDA for an adult woman at 44 grams of protein a day. So Jennifer's 63 grams is well above this minimum—in fact, almost 50 percent more protein.

Suzanne Havala, a Registered Dietitian and a co-author of the American Dietetic Association position paper on vegetarianism, considers protein a non-issue. She notes that as long as you eat a variety of foods and enough calories to meet energy needs, you'd have to work hard not to get enough protein. (More details on the ADA's position on vegetarianism can be found at their Web site, www.eatright.com.

Sufficient protein thus is not an issue for vegetarians. Just remember these two rules:

- Choose foods every day from each of the four basic plant food groups.

- From within each group, choose a variety of foods.

Unofficially...
Benjamin Spock, the guru on raising children, at age 91, became a vegetarian. In his latest (7th) edition of *Baby and Child Care,* Spock urged a vegan diet for children after age 2.

Plant foods with protein—not just soy products

Vegetarians have to adopt an open mind towards protein. Don't think of your protein as coming from one or two main sources. All plant foods provide protein—some more, some less, but every food contributes. And as we see in both Cynthia's and Jennifer's diets, the protein adds up at the end of the day.

Meat eaters, in contrast, think of the entire day's protein coming from meat or dairy foods. So be it, but meat eaters, when they switch to vegetarian eating, often bring along that single-source focus. It's a serious blunder. The result of single-source thinking is that individuals ask how they can replace meat. Such individuals mistakenly turn to a single plant source they believe to be the best substitute for meat—soybean products.

True, soybeans have a high protein content, more than other beans (but not much more). A downside for home cooks is that, compared to other beans, soybeans are bothersome to prepare and cook. Consequently, people buy commercial soy products: tofu, tempeh, isolated soy protein, and TVP (textured vegetable protein). Incidentally, you also see TVP defined on product labels as textured soy flour. Chapter 3, "Grains, Legumes, and Nuts," touched on issues of eating soy products. We recapitulate two:

- Soy products undergo commercial processing that lowers their nutritional value. You don't get full nutritional value compared to cooking up a dish of dried navy, lima, or other beans. When you eat a soy product, you eat a partial plant food.

- Soy products contain isoflavones, which mimic the female sex hormone, estrogen. These substances can have physiological effects on individuals who consume large amounts of soy products. Whether or not the effects in the long run are good or bad is unclear. More research must be done to answer the question.

Nevertheless, you don't need to avoid soy products altogether. Just don't eat a big slab of tofu or a TVP burger every night as a substitute for steak. Put soy products into an overall vegetarian context, one of dozens of foods from which to choose your menu.

What about pregnancy and breast-feeding?

Can a vegetarian diet provide the high level of nourishment demanded by mother and fetus? The answer is clearly yes. The American Dietetic Association, in its position paper on vegetarianism, says that both lacto-ovo vegetarian and vegan diets meet the nutrient and energy needs of pregnant women. One proof is birth weight. Infants born to vegetarian mothers are in the same range as babies born to nonvegetarian mothers. There are, however, things a vegetarian woman should keep in mind.

Watch Out!
The mold *Aspergillus flavus*, which produces the poison aflatoxin, loves peanuts. Stores that have do-it-yourself peanut grinders are at risk from *Aspergillus* growing on peanut residues. Such machines should be cleaned every day. Check with store management to see if this is the case.

- **Whole foods.** It's imperative to choose fresh, whole foods and follow the basic rules of vegetarian eating, including a selection of foods from all four food groups. Lacto-ovo vegetarians should favor low-fat or nonfat dairy products and not go overboard on cheese—too much saturated fat.

- **Protein.** The protein RDA for a pregnant woman is 60 grams a day, a 16-gram increase over the needs of a nonpregnant woman (44 grams). Keep in mind that the appetite goes up and protein intake goes up correspondingly. Take Jennifer's vegan diet as an example. She eats 1,860 calories, which is her normal level of food intake. If pregnant and in her second and third trimester, she would be eating 350 more calories a day, or 2,210 calories.

  Assume her general diet stays the same and she just eats more. Her protein intake goes up—from 60 to 71 grams, well over the RDA value. The same reasoning applies when a mother breast-feeds her infant. The protein RDA during lactation is 65 grams. But because a mother eats more (600 to 800 extra calories a day), she takes in plenty of protein.

- **Vitamin B_{12}.** The American Dietetic Association recommends that vegans take a B_{12} supplement of 2.0 micrograms a day. And when a mother breast-feeds, she should increase the supplement to 2.6 micrograms a day.

- **Vitamin D.** A supplement may be in order unless there is adequate exposure to the sun. Lacto-ovo vegetarians who drink milk will get vitamin D from that source.

CHAPTER 9 ■ VEGETARIANISM: SHOULD YOU MOVE
TOWARDS A PLANT-BASED DIET?

261

When breast-feeding, keep in mind that a lot of the nutrients a baby needs come from the mother's diet. Yet the vegetarian mother eating a well-balanced, high-level diet (making sure about vitamins D and B_{12}) need not worry. Everything a baby needs will be in the milk.

Babies of vegan mothers, incidentally, get an added bonus. Their milk is less contaminated. Most of the pesticide residues and industrial waste chemicals that people ingest in their food are located in meats and animal products. These chemicals lodge in body fat. When a woman lactates, the accumulated chemicals flow from the fat into the milk. Vegan mothers with their cleaner bodies deliver cleaner milk.

Macrobiotics, a way of life

The macrobiotic diet falls into the general category of vegetarian diets, but it is about more than food. Macrobiotics is a way of life in which followers take responsibility for their health and actions so that the overall effect on the world is positive. Macrobiotic followers choose natural, organically grown, whole foods, natural cleaning and body-care products, and clothing made out of natural materials.

While basically a vegan diet, macrobiotics is more restrictive than this book recommends for a balanced vegan diet. It places great emphasis on grains, between 50 and 60 percent of the diet. The proportions of the standard macrobiotic diet are shown in the table on page 262.

The macrobiotic system has its advantages:

■ It emphasizes organically grown foods, which minimizes stress on the environment.

Bright Idea
If you are a meat eater thinking of turning vegetarian, do it thoughtfully. If you decided to take up rock climbing, would you immediately hurl yourself off a cliff? Not likely. You would read up on the subject, consult experienced climbers, and start gradually. Do the same when you make the switch to vegetarianism.

TABLE 9.3: THE STANDARD MACROBIOTIC DIET

Food	Percent (calories)
Whole grains, such as brown rice, barley, millet, oats, corn, rye, wheat, and buckwheat. A small percentage may be noodles and unyeasted breads.	50
Vegetables, preferably fresh, locally grown, lightly steamed, boiled, or sautéed. About one-third may be eaten as fresh salad or pickles. Vegetables to be avoided are potatoes, tomatoes, eggplant, peppers, spinach, beets, and zucchini.	20–30
Cooked beans and tofu. Sea vegetables, such as nori, wakame, dulse, kombu.	5–10
Soups. 1–2 bowls every day made with miso, tamari, soy sauce (fermented soy products), plus sea and land vegetables.	5
Occasional use: Fish and seafood, raw or cooked fruit 2–3 times a week, nuts, seeds, and other natural snacks.	

(For more details go to the Kushi Institute Web site, www.macrobiotics.org)

- It emphasizes locally grown produce, which cuts down the costs, both financial and ecological, of long-distance transport.

- People on a macrobiotic diet are rarely overweight.

The standard macrobiotic diet, on the other hand, has weaknesses you should be aware of:

- Grains are overweighted at the expense of vegetables. When you eat grains, you eat seeds, which are mostly starch. Vegetables, in contrast, provide a rich spectrum of substances coming from all parts of the plants: roots (carrots, parsnips), stems (asparagus, broccoli), leaves (lettuce, spinach), and fruits (peppers, tomatoes).

- Except for the small salad, the macrobiotic diet is all cooked. Cooking, even under the best of conditions, destroys some nutritional value of the foods.

- While the standard macrobiotic diet may work for adults, it is less advantageous for infants and growing children. They may suffer from a deficiency of certain vitamins and minerals, insufficient protein, and a dearth of calories. Growth consequently suffers.

- There is risk of an overload of sodium because of the large amount of fermented soy products.

- Where's the fruit? You don't see any emphasis on fruit in the standard diet. Fruits are omitted from the standard macrobiotic diet but allowed as occasional foods a couple of times a week, preferably cooked or dried.

In spite of these negatives, in fairness we ought to ask: How does the standard macrobiotic diet compare with the standard American diet of fast foods, chicken-fried steak, potato chips, and pie à la mode? The answer is that the person following the macrobiotic diet will probably be healthier in the long run.

In saying that, it is like watching a second-class race horse race against a nag. The second-class horse obviously wins. Well, how about a first-class race horse? Is the standard macrobiotic diet on a par with the balanced four-group diet of the vegan, which includes fruits as a major component and emphasizes a higher percentage of raw foods? The answer is no.

The Mediterranean diet

The Mediterranean diet is eaten by peoples of the olive-growing areas of the Mediterranean region. The diet first came to the attention of Americans from studies conducted by Ancel Keys at the

Watch Out!
The five most common vegetables on American plates are french fries, baked potatoes, tomato ketchup and sauces, iceberg lettuce, and onion rings. Not exactly vegan heaven. Except for the baked potato, dump the rest in the trash can.

University of Minnesota in the late 1950s and 1960s. The peoples of that region, he discovered, had overcome the privations of the Second World War but had not yet accepted the American fast-food culture.

The diet varies among the countries of that region. The Italians eat more pasta, the Spanish more fish. The Greeks eat more fat, about 40 percent of total calories. The Greek version is also the best studied. It has the following features:

- About 40 percent of calories from fat (but because much of the fat consumed is olive oil, there is a high ratio of monounsaturated fat to saturated fat).

- Moderate alcohol consumption—mostly red wine.

- High consumption of legumes.

- High consumption of grains, including large quantities of whole-grain bread.

- High consumption of fruits and vegetables. Adult Greeks consume about a pound of vegetables a day.

- Rare consumption of meats. When eaten, meat is used more as a condiment.

- Moderate consumption of milk and dairy products.

- Big Greek salads with lots of feta cheese.

- Finally, daily exercise is a must to gain the full benefits of the Mediterranean diet.

The high consumption of fresh fruits and vegetables and cereals, plus liberal use of olive oil, guarantees a high intake of vitamin C, beta-carotene, and other phytochemicals. The diet is rich in the other vitamins and essential minerals.

It is difficult to find any fault with the traditional Greek diet. The bottom line, of course, is health. It was the robust health of the Greeks that first attracted the attention of Keys. The researchers found the Greeks had a low rate of heart disease and an extraordinarily long life. In 1965, the remaining life expectancy of a 45-year-old American male was 27 years. That of a 45-year-old Greek male was 32 years. Also keep in mind that the Greeks had limited medical care compared to that available in the United States. The Greeks were not getting sick.

While we can learn much about the benefits of the traditional Mediterranean diet, it is rapidly fading into history. Why? Affluence, a changing culture, and a desire for convenience. The traditional Greek diet was shaped by poverty, climate, and hardship rather than by any nutritional insight. The health benefits were a by-product. As affluence spreads to Greek villages, the diet is being replaced by the fast-food culture of America.

Fortunately, the benefits of the traditional Mediterranean diet can be recaptured in the lacto-ovo and vegan vegetarian diets described in this chapter.

FAQs: Frequently asked questions

A vegetarian in a nation of barbecues and beef eaters is like a left-handed person going into a sport shop that sells right-handed golf clubs. All the nutrition advice and meal planning you see on TV and in magazines is directed at the majority of the population—meat eaters. As a result, there is a lot of uncertainty about key vegetarian issues. Here are 12 frequently asked questions (FAQs) about vegetarian diets and health.

Unofficially...
The late health-food writer Adele Davis did much to perpetuate the myth that you can only survive by eating a high-protein diet. In her book, *Let's Eat Right to Keep Fit*, she wrote that ignorance of protein was the greatest hindrance to health. She recommended eating 150 grams of protein a day.

1. **Question:** I am currently eating a meat diet but would like to change to a vegetarian diet. However, I find the thought of making the switch daunting. What do you recommend?

    Answer: Here are tips for easing the transition to a meatless diet.

▪ Do it gradually over a period of weeks. Cut out meat 1 day a week, then 2 days and so on. As you do, substitute meatless dishes. Some people make the transition by cutting out meat in a progression—first beef and pork, then chicken and turkey, and finally fish.

▪ Don't make the mistake of substituting eggs and cheese as you cut down on meat. Replace meat with plant foods.

▪ Inexperienced in making meatless dishes? Frequent vegetarian restaurants and pick out dishes you like. Ask the chef for recipes. Buy vegetarian cookbooks. Several excellent ones are listed in Appendix B, the resource section.

▪ Put a big bowl of fresh fruit on the kitchen counter where the family can see it.

▪ Turning vegetarian ought to be a shared experience, with the whole family involved. Don't insist the children turn vegetarian while the parents eat steak.

▪ Make the transition first to a lacto-ovo vegetarianism. Then, when comfortable with this style, consider making the transition to vegan. Many vegetarians, unless they are strict vegans for religious or other reasons, oscillate between vegan and lacto-ovo vegetarianism.

▪ Consult a nutrition professional for help in adjusting to a vegetarian diet.

2. **Question:** Is a vegan diet suitable for preteen and teen children?

   Answer: A high-quality vegan diet as described earlier in the chapter provides children with the nutrition they need to grow and develop healthy bodies. Keep in mind that, because of their active life, children need more calories. You can solve this problem by increasing the proportion of energy-dense foods, like avocado, nuts, nut butters, and dried fruit.

3. **Question:** I have a teenage son active in sports. Does a vegan diet supply enough protein for his needs?

   Answer: Teenage boys should have 0.4 grams of protein per pound of body weight. So a 16-year-old boy weighing 150 pounds needs 60 grams a day. But teens tend to eat more. Boys at a high level of physical activity may consume as much as 3,000 calories a day. Supposing a boy ate the typical vegan diet shown in the table earlier in this chapter. At the 3,000-calories level, he would take in 100 grams of protein.

4. **Question:** My teenage children like to snack on the run. What are good vegan snacks?

   Answer: Fruits, like bananas, apples, and oranges, are easy to stuff in a pocket. Dried fruits and nuts, like trail mixes, are energy-dense, nutrient-dense snacks. Bean burritos, tacos, and a hummus, whole-wheat sandwich are also energy-rich.

5. **Question:** Should soy milk be used to feed infants?

   Answer: No. Soy milk is made by pureeing soybeans with water, straining off the liquid, and

Watch Out!
Don't eat the peels of citrus fruits or put them in drinks unless you buy pesticide-free fruit. Citrus fruits are sprayed with very high amounts of pesticides that are difficult to wash off.

cooking it. The liquid is filtered and may be sweetened with corn syrup or other sweeteners. While suitable for older children and adults as a drink, soy milk lacks the vitamins and minerals and the protein balance needed to support growth and development of an infant.

6. **Question:** What about fish? Should a vegetarian eat fish?

   Answer: Fish represent another variation on vegetarianism. Some vegetarians, while excluding meat and dairy products, eat fish. This is a personal decision. While fish are inherently a splendid food, practical issues exist: water pollution and the problem of moving a highly perishable product from sea to consumer (see Chapter 5, "Meats, Fish, Poultry, and Eggs"). In any event, fish should represent only a small portion of the diet.

   Fish are recommended by many nutritionists because of the essential fatty acids they contain. But a diet high in vegetables delivers plenty of those essential fatty acids.

7. **Question:** Do foods that complement each other with respect to protein, like rice and beans, have to be eaten together?

   Answer: No. You benefit from the protein complementary effect of different plant foods if you eat one food, for example, at noon and the other at the evening meal.

8. **Question:** What is seitan and how can it be used?

   Answer: Also known as wheat meat, *seitan* is the protein, gluten. Whole-wheat flour is mixed with water and made into a dough, which is

CHAPTER 9 ■ VEGETARIANISM: SHOULD YOU MOVE
TOWARDS A PLANT-BASED DIET?

269

boiled in water to remove the starch. This glutinous dough is called kofu. Kofu can be processed in many ways, one of which is seitan. Kofu is made into seitan by simmering in a stock of tamari, soy sauce, and kombu sea vegetable. You find it packaged in the refrigerated sections of natural food stores. Use it in stir frys and stews. The protein content is comparable to steak—18 percent.

9. **Question:** Are TVP burgers good nutritional value?

Answer: TVP (textured vegetable protein) is a soybean product. As described in Chapter 3, TVP ranks at a nutritional quality level of 4 (bottom). TVP is a highly processed food, high in chemical additives, salt, and often fat. TVP is low in the spectrum of nutrients found in whole beans or meat. It has limited nutritional merit. If you fancy veggie burgers, look for ones that don't contain TVP.

10. **Question:** Is vitamin B_{12} an issue for lacto-ovo vegetarians?

Answer: Not generally. Authorities recommend 2 to 3 micrograms a day. A half glass of skim milk or half cup of cottage cheese gives about 1 microgram. An egg provides 0.7 micrograms.

11. **Question:** Should vegetarians take vitamin and mineral supplements?

Answer: Individuals eating a high level lacto-ovo or vegan diet will obtain a superior spectrum of vitamins and minerals compared to individuals eating the standard American meat diet. Nevertheless, as pointed out in Chapter 8, "To Supplement or Not to Supplement Is No

Longer the Question," there is merit in taking extra vitamins and minerals. Follow the advice in that chapter (100 percent DV supplementation of most vitamins and minerals, extra quantities of vitamins C and E).

12. **Question:** Is a vegetarian diet low in saturated fat and cholesterol?

    Answer: Plant foods don't contain cholesterol. The lacto-ovo vegetarian will get some cholesterol in dairy products and eggs, but since these represent a small part of the diet, the amount of cholesterol is insignificant. The vegan eats no cholesterol. The fats of plant foods are mainly mono- and polyunsaturated. The vegetarian diet consequently is naturally low in saturated fat.

Vegetarianism: A wrap-up

The mere fact of being vegetarian does not automatically serve up health on a platter. Following a vegetarian style of eating is like following any other type of diet. You can do it badly or you can do it well. Remember, don't let the following blunders cancel your health rewards:

- Eating quantities of processed foods, believing just because they don't contain meat, they are okay. Choose upper-level foods, ranking at levels 1 and 2 in the guides presented in chapters 2 and 3.

- Thinking you have to include a nonmeat substitute for meat in your meals. The meat substitutes on the market shaped to look like hot dogs, fish sticks, or meat patties are manufactured foods of limited nutritional value.

- Putting undue emphasis on one group of plant foods, like grains or fruit. The key to high quality vegetarian diet is balance among all four plant food groups.

- Eating too much cooked food. Eat raw fruits and vegetables (salads) every day.

- Failing to supplement with vitamin B_{12} (vegans).

- Compensating for lack of meat by increasing the amount of dairy products and eggs (lacto-ovo vegetarians). You replace one fiberless food with another. The trick is to keep dairy and eggs in balance. Replace meat with plant foods.

A final word: Being a good vegetarian requires thought, attention to details, and patience in getting through the supermarket checkout as the clerk struggles to ring up the items of fresh produce.

Just the facts

- Lacto-ovo vegetarians eat eggs and dairy products. However, the main emphasis is on plant foods.

- Vegans eat only plant foods. They should eat a balance of foods from the four plant groups: vegetables, fruits, grains, and legumes/nuts.

- Vegetarians as a group are healthier than non-vegetarians. Their rates of heart disease, adult-onset diabetes, and cancer are lower; they live longer. To reap the full health benefits of vegetarianism, however, it is necessary to eat upper-level foods: whole grains, fresh vegetables, and raw fruits.

- A balanced vegetarian diet supplies the full spectrum of vitamins (vegans must supplement vitamin B_{12}) and minerals, plus more than adequate amounts of protein.

- Vegetarian diets are suitable for all stages of life, from pregnancy to golden years.

- Macrobiotics is a form of vegetarianism that emphasizes a concern for ecology by eating whole foods, locally grown. The diet is heavily weighted towards the grain group and cooked foods.

GET THE SCOOP ON...
Fast-food restaurants ▪ Secrets of restaurant
kitchens ▪ How to rate a restaurant ▪ Home
meal replacements

Dining Out: Smart Eating in Restaurants

Chapter 10

If you are an average citizen, you eat four meals a week in a some kind of restaurant. It could be a fast-food restaurant, workplace cafeteria, family-style chain, or an owner-operated restaurant. Whatever the style, you eat food prepared by someone else, whether a minimum-wage cook at the grill or a chef trained at a culinary school. In addition, for every meal you eat in a restaurant, you buy a takeout or a packaged meal from the frozen food case of a supermarket and bring it home to eat. The industry calls the trend of bringing meals home *home meal replacement*. In short, for all these meals, your nutritional well-being passes to the hands of others.

How do you judge the nutritional quality of a restaurant meal or a complete meal that comes in a frozen package? This is a pressing issue, because the amount of food people buy from restaurants is rising. At one time dining out was reserved for special days. Nutritional quality was of less interest than the enjoyment of the experience. But now restaurants,

273

> **"**
>
> Persons of under-standing like food which increases vital force, energy, strength, and health. Persons of ignorance and inertia order foods which are stale, tasteless, rotten, and impure.
> —From the *Bhagavad Gita*
>
> **"**

caterers, and home meal replacements have become a major source of our nourishment. In fact, sales of restaurant food, whether eaten in or taken out, surpass total supermarket sales!

In the 1980s the government recognized the importance of providing information about a food's nutritional quality. This led to the food labeling law of the 1990s. Nutrition information on the labels of packaged foods, while incomplete, is nevertheless helpful. But when it passed the labeling law, Congress left a big void, exempting labeling of foods sold in restaurants and takeouts.

You have no guidance about the basic nutrition facts of meals ordered in restaurants. Moreover, you probably won't get very far asking a restaurant manager to provide you with such information. The law states that a restaurant is under no obligation to give you any nutrition information about the meals it serves. The meal can be loaded with hidden fats, contain ingredients to which you might be allergic, or weighted down with a baggage of chemical additives. You will not easily find out.

As you've seen, Part II of this book provides a basis for ranking the nutritional value of foods—the four quality levels. The system rates level 1 at the top and level 4 at the bottom. The system is not based on nutritional absolutes but rather on a relative scale. A food ranked at quality level 3 offers better nutritional quality than one ranked at level 4. A food ranked at level 2 is better than a food ranked at level 3, and so on.

This system works well for foods you buy in a supermarket or other food market. You see what you are buying. You know whether the carrots are fresh or in a frozen package. Fresh carrots rank at quality level 1. Frozen carrots rank at quality level 3. But when you order a meal in a restaurant, the carrots in the entree arrived already cooked, and so you can't be sure how they started out: fresh, frozen, or even canned (quality level 4).

Moreover, in a restaurant, we need to judge the nutritional merits of the entire meal. Clearly, the concept of quality levels takes us only so far. To judge the nutritional quality of a prepared meal set before us, we need additional clues.

Just a reminder. This is a book on nutrition. Don't expect a professional restaurant critic's guide to restaurants. Restaurant critics look for taste and sensory enjoyment. Still, some of the things they look for serve as useful clues. They look, for instance, for the freshness of ingredients. Is the food a trifle mushy, the lettuce wilted, or the meat tasteless? Critics also look for quality of service. Does the food sit under a heat lamp or warming table for a long period, slowly deteriorating in both quality of taste and quality of nutrition? These are all clues to the nutritional quality of the meals you are served.

For starters, the first clue to nutritional quality you can use is the class of restaurant. But this clue alone is insufficient, because within each class of restaurant, nutritional quality varies with menu items. You can find menu items ranked at level 4 in upscale restaurants, whereas items ranked higher, at levels 1 and 2, can sometimes be found in fast-food restaurants. Nevertheless, noting the class of restaurant is a start.

Keeping this variation in nutritional quality in mind, this chapter looks at three main classes of restaurants:

Watch Out!
Portion sizes in American restaurants are huge compared to portions in English restaurants. A pasta dish in an English restaurant weighs 8 ounces. The same dish in a New York restaurant weighs 1 pound.

- Fast-food restaurants.

- Chain restaurants with table service.

- Independent, owner-operated restaurants with table service. Such restaurants vary in price and style of food, from mid-range to upscale restaurants.

The chapter takes a behind-the-scenes look at the way each class of restaurants operates and how that affects the nutritional quality of the meals they serve.

Eight tips for judging restaurant nutrition quality

Before discussing specific classes of restaurants, let's consider some general clues when you go into a restaurant. What things tip you off immediately about the quality of the food you are about to get there? Here are eight tips:

1. The lettuce in the salad bar. Only iceberg? The nutrition you get from iceberg is not much different than from green leafy lettuce. The difference is quantity. Iceberg is mostly water. You get about half the nutrition from a leaf of iceberg as a leaf of romaine. But iceberg also signals a lack of imagination and interest on the part of management in providing a varied, fresh salad bar.

2. At the salad bar, check the number of items that are genuinely fresh, such as sprouts, pepper slices, fresh tomatoes, and so on. Are most items out of cans, like bean salad, pasta salad, baked beans, and pickled tomatoes? A salad bar loaded with fresh items indicates that restaurant management takes an interest in nutritional quality. Look for an added plus: Does the restaurant offer local fresh produce in season?

3. If salad is served at the table, does it arrive drenched in dressing? This may mean the salad is prepared long in advance, possibly at a central factory. Order dressing on the side. (Of course, some types of salads are typically served already mixed.)

4. Look at the menu's selections for kids. Do the selections consist of fried food and french fries, with no items of better nutritional quality? It is unlikely the restaurant's main selections will offer you any better quality.

5. Does the restaurant offer a choice of rolls or bread, including whole-grain breads? Or do they restrict your choice to a white, exceedingly soft roll or mini-loaf? In this case, the restaurant is almost certainly giving you a chemical-laden, frozen-dough bread, fourth rank nutritional quality.

6. Does the restaurant microwave hot items? This fact is generally hard to tell unless you can see the kitchen. Sometimes, a cooperative serving person will tell you. In any event, microwaving indicates you are getting warmed-over food, prepared goodness knows where or when—ranked at quality level 4.

7. Details. A good restaurant pays attention to details. Likely, you won't see butter pats in wrappers or crackers in cellophane.

8. Finally, you need to exercise common sense. While each tip by itself is indicative of the quality of the food a restaurant is prepared to serve, you have to consider all factors. Many times, you are unable to make a final judgment until you have eaten in the restaurant at least once.

Moneysaver
Order less food in a restaurant. Women who eat frequently in restaurants generally eat more—on average 300 calories more a day—than women who eat at home, most of it extra fat.

This fact brings us to the nutritional quality of the foods you find in different classes of restaurants.

Fast-food restaurants

The fast-food industry started in 1954 when Ray Kroc, an aggressive salesman of milkshake machines, met the McDonald brothers at their hamburger stand in San Bernardino, CA. The McDonald brothers, stolid New Englanders from Bedford, NH, had come to California to make their fortune in the movies, but instead opened a highly successful hamburger stand. When Kroc met them, the stand was grossing an estimated $250,000 a year, at a time when $5,000 a year was considered a respectable annual salary.

The McDonald brothers had worked out all the details of what has become the bedrock of the fast-food system. There was nothing to steal—everything was served in or on disposable containers. Food was simple and appealing to all tastes—a hamburger patty, a bun, fries, and a shake. Service was quick. The McDonald brothers had solved the problem of pesky teenagers who normally hung around hamburger outlets. Fast service, uncomfortable chairs bolted to the floor, and an unappealing decor gave them no reason to stay.

Kroc was impressed and decided this concept would work anywhere. In due course, Kroc bought out the McDonald brothers, their concept of fast food, their name and, most important, the golden arches the brothers used to distinguish their San Bernardino hamburger stand. The McDonald's empire was launched.

It didn't take long for other companies to copy the McDonald brothers' fast-food idea. In the last

50 years, major chains like Arby's, Burger King, Wendy's, Hardee's, International House of Pancakes, and Jack-in-the-Box have grown along with McDonald's. McDonald's races ahead in sales, however, dominating the fast-food restaurant market with 30 percent of total sales. The next largest chain, Burger King, has only about 10 percent of the market. The rest trail in the distance.

The country is blanketed with fast-food outlets in every community and, in cities, every few blocks. Market saturation makes it difficult for the chains to grow. The fast-food chains can only steal market share away from each other. Interestingly, as competition for the burger market has tightened, the foods the chains offer have grown similar. Menus, looks, styles of presentation, and tastes of the foods each chain offers are almost identical.

Fast-food chains cater to impulse eating. When people feel hungry, they want food now. With the availability of fast food, they get it—sometimes as quickly as a minute or so after ordering. The food is consistent, with no surprises. Customers know exactly what they will get when they order.

Economics drives the fast-food business. Nutrition, if it plays a role at all, is incidental. The big question: Can you eat both fast and healthy? The answer to that question has to be "only with difficulty." Fast foods thrive on three ingredients: fat, salt, and sugar. It's what customers want. Take, for example, a typical fast-food meal of hamburger, fries, and chocolate shake. Here is an analysis of such a meal served at McDonald's.

> **"**
> Why do people eat at fast-food restaurants? It's pretty good food and you fill up. It's like going to a filling station.
> —Marvin Greenberg, Toronto-based restaurant consultant
> **"**

TABLE 10.1: A MEAL AT MCDONALD'S

Menu Item	Calories	Fat, grams	Protein, grams	Carbohydrate, grams
Big Mac	560	32.4	25.2	43
French fries, large	400	21.6	5.6	46
Shake, chocolate	320	1.7	11.6	66
Totals	1,280	55.5	42.4	155

(Source: McDonald's and USDA databases)

This meal provides 1,280 calories, two-thirds of the daily calories an average woman needs with the calorie proportions skewed towards fat. The calorie breakdown is:

- Proportion of calories from fat, 39 percent
- Proportion of calories from protein, 13 percent
- Proportion of calories from carbohydrate, 48 percent (half from added sugar)

This meal provides a good proportion of protein. Generally with fast food, insufficient protein is a nonissue. The main nutritional problem with this meal lies in the fact that 63 percent of its calories come from two impoverished sources, fat and sugar. The consumer gets calories, but few if any nutrients the body needs to digest and metabolize the food. In addition, the fat, mainly from the french fries, consists partly of the unnatural trans fats.

From a cell's-eye perspective, a meal of this type puts an enormous strain on the body's resources. First, the meal is difficult to metabolize. Second, the spectrum of essential building blocks the body needs for tissue renewal is incomplete. It's equivalent to repairing a leaking roof on your house when there aren't enough new shingles to complete the job. The roof functions, but the leaks don't stop.

The counterargument to this concern about impoverished calories is that the individual will

Unofficially...
A core of super-heavy users constitutes 75 percent of McDonald's business. According to the company, they are young males, age mid-teens to early 30s, who eat at a McDonalds at least four times a week.

balance her or his nutrition through the rest of the day's food. It's an argument that says, in essence, that the fast-food restaurant doesn't have to supply top-level nutrition because the customer will get needed nutrition elsewhere. The argument doesn't wash, however—much of the food the average American eats the rest of the day is not much different from the fast-food meal.

In fairness to McDonald's, they did listen to criticism about too much fat, and in the early 1990s introduced a low-fat burger, the McLean. McDonald's promoted this trimmed-down burger with great fanfare for those customers who wanted their food healthy and fast. A McLean Deluxe contained 310 calories, 29 percent derived from fat. This compares with the regular Quarter Pounder, weighing in at 410 calories, 44 percent from fat. The McLean survived until 1996, when McDonald's canceled it—not enough customers.

> People who choose to eat our pizza have decided to make an indulgent choice. They can balance out their calories or nutritional needs across the week.
> —Bill Cobb, executive, Pizza Hut (*USA Today*, Feb. 21, 1996)

Chicken healthier than beef?

Chicken has long been advertised as the white meat, healthier than red meat (beef). But in the hands of fast-food chains, a chicken meal doesn't look much different from a beef meal. The following table gives a breakdown of the nutritional components of a meal from Kentucky Fried Chicken.

TABLE 10.2: A MEAL AT KENTUCKY FRIED CHICKEN

Menu Item	Calories	Fat, grams	Protein, grams	Carbohydrate, grams
Chicken, Original Recipe	400	24	29	16
Corn bread	228	13	3	25
Potato salad	230	14	4	23
Coca-Cola, 12 ounces	146	–	–	41
Totals	1,004	51	36	105

(*Source: Kentucky Fried Chicken and USDA databases*)

The proportion of fat calories from this meal approaches the 50 percent mark. Here is a calorie breakdown:

- Proportion of calories from fat, 46 percent
- Proportion of calories from protein, 13 percent
- Proportion of calories from carbohydrate, 41 percent (almost 60 percent of that from added sugar)

Like the McDonald's hamburger meal, the proportion of calories from protein is good. But the proportion of calories from fat and sugar is no better than that of the hamburger meal. The calorie breakdown for the chicken meal is similar.

One of the nutritional issues about fast-food meals is the large amount of salt they contain. The Kentucky Fried Chicken meal, for instance, contains 1,850 milligrams of sodium. This amount is almost 80 percent of the 2,400 milligrams health authorities consider maximum. The 1,850 milligrams of sodium translates into one level teaspoon of table salt.

You should consider three aspects about the huge amounts of salt in fast food:

1. You don't need added salt whatsoever in the diet. Your body requires very little salt, obtaining sufficient amounts from the natural amount in foods.

2. The reason health authorities warn against eating too much salt is that it contributes to high blood pressure (hypertension).

3. Salt enters fast food in large amounts because it masks unusual tastes and the fact that basic ingredients are often bland and tasteless.

Fast food, regardless of the chain, embraces a certain sameness, although a fast-food devotee might believe there is variety in eating a burger meal one day and a chicken meal the next. From a cell's-eye view, this is not variety. It's the same impoverished set of calories arriving in the body, stressing the body's reserves. Stress chills immune defenses and, in the long run, contributes to premature health breakdown.

Upgrade your nutrition in a fast-food restaurant

Is it possible to do better for your body's cells? The answer is yes. In most fast-food restaurants, you can put together a selection of menu items that upgrade your nutrition. Here is an example of a selection at Wendy's.

TABLE 10.3: A MEAL AT WENDY'S

Menu Item	Calories	Fat, grams	Protein, grams	Carbohydrate, grams
Plain potato with pat of butter	346	4	7	7
Deluxe garden salad	110	60	7	10
Hidden Valley Ranch dressing, 2 T	90	10		1
Milk, 1%, 8 ounces	102	2.6	8	12
Totals	648	22.6	22	94

This meal has fewer calories than the burger and chicken meals, and the proportion of calories is better.

- Proportion of calories from fat, 31 percent

- Proportion of calories from protein, 13 percent

- Proportion of calories from carbohydrate, 56 percent

Unofficially...
Half the food sold in fast-food restaurants is sold at the drive-up window. The chains design their meals so they can be eaten in a car. The french fries are coated with starch to hold in the heat and retain crispiness longer. Entrees are less greasy, because customers dislike driving with greasy hands on the steering wheel.

Bright Idea
Be a fat detective. Avoid the hidden fat in foods like stuffed potato skins, Mexican chimichangas, cheese sauce, sausages, bacon, salad dressing, most sauces, buffalo wings, and any fried food. Go for roast chicken over the fried. Discard the skin.

This meal features more carbohydrate calories and fewer fat calories. We should not judge meals solely on the merits of low fat versus high fat. In general, however, as fat calories go down, nutrition goes up. This is because the lower fat meal contains less processed food.

The Wendy's meal differs from the burger and chicken meals, for example, in two ways. First, the meal contains raw food—in the salad. Second, most of the meal consists of foods minimally processed. The potato has been merely baked, with no additives or excessive handling. The milk is milk, not sugar water.

Are wraps more nutritious?

Attempting to upgrade nutritional quality and yet still provide fast, cheap food, fast-food chains have come up with wraps. These are pita pockets stuffed with chicken, cheese, and vegetables.

However, there are good wraps and there are bad wraps (nutritionally, anyway). The following table shows the calorie breakdown of three different wraps.

TABLE 10.4: WRAPS—SANDWICH FILLINGS IN A PITA POCKET

Menu Item	Calories	% Fat calories	% Protein, calories	% Carbohydrate, calories	Sodium, milligrams
Jack-in-the-Box, chicken fajita pita	290	25	34	41	700
Wendy's chicken Caesar pita	490	31	30	39	1,300
Taco Bell, chicken fajita wrap	461	41	16	43	1,214

(Source: The fast-food chains and USDA database)

Of the three wraps, the Jack-in-the-Box wrap wins the fat race, mainly because it comes without dressing. You add as little as you like. The rich dressing in both the Wendy's and Taco Bell wraps drives up fat calories. Note the high amount of sodium (salt) in each of the three. The fast-food chains can't break their love affair with salt.

Better choices at fast-food restaurants

In comparison to food you prepare at home from fresh ingredients, fast foods rank low. The big sellers—burgers, chicken sandwiches, pizza, fries, shakes, and soft drinks—rank on a nutritional quality scale of level 4, the bottom level. The trick in a fast-food chain is to find items that are nutritionally better than the bottom-ranked items. The Jack-in-the-Box wrap, for example, ranks at level 3. The salad and baked potato combination raises the meal to a level 2.

Here are seven tips for surviving a trip to a fast-food restaurant:

1. Ask the server to delete sauces, like the mayo on the burger and the tarter sauce with the fish. Ask for salad dressing on the side. The sauces are loaded with fat and salt but have no nutritional value.

2. Order healthier pizza toppings and garnishes like sweet pepper, mushrooms, spinach, and onion.

3. Avoid the processed meats on pizza toppings or in sandwiches, like pepperoni, sausage, ham, bacon, and hot dogs.

4. Avoid anything deep-fried. That includes french fries.

5. Go easy on pickles, mustard, and ketchup, all high in salt.

6. Avoid American or processed cheese. Ask for cheddar, provolone, Swiss, or other hard cheese.

7. At the salad bar, look for genuinely fresh items, such as a variety of lettuce, pepper slices, sprouts, fresh mushrooms, grated carrots, tomatoes, scallions, raw nuts or seeds, and fresh fruit.

If you follow these tips, you'll upgrade your nutrition, not to a top level, but at least to a nutritional level better than the burger-and-fries combo.

The full-service, casual dining chains

A cut above the fast-food chains are restaurant chains that provide table service or buffet grills. They offer casual, sit-down dining with unbolted chairs. Customers like them for their more relaxed atmosphere, and are willing to pay the slightly higher prices.

The chains can be classed as:

- **Grill and buffet.** Customers select items from a standard buffet plus something from the grill.

- **Family chains.** They offer table service and are open for breakfast, lunch, and diner, but typically serve no alcohol.

- **Dinner house chains.** They offer table service and are open for lunch and dinner. They serve alcohol.

Whatever the class, the behind-the-scenes food service is the same. These chains copy the operating techniques of the fast-food chains. They have a standard menu for all restaurants in the chain. The menu, which remains the same year after year, is generally broader than menus of the fast-food chains. They serve the burgers, the french fries, and the chicken sandwiches, plus other food items that can be mass-produced.

The food is produced in a central factory, portioned, frozen, and shipped to each restaurant of the chain. Steaks, for example, are not solid meat. They have been flaked and formed into artificial steaks. In this process deboned meat is cut into fine flakes, chemical binders and extra fat are added, and the gummy mass is formed under steamroller pressure into an artificial steak. The same process can be used to make artificial chicken breasts, each of identical size. As a final touch, the automatic machinery paints on grill marks.

Cooking in such a restaurant requires no skill. When a customer orders an item, the minimum-wage "cook" pulls the frozen meat out of the freezer and puts it on the grill for a set number of minutes. There's no guesswork, because each portion is identical. Cooking time is standardized.

By the time the meal reaches the customer's table, many hands have manipulated the food, added chemicals, sprinkled on taste enhancers, and dumped in salt—plenty of salt. The food has been frozen and thawed, perhaps more than once.

In terms of nutrition, the food is no better than what you get in a fast-food restaurant. On a nutritional quality scale, this food, in general, ranks at level 4, the bottom.

The menu items are high in fat, salt, and additives. The following table gives three examples.

Watch Out!
Half the food sold in restaurants is takeout. The customer receives the meal hot. Follow the 2-hour rule. Either eat the food or refrigerate it within 2 hours. Cooked food spoils fast.

TABLE 10.5: CALORIE BREAKDOWN OF SELECTIONS FROM CASUAL DINING CHAINS

Menu Item	Calories	% Fat, calories	% Protein, calories	% Carbohydrate, calories	Sodium, milligrams
Chicken pot pie	840	51	9	40	1,030
Chicken Caesar salad	520	45	21	34	1,050
Cream of asparagus soup	310	47	16	37	2,050

(From USDA database)

You see from these selections that each item obtains almost half its calories from fat. The amount of sodium is also extraordinary, especially in the soup. The large amount of salt is a tip-off of extreme processing. The salt restores a semblance of the lost flavor, but it can't restore lost nutrition.

In fairness to these chains, like in the fast-food chains, you find menu items that provide better nutrition than the bottom-ranked items. Most of these restaurants offer salads and vegetables. Use these items to round out a meal.

Finally, to upgrade your nutrition, follow the same survival tips given earlier for eating in a fast-food restaurant.

Independent, owner-operated restaurants

By far the greatest number of restaurants are independent and owner-operated. The restaurant business is probably the easiest business to start. You don't need cooking skills—as we'll see in a moment—and there's a ready-made customer base. People need to eat. But keeping customers and staying in business is another matter. Only those owner-operators who find a winning formula and have good business skills survive.

Unofficially...
Las Vegas, Nevada, tops the field in mega-buffets. Casinos outdo one another in offering their clients gigantic buffets at fast-food prices. The buffet at the Rio Suites Hotel and Casino stretches a whopping 50 yards and includes a selection of foods of seven ethnic cultures.

Independent restaurants vary enormously in the quality and kinds of meals they offer. They range from the low-price, family-style to the upscale, expense-account restaurant with a kitchen run by a chef, a graduate of a culinary institute.

Assessing the nutritional quality of food in an independent restaurant is not straightforward. At least in a fast-food restaurant, you know most of the items rank at quality level 4. But for an independent restaurant you don't know if the cook is merely pulling frozen meals out of a freezer (level 4 meals) or actually making better-quality meals from scratch using fresh ingredients.

At the beginning of the chapter, you saw a list of seven tips for judging the nutritional quality of a restaurant's food. One tip was to look at the quality of the fresh foods sitting in the salad bar or the salad served at the table. You generally have no access to the kitchen. What goes on there is a mystery. But a "fresh" salad is a naked food, exposed to view. It can't be manipulated with salt and chemical additives. The freshness and quality of the salad is a good indicator of the attention the restaurant gives to its cooked menu items. With this in mind, here is a more detailed look at the restaurant salad bar.

Restaurant salad bars

From a restaurant's perspective, salad bars are profit centers. The ingredients are relatively inexpensive and cheap to prepare. Customers serve themselves. But are the customers' best interests being served?

No government regulations specify how long a food can remain on a salad bar. No regulations prevent leftover food items from being recycled one day to the next. The restaurant staff generally doesn't police customers who stick their fingers into the dishes for a taste. Small children are particularly menacing.

Restaurants often keep refilling containers without ever washing them. The old food residues become breeding grounds for germs.

Temperature is another problem. Cold food should be kept cold at 40°F (4.5°C). If the salad bar includes hot items, they should be kept hot at 140°F (60°C). In many restaurants, the salad bar is at room temperature, and the hot items are lukewarm—temperatures bacteria love.

Apart from the growth of germs, the nutritional quality of cold foods not held at proper temperature deteriorates quickly.

Here are other things to watch for:

Watch Out!
People do a better job of maintaining food safety at home than food professionals do. Four out of five foodborne illnesses result from food eaten outside the home.

- Is the salad bar busy? If it is, that means a high turnover with fresh supplies flowing from the kitchen cooler. If the salad bar is not busy, the fresh items may sit there a long, long time.

- Are the containers iced or in some way refrigerated? Beware of warm salad bars.

- Are there dead or live flies or other insects present?

- Be cautious about mixed salads containing protein, such as chicken or tuna salad. If these dishes have been kept at improper temperature, they breed food-poisoning germs. Sprouts may be another danger point, because they are difficult to wash.

- Pass up hot foods that look crusted or dried out. Once a food is cooked, nutritional quality sinks. The longer the food sits in a hot pan drying out, the less the nutritional value.

Running a clean, fresh, and appealing salad bar is not easy. But restaurants that succeed at their salad bars will also do the same in their kitchens.

Behind the scenes in the restaurant kitchen

Labor represents the major cost for restaurants. Preparing food is labor-intensive. Thus it isn't surprising that restaurants save on labor any way they can. Food technologists have obliged and invented hundreds of labor-saving food products, especially for restaurants. These products basically remove the skill from food preparation in a restaurant kitchen. Here are some examples.

Soups and sauces

In a traditional restaurant, the most skilled chef is assigned the task of making soups and sauces. A high-salaried chef is an expensive way of making soups or sauces. Near-identical and cheap soups can be bought in cans or as powders that require only the skill of adding water. The restaurant chef may add a touch of some sort—a sprig of parsley, a touch of a spice—to give the soup a "prepared-by-our-own-chef" flavor.

Such soups are manufactured in a factory. The extensive processing requires chemical additives, taste enhancers like MSG, and lots of salt. Their nutritional value falls to quality level 4, the bottom.

There are canned or powdered sauces that can turn a minimum-wage kitchen helper into a classic French or Italian chef. Take, for instance, alfredo sauce used in the Italian dish fettuccine alfredo. A genuine chef would make this sauce with butter, heavy cream, and parmigiano-reggiano cheese. Sounds simple, but it takes experienced hands to make the sauce properly.

A kitchen helper can make this sauce by merely adding cold water to a powder. The fake alfredo sauce consists of powdered sour cream, nonfat dry milk, dehydrated cheese, a whey, concentrated butter, butter flavor, powdered onion and parsley, and salt. But that's not all. In addition, the alfredo powder contains cellulose gel and chemically modified food starches. These latter ingredients give the powder, when mixed with water, the approximate consistency and "mouthfeel" of genuine alfredo sauce.

According to directions, all the kitchen helper needs to do is mix the powder with water, heat for 3 minutes, then pour over pasta.

One might cringe at the amount of fat in a real alfredo sauce. But do you wish to burden your body with the ingredients of fake alfredo sauce, even though the menu might advertise it as "light" alfredo?

Fake meats

Soy protein is a highly versatile product that can be fashioned into meatlike products, such as textured vegetable protein (TVP). From the point of view of the food technologist, the manufactured soy protein has the virtue of having a similar "mouthfeel" to meat. It can be flavored and textured to resemble a piece of beef, a slice of ham, or a fish fillet.

Restaurant owners love these products because they are cheaper than real meat or fish and easy to incorporate into dishes. They are used mainly to extend a meat or fish. A cynical person might describe such use as adulteration. Why? Because the tuna in the tuna salad is extended 30 percent with soy protein, which goes unmentioned on the menu.

The soy-fish is also used in fish sticks and fish that is battered and deep-fried. Similarly, meat loaf, hamburger, meatballs, and any number of dishes containing meat can be mixed with a soy taste-alike.

Nutritionally, the textured soy protein ranks at quality level 4. Moreover, the customers eating the

Unofficially...
Are foods you see in food ads real? Well, sort of. The Federal Trade Commission, which requires truth in advertising, stopped the practice of filling a soup bowl with marbles to force the vegetable chunks to the top. However, the Commission didn't object to nectarines coated with anti-fungal foot spray to resemble fuzzy peaches. And those nicely arrayed slices of meat you see in ads may be pinned or glued together.

dishes with the fake meats are denied the full nutritional value they would get from the meat.

Complete entrees out of the freezer

Restaurants have the same access to frozen meals as you do in the supermarket. But whereas supermarket frozen meals are packaged in a plain aluminum tray, frozen meals for restaurants are artfully presented. When the meal arrives steaming hot at your table, it looks professionally arranged by a skilled chef. In point of fact, a kitchen helper could have taken the dish out of the freezer 5 minutes before.

These professional, precooked meals, complete with meat, vegetables, sauce, and garnish, arrive at the restaurant frozen, each meal in a vacuum bag. When an order for a meal comes into the kitchen, a helper removes the frozen bag from the freezer and pops it into boiling water. In a few minutes, the helper takes the bag out of the water, opens it, and slides the meal onto a dinner plate.

One restaurant supply company sells 350 different entrees. They include duck breast, grilled salmon, roast beef au jus, chicken Kiev, squab, every imaginable pasta dish complete with their sauces, and a complete range of Chinese stir-fry dishes.

The skill of the food technologists who create these frozen meals is extraordinary. The trick is achieving that final look. When the kitchen helper slides the meal from the hot bag onto the customer's plate, the meal has to look as if it has taken a skilled chef all afternoon to prepare and arrange it. Depending on the food, special chemicals are added to preserve the fresh look throughout factory processing, freezing, warehousing, and thawing.

What about nutritional value compared to a similar meal made from scratch in the restaurant kitchen? If the meal is made from fresh ingredients,

> 66
> The best restaurants are operated by people who like food better than money. The worst ones are run by people who don't know anything about food or money.
> —Andy Rooney, *A Few Minutes with Andy Rooney*, Warner Books, 1981
> 99

then cooked and served immediately, you get a meal that ranks at quality levels 1 or 2.

The precooked and vacuum frozen meal, on the other hand, may look great and please the customer, but it's nutritional quality ranks at level 4. In short, the nutrition is no better than what you get in a fast-food restaurant.

How you know what goes on in the kitchen

The key question for the customer is: How do you know if your meal is precooked, vacuum frozen, or cooked from scratch with fresh ingredients? The answer is not straightforward. For upscale restaurants with a name chef, you'll likely get freshly prepared food using fresh ingredients. Nutritional quality is upper level (ranked 1 or 2).

For the great mass of mid-range restaurants, you don't know for sure. The restaurants have many options, none of which improve nutritional quality:

- They can use entirely the precooked, vacuum-bagged meals. A tip off for such a restaurant is the large number of entrees on the menu. You might wonder how the kitchen staff manages to cook so many different meals. They don't.

- The kitchen may use preprepared ingredients, such as the canned or powdered sauces. An Italian restaurant, for instance, might cook pasta as you would at home and add heated, canned sauce. A rosemary sprig gives the dish the appearance of an original creation. Such cooking, if you call it that, can be done by an unskilled person.

- The restaurant mixes and matches. The basic ingredients arrive in the kitchen canned, powdered, or frozen in vacuum bags. The chef mixes and matches to vary the menu. One day he or she serves roast duck with pasta, the next day duck with roast potatoes.

There is no kitchen waste in such an operation. Nothing is pulled out of the freezer until a customer orders the meal. But, no matter how the kitchen help mixes and matches, nutritional quality remains at the bottom, level 4. Nevertheless, you can improve your overall nutrition in such restaurants by including a fresh salad in the meal. This is one reason why you should look for a restaurant that serves a good salad. In terms of nutritional quality, the salad is the only upper level food on the premises.

It's worth looking for a quality restaurant

Perhaps you only dine out on special occasions. There is a temptation to let down your nutritional guard and not worry about quality. You prefer to concentrate on the occasion. That's okay. A nutritional lapse from time to time won't make much difference to your nutritional well-being and health. But if you dine out frequently, it's worth your health to look for a quality restaurant. Quality in this instance means nutrition.

Few of us can afford to eat several times a week in an upscale restaurant with a real chef cooking from scratch—assuming there is such a restaurant in your neighborhood. So setting aside that option, here are two examples of mid-range restaurants that offer quality both in dining pleasure and in nutrition.

The minimalist restaurant

The best cooking from a nutritional standpoint is minimalist. The less cooking, the better. That's why foods that rank on the nutrition quality scale at level 1 are raw fruits and vegetables or items that require

Unofficially...
Alice Waters, author and co-author of six cookbooks, owner of Chez Panisse in Berkeley, CA, and a role-model for professional chefs, sees one's dining table in the larger sense of the community. Her restaurant buys from and encourages organic growers. She would like all Americans to have access to organically grown fresh produce. It would be good for the environment.

light cooking, like brown rice and lightly steamed or baked potatoes. Lightly cooked, fresh vegetables other than potatoes rank at level 2, still upper-level nutrition.

You'll find such foods in a restaurant that offers a simple menu. For example, the restaurant has a gigantic salad bar with many fresh items. The cooked items are a baked potato and/or steamed vegetables and a freshly grilled solid piece of meat: steak, chicken, or fish fillet.

You can't do much better at home than in a restaurant like this. Nutritional quality ranks between levels 2 and 1.

Natural foods restaurant

Most communities have one or more restaurants that serve meals prepared from organically grown produce. Since these restaurants are owner-operated, they vary in set up and in their menus. Most serve a vegetarian menu. Because they take pains to obtain organic produce, these restaurants also tend to practice minimalist cooking. Thus, in general you get meals whose nutritional quality is upper level.

Home meal replacements

The growing trend to spend less time in the kitchen has spawned a new sector of the food business—complete meals known as home meal replacements. People buy complete meals hot or cold, and bring them home to eat. It's the modern equivalent of a live-in cook. At first, home meal replacements or HMRs were an offshoot of restaurant takeouts. But the takeout side of the business has grown, so now half the food sold in restaurants is takeout.

Supermarkets and delis have also gotten into the act, offering hot meals and complete boxed meals located in the frozen food section of the store.

Bright Idea
For nonvegetarians, don't let the idea of a strictly vegetarian menu in a natural foods restaurant put you off. Such restaurants often concentrate on serving delicious food that appeals to everyone.

If you buy HMRs frequently, you should be aware of the following:

- Whether for takeout or not, restaurants and caterers employ the same tricks in meal preparation described for the restaurant kitchen. Your takeout meal may have started out as a canned product or powder or a complete meal, vacuum frozen in a plastic bag.

- Several companies make complete, boxed meals you can find in the frozen food section of supermarkets. In order to make the meal look presentable when removed from the box and heated, the food has to be supported with chemical additives, colors, flavors, and salt. Without such cosmetics, the food would look unappetizing and taste mushy. That is a sign of how poor the true nutritional quality is.

- All these foods, whether you buy them hot or buy them in the frozen food case, by virtue of the heavy industrial processing have the same nutritional quality. On a nutritional quality scale, they rank at the bottom, level 4.

On the bright side, you can upgrade your meal if you include a salad or other raw vegetables or fruits.

Moneysaver
When buying complete meals from the frozen food case of a supermarket, look for the ones with the shortest list of additives. Save your money on those with long lists.

Just the facts

- Restaurant sales have surpassed supermarket sales and become the dominant source of American food. The laws that mandate nutrition labeling on packaged foods do not apply to foods sold in restaurants.

- The salad, either from a salad bar or served at the table, is one of the best clues to the nutritional quality of a restaurant's food.

- Fast food in general is high in fat and salt. On a nutrition quality scale of 1 to 4, these foods rank at the lowest level, 4.

- Casual restaurant chains offer foods similar to the foods of the fast-food restaurants but with table service. The nutritional quality of the food often is no better than fast food.

- Independent restaurants have a large industrial-support network that precooks the meals. Restaurants are able to buy complete meals, frozen in a vacuum bag. Nutritional quality ranks at level 4.

- Not all independents operate with precooked meals. Some have a salad bar and offer cooked vegetables and freshly grilled meat. Some have skilled chefs who cook from scratch and some prepare meals using organically grown foods.

- You can upgrade your nutrition in any restaurant by selecting a salad or raw fruit with your meal.

Nutrition Pitfalls

GET THE SCOOP ON...
Foods that complement your fitness program ▪
Foods that create energy, not fat ▪ Products
that waste muscle ▪ Snack food and drinks for
prolonged exercise ▪ Sports drinks

Don't Let Bad Food Habits Cancel Fitness Benefits

Chapter 11

The world of exercise and nutrition abounds with myths. "You shouldn't eat before exercising." How often have you heard that myth? Or how about the claim that physical performance depends on high protein intake? Yet another myth. To be sure, some of these false assumptions are based on fact, but the facts are carried to an extreme.

No, you shouldn't engage in strenuous exercise after eating a Thanksgiving feast. But a smaller amount of the right foods before exercise can enhance performance and give your body a bigger fitness reward. As for protein and exercise, protein is hard to digest. It is expensive in the sense that the body has to work hard to extract the energy—hard work that would be better spent on the exercise itself. There are better choices for fuel.

Unofficially...
A Harvard University study of its own alumni found that men who exercised regularly had one half the rate of colon cancer as those who didn't exercise. The study's directors concluded that exercise speeds up passage of food through the intestinal tract.

Common misconceptions

Here are seven mistakes athletes commonly make about nutrition and exercise.

1. "I don't need to eat after a workout."
   Individuals make the mistake of working out, taking a shower, and going to bed. Or if it's the middle of the day, they go about the day's business and several hours later have their evening meal. Muscles right after a workout are vulnerable, saturated with lactic acid and depleted of glycogen. *Glycogen* is the starchlike substance stored in muscles that provides the energy for muscle contraction. It's important to eat a snack after the workout in order to recommence glycogen buildup in the muscles.

2. "I have a teenage daughter who is a dancer, worried about weight. She says salads are all she needs to eat." Nothing wrong with salads, but she is still growing. As a dancer, this teenager expends a lot of energy, and she needs fuel. Energy she doesn't replace drains her still-developing body. She is setting herself up for problems later in life. Salads as part of the day's nutritional balance are great, but this young woman needs to include energy-dense foods as well.

3. "I'm a wrestler. Before a match, I put two garbage bags over my upper body and then run to sweat. I need to lose weight in order to meet my weight class limit." Individuals who compete in weight-restricted sports often do tricks like this to creep under their weight limit. But forced dehydration is self-defeating, because it causes fatigue and diminishes performance.

Better to compete at your natural weight with your body performing at its peak.

4. "I like to roll out of bed and go for a 5- or 6-mile run, then have breakfast." This person hasn't eaten for 10 hours or so. Where's energy for the exercise coming from? The answer may be a shock. Little energy comes from fat stores. Energy for heavy exercise on an empty stomach comes partly from stored glycogen in the muscles and partly from the breakdown of the muscles themselves. Muscle protein is broken down to be used to make blood glucose, needed by the brain. This person can avoid this by having a light meal (a bowl of cereal or some fruit) before the run.

5. "In hot weather, I tank up on sports drinks before my workout." Yes, you should have liquid, but sports drinks with their high sugar content can provoke an insulin shock, according to some. The athlete experiences a temporary sugar high. But the body in response releases insulin, which within a few minutes causes blood sugar (glucose) to plummet, with a consequent energy drop. Plain water is best.

6. "Exercise is fine for young folk, but I'm in my 60s and I don't see any need to exercise." Big mistake. Your body needs exercise in the way it needs food. Any exercise is beneficial, whether walking, swimming, calisthenics, or weightlifting. It is important to engage in some exercise every day. Continuing exercise is essential for continuing health.

7. "I've heard caffeine improves athletic performance." The use of caffeine to enhance sports

Moneysaver
Save money on medical bills. Evidence abounds that an active lifestyle works in synch with an upper-level diet (quality levels 1 and 2 foods) to pump up the immune system and ward off disease. Start early in life. Preteens should engage in at least 60 minutes of physical activity every day.

performance is questionable. Caffeine seems to increase endurance, but that applies only to vigorous exercise lasting more than $1\frac{1}{2}$ hours. The downside, however, cancels any supposed benefit. Caffeine increases heart rate, and stimulates excessive urinary output, with subsequent risk of dehydration.

Kids, nutrition, and sports

We hear a lot about soccer moms. What about soccer kids? Children playing organized sports have nutritional needs like those of adult athletes—with a difference. The child has two needs: the energy demands of the sport and the nutritional needs of a growing body. So for parents, it's a challenge to satisfy both the energy and nutritional needs of sports participation.

As a parent, you can protect your child three ways:

- Good nutrition throughout the day
- Bracket the workout or sport event with before and after snacks
- Adequate hydration

In the following sections we look at the nutritional needs of preteens, teenage girls, and teenage boys.

Preteens: The time to instill good eating habits

The early years of a child's life are the best years to instill good nutritional habits. It's an opportunity for the parent to tie the child's enthusiasm for a sport into eating right. Good nutrition enhances stamina, energy level, and performance. With your help, your child can easily make the connection.

Good nutrition for the sports-minded child rests on the day's regular meals and snacks. Start first thing in the morning. Too often children are in a hurry to get to school and don't feel like eating, so they skip breakfast. Big mistake. The child will lack the stamina and alertness to get through the morning. Worse, the famished child may head for the nearest vending machine or convenience store for a candy bar or bag of chips and fill up on empty calories. Here are some suggestions for the child's first meal:

- Hot cereal. Cook with pieces of an apple or pear. Kids like those fruity lumps.

- Whole-grain, ready-to-eat cereal or granola. Add sliced banana or strawberries.

- Grilled cheese on whole-grain toast. Make sure cheese is not American or processed.

- Whole-grain bagel spread with peanut butter, tofu spread, or cream cheese.

- Whole-grain pancakes containing a fruit, like blueberries or banana, with a small amount of maple syrup.

Finally, arrange your own schedule to eat breakfast with your child or children. They appreciate the attention, and your own eating habits will reinforce the child's.

On days of either a workout or game, make sure the child has a pre-event snack. This snack should be easily digested and should be eaten just before the event. Fruit is the best choice. The post-event snack can be more substantial:

- A whole-grain sandwich with peanut butter and jam (easy on the peanut butter)

- Low-fat yogurt with fruit pieces, or a whole-grain cookie with raisins

Watch Out!
If your child plays in an all-day tournament in which she or he plays two or more games, watch out for dehydration and glycogen depletion. Make sure your child has plenty of fluid and snacks throughout the day.

- Granola bar, loose granola, or breakfast cereal
- Vegetable sticks (carrot, zucchini, broccoli, cauliflower, sweet pepper) with yogurt or tofu dip

Quality nutrition is important at this moment. After vigorous exercise, the child's muscles are low on glycogen, blood sugar has fallen, and the child feels tired. The body's natural course is to start recovery, for which it needs nourishment. The body has two choices. It draws on the snack the child eats, or it starts to "cannibalize" itself. So keep the snacks coming.

Make sure your child engages in physical activity

If your child is not involved in organized sport, he or she still needs physical activity. Children should be physically active at least an hour a day. Here are some suggestions:

- Restrict TV viewing
- Walk instead of ride to school or bus stop
- Enroll in tennis classes
- Take up roller-blading
- Walk the dog, either yours or the neighbor's
- Take a long walk
- Take swimming lessons
- For young girls, take skipping rope to school to use at recess

Whatever it takes, keep your child moving.

The female athlete triad: How to avoid it

The pubescent growth spurt takes place in girls roughly from the ages of 9 to 13, with slowed but continued maturing for some years thereafter. The young woman athlete has to accommodate these growth changes along with the physical demands of her often strenuous sport. Some young women fail to accommodate both needs and sink into three problems:

1. Disordered eating habits, with wild weight swings

2. Cessation of menstrual cycle (amenorrhea)

3. Premature bone loss and, in some cases, subsequent stress fractures

The underlying problem of the triad can be summed up in one word—weight. And with weight goes body image. A normal-size young woman carries 20 to 22 percent of her body weight as fat. A thin woman still carries about 18 percent fat. From an athlete's perspective fat is dead weight, contributing absolutely nothing to performance. It's muscles that move her about. So as a result, young female athletes are desperate to shave off fat. Many coaches, in fact, tell their charges to reduce body fat to 10 percent or less.

Nature, on the other hand, has a different perspective on body fat. In reasonable amounts, it's there for a purpose, part of the healthy body's function. Fat protects vital organs, is a reservoir for essential fatty acids, and is available as a muscle fuel. The heart, for instance, runs almost exclusively on fat.

Low body fat sends the wrong signal to the body. When a woman drops her body fat towards the 10 to 13 percent mark, the body flips into starvation mode. It hunkers down. Athletic efficiency no longer takes priority. Like a person going around the house at night turning off lights one by one, the body starts shutting down nonessential body functions. The reproductive system is the first to go.

Watch Out!
Watch out for liquid meals. They are touted as high-carbohydrate foods, but the carbohydrate comes from refined sugars. The meal in a can is a level 4 food. You can do better. Make a fruit smoothie: Blend fresh fruit with ice cubes and low-fat yogurt.

Menstruation ceases—amenorrhea. This is the most obvious effect, but other nasty events also occur. The body wastes muscle mass, converting muscle protein to glucose to keep the brain operating. The female athlete sees the needle on the scale dropping and thinks: "Oh great, I'm losing body fat." But, in fact, she's losing muscle mass along with the fat. It's ironic, because she's losing the very part of her body she needs for physical performance.

That's not all. The normal menstrual cycle produces estrogen, which is involved in bone formation. In effect, estrogen stops bones from dissolving. The female athlete who is not menstruating has a hormonal balance similar to that of a post-menopausal woman. Lack of estrogen causes bones to lose density. The result? The athlete is more susceptible to stress fractures.

The sad part of bone loss during teen years is that bone density is largely not recovered. The individual sets herself up for the risk of serious fractures later in life.

At one time amenorrhea was accepted as a part of a female athlete's training program. No longer. Medical authorities consider suspension of menstruation for whatever reason as abnormal and undesirable.

The sports where the participants are most likely to fall into the female athlete triad are those where a slim figure is highly desired, such as gymnastics, figure skating, swimming, and long-distance running.

While eating disorders in young girls is a complex topic, involving both bulimia and anorexia, these disorders often result from a girl's desire to lose weight. The individual loses weight by starving herself. Then she can no longer resist food and pigs out; this is followed by another round of weight loss. Her weight yo-yos, while through it all her body is under stress from inadequate nourishment.

It's a case of the athlete focusing on the wrong thing (weight). The foundation of superior performance lies in superior nourishment. To perform at the top level, a female athlete should heed these four tips:

Bright Idea
Allow younger children to participate in food selection for meals and snacks. Parents should guide, but make the child part of the nutrition team.

- Eat nutrient-dense foods. We talk of burning fuel as if our bodies were an engine burning calories. The truth is that muscles generate energy only when supplied with the full complement of vitamins and minerals. Eat foods that supply not only calories but nutrients. Examples: whole-grain breads and pastas, fresh fruits and vegetables, upper-level meats (levels 1 and 2: See Chapter 5, "Meats, Fish, Poultry, and Eggs"), yogurt, cottage cheese, and unsalted nuts.

- Avoid calorie-dense, nutrient-light foods. Examples: soft drinks and sugary sports drinks, french fries, fast-food hamburgers, hot dogs, bologna and other luncheon meats, processed cheese, potato chips, and any fried foods. These foods overload the calories, but instead of energizing the body, burden it. Without the spectrum of nutrients, they are either poor or useless foods for building what the athlete needs most—glycogen.

- Adequate energy. A female athlete who expends 2,000 calories in normal daily activities may expend 1,000 calories during workouts. She may have to consume 3,500 calories a day. One indicator of getting sufficient calories is weight. The weight of an athlete consuming enough calories should remain constant or increase or decrease slightly as muscle mass increases and body fat is reduced. Large decreases are a bad sign.

■ Pace your food intake. Spread your food over the day, hinging your menu for the day on a good breakfast. Practice snack bracketing around your workouts (more about snack bracketing in a moment). For a small woman, eating this much food can be daunting, but by eating small amounts frequently, she keeps up with her body's energy demands. She doesn't exhaust her muscle glycogen, and what glycogen she uses is replaced.

Adolescent boys (and girls) want to bulk up

The adolescent male athlete, like the female athlete, faces the same nutritional challenges: supplying nourishment for a growing body and energy for an intense sport activity. The typical teenage boy, however, instead of wanting to slim down, wants to bulk up. Teenage boys want to look bigger and be stronger. Because they are interested in larger muscles, they think about getting more protein in their diets. They make the mistake of believing that by taking in more protein their muscles will automatically balloon.

True, the teenage boy needs more protein, but how much more? And will a regular diet supply enough? Boys hit their pubescent growth spurt from about age 12 to 16, with maturing ongoing for a few more years. During these years their protein requirement goes up slightly.

The National Research Council of the National Academy of Sciences recommends an amount of

Moneysaver
Don't buy dietary supplements touted to build muscles. What builds muscles is repeated, hard exercise.

dietary protein based on body weight: 0.4 grams per pound of body weight. For a 150-pound boy, that amounts to 60 grams.

This amount of protein is for an individual with normal activity. But the teenage boy engaged in strenuous sports requires more protein. The American Dietetic Association recommends a protein intake of 0.45 to 0.68 grams per pound of body weight for athletes. For our 150-pound athlete, those values translate into a protein intake between 68 and 102 grams.

The next question: How easy is it to eat that much protein? The answer—surprisingly easy. The teenage athlete, by virtue of intense physical activity, eats a lot of food—easily 3,500 calories a day. Supposing a teenage boy ate the high-carbohydrate diet similar to that of Tom S. (see the table in the section on high-carb foods later in this chapter), which is 12 percent protein. At 3,500 calories, he would consume 105 grams of protein.

The point is that the teenage male athlete eating quality foods doesn't have to make a special effort to eat extra protein. This individual doesn't need to eat steak and potatoes. He needs the energy, not a surplus of protein. The excess, in fact, is a drag on the body.

In summary, here are two tips for teenage male athletes:

- By eating a high-carbohydrate diet consisting of quality level 1 and 2 foods, your body will get the protein it needs without having the extra work of disposing of excess protein.

- Forget about fast-food hamburgers and french fries. This kind of food is like putting low octane fuel in a racing car's engine. Your

Watch Out!
Remember, more is not always better. When you eat too much meat and starchy food, your body has to work to store the food as fat and dump excess nitrogen in the urine. This excretion pulls water out of the body, increasing the risk of dehydration.

athletic, fine-tuned body needs high-octane fuel—upper-level foods.

Bracket your workout with snacks

A principle of smart nutrition highlighted in this chapter is matching food intake with energy expenditure. When you exercise, the body's energy demand goes up, often way up. Just like kids engaging in physical activity, adults too need to eat.

To get full benefit from exercise, you must pre-fuel with the right kind of snack. At the end of the workout, your body immediately enters into a recovery phase, and you need to provide the right nourishment to enhance recovery. In effect, you should bracket your workout with before and after snacks.

Take, for example, Marge M. She has a regular tennis workout every morning. In her early 50s, Marge is an independent businesswoman whose children are grown. She sets her own schedule and arranges the daily tennis workout in mid-morning, which comes halfway between breakfast and lunch. To gain maximum health benefit and play her best tennis, she needs to bracket the tennis game with suitable snacks.

Playing tennis requires a big increase in energy. Going about her regular daily activities, Marge burns about 115 calories per hour. During 1 hour of singles tennis, she expends about 400 calories, almost a four-fold increase. That amount of energy is enough to bring 5 quarts of cold water to a boil. Where is the fuel coming from to generate that much energy? The body stores two sources of fuel for such situations.

- **Glycogen** is stored in the muscle right where it is used, and is available to power the arm at the first tennis stroke.

■ **Body fat** can be mobilized. Fat from the midriff dissolves into the bloodstream, where it is conveyed to the muscles. But fat mobilization can take time, as much as 30 to 45 minutes of continuous exercise. Thus for Marge, who plays about 1 hour, glycogen largely powers her muscles during the first part of the match. In the latter part, her muscles are able to draw on both glycogen and fat, although glycogen still remains a key fuel.

Marge has plenty of stored glycogen and body fat to fuel a 1-hour tennis match. So why is a pregame snack so critical? There is a small complication. Muscles aren't the only body tissue demanding energy. The human brain runs flat out, every second, every hour of the day. It can't slow even for a moment, otherwise the body shuts down and permanent brain damage results. Not to worry, though. This won't happen, because the body has ways to protect against even momentary brain slowdown. This protective system is the reason the brain's energy demands complicate Marge's tennis match.

The brain can't use the body's two big energy stores, muscle glycogen and body fat. The brain runs on glucose drawn from the blood. You might consider this fact a flaw in the design of the human body—two big stores of fuel and the brain can't use them. But the body has other tricks for keeping blood glucose at a level to satisfy the brain. First of all, it has a small reserve of glycogen in the liver which, however, is soon depleted.

Second, to keep blood glucose flowing, the body now converts muscle tissue into blood glucose by way of the liver. Yes, that's right. The liver draws on the protein of muscles and converts it into glucose,

Bright Idea
Which half of the population are you in? The President's Council on Physical Fitness and Sports estimates that half of adult Americans never engage in activity more strenuous than sitting in front of the TV. For the other half of the population, regular walking is the most popular form of physical activity.

which is shunted by the blood to the brain. Who wants to lose muscle mass during a workout? Probably no one. So how do you prevent the body from cannibalizing muscles to fuel the brain?

The answer: the pregame snack. A suitable snack eaten just before the workout puts food in the intestinal system. Over the next hour or so, the digestive process trickles glucose into the blood. Glucose fuels the brain and, thus, spares the muscles. And there is an added bonus. Playing tennis requires coordination and focused thought, all directed by the brain. A brain not struggling for fuel is a brain that gives you the edge in coordination and strategic thinking.

The preworkout snack

The preworkout snack should be eaten in the locker room just before going out to play tennis. It shouldn't be heavy—that is, it shouldn't contain too much fat. It should be a snack high in carbohydrates and easily digested. Katerina Witt, the Olympic gold medalist figure skater, would suck a piece of orange or other fruit just before she stepped on the ice. She and her coaches knew that the last-minute fruit would give her an edge, keep her energy level at a high pitch during her performance.

Here are two preworkout snack suggestions:

■ Eat one or more pieces of fruit. Eat the whole fruit, rather than drinking the juice. What's wrong with juice? With a meal, juice is fine, but as a snack it presents the same problem as a sports drink—too much sugar enters the blood too quickly. The fruit sugars in the juice race through the intestinal system and into the blood. You get a momentary bolt of blood glucose, but it doesn't last, and you risk that blood-sugar plunge because of insulin release. A whole fruit, however, contains fiber, which slows the digestion and absorption of glucose into the blood. The whole fruit acts like a sustained release capsule of glucose.

■ Eat nonfat yogurt. Yogurt contains carbohydrates: the milk sugar, lactose, plus (in some brands) added sugar as a sweetener. Try mixing fruit with plain, nonfat yogurt.

Remember, the key to an effective, preworkout snack—whether it's tennis, running, or other intense activity—is eating the snack just before you start. You may have to experiment to find what works best. You want that glucose trickling into the blood during the workout, not before. Otherwise its value is wasted.

The postworkout snack

Marge finishes her tennis workout at 11:00 a.m. and doesn't usually have lunch until 1:00 p.m. At the end of the workout her body is crying out for immediate attention, needing fuel to replace the glycogen in depleted muscles and for her brain. One hour of intense singles tennis will deplete much of Marge's available muscle and liver glycogen stores.

The pregame snack will be used up by now, and unless she eats something soon, her liver will start wasting muscle mass to maintain blood glucose. The answer is a snack to tide her over until lunch.

Here are six suggestions:

■ Nonfat yogurt and fruits.

■ Whole-grain bagel, with thin coating of tofu, jam, or hummus.

■ Home-baked oatmeal cookies with raisins.

Timesaver
The most important time for glycogen restoration is during the first few hours after exhaustive exercise. During this time, high-carbohydrate food is most effective in replenishing liver and muscle glycogen, such as whole grain bread and pastas, fruit salad, potatoes (not fries), and vegetables.

- A whole-grain breakfast cereal, including granola, with skim milk.

- Vegetable sticks (carrots, broccoli, cauliflower, celery, zucchini) with a yogurt or tofu dip.

- Figs, dates, prunes.

The idea that one must exercise on an empty stomach comes from days when athletes ate fat-laden meals of meat and few vegetables. The body strains to digest such meals. Athletes waited long after a meal before exercising so digestion would not draw blood and energy from physical performance.

Bracketing workouts with before and after snacks requires a little finesse. You don't want to overload the digestive system and draw blood away from exercising muscles, but you want to provide enough fuel during workout to supercharge muscles.

Eat high-carb foods to replenish glycogen

Let's consider the situation where the athlete engages in sustained exercise almost every day. Such individuals have to think not only of today's food but also of refueling for tomorrow's exercise.

Tom S. is a long-distance runner. He runs $1\frac{1}{2}$ to 2 hours, almost every day, burning about 1,500 calories during the run. Altogether, Tom expends some 4,000 calories a day. How does he fuel his body in such a way as to remain in top physical shape? The key is a high-carbohydrate diet.

You've heard endurance athletes talk of getting their carbs, of eating a big pasta meal before a competition. Yes, getting carbs is critical, but the big pasta meal has taken on a mythic dimension that is unjustified. To understand why, we need to delve into a little muscle physiology—in particular, a look at the glycogen muscles use for fuel.

As mentioned, exercising muscles run on two fuels—glycogen stored in the muscle and fat arriving via the bloodstream. In a long-distance run, muscles mainly use glycogen for about the first hour, then gradually increase the proportion of fat. In any event, muscles continue to burn glycogen until stores are exhausted. At this end point—if he pushed himself this far—Tom would collapse. Well-trained endurance athletes know when their glycogen stores are approaching the end, and Tom is experienced enough not to push the end point.

You might wonder, what about fat as a fuel? The body's fat stores are 20 to 30 times greater than its glycogen stores, so why can't muscles switch completely to fat when muscle glycogen is exhausted?

Nature doesn't work that way. Muscles can't operate on fat alone. They need some glycogen in order to burn the fat. This fact makes glycogen the limiting fuel in any endurance sport.

What is glycogen?

We've been talking about glycogen. It's time to provide more detail about this key energy fuel.

Glycogen is a polymer of glucose, the animal counterpart of starch in potatoes and grains. If you peered at a slice of muscle tissue through a microscope, you'd see little granules dotted throughout the muscle. These are glycogen granules, a compact way of storing glucose. Muscle design is remarkably efficient. The glycogen granules are located alongside the contractile fibers, the shortest possible distance from where glycogen is "burnt" in a working muscle. Because glycogen is stored inside muscle cells and is instantly available, muscles use glycogen as the preferred fuel (though fatty acids are used as well).

Unofficially... Persons who exercise and remain lean hang onto their aerobic capacity. Aerobic capacity refers to the amount of exercise one can do without running short of breath. Technically, it is a measure of the amount of oxygen your lungs absorb and the body can use. Nonexercising individuals lose half of their aerobic capacity by age 70. They are able to climb fewer stairs without having to stop to catch their breath.

Glycogen recharges slowly

At the end of a 2-hour run, the legs muscles of a runner like Tom S. have pretty well used up their stored glycogen. The problem the runners faces is recharging those muscles before a run the following day.

One thing to keep in mind is that muscles recharge with glycogen slowly. A resting muscle takes in glucose from the blood and converts it to glycogen, a slow process. Tom's leg muscles take almost 24 hours to recharge fully with glycogen. That means the muscles are busily recharging while Tom goes about his normal day's activities and while he sleeps.

This slow recharge rate explains why an enormous meal of pasta and not much else doesn't work as well as you might think. The carbohydrate of the pasta is digested and converted to glucose. A big slug of glucose arrives in the blood from the meal. But the leg muscles can use only a small part of this huge influx of carbohydrate. The body is stuck, so to speak, with a glucose excess, so it shunts the excess into body fat. The stored fat won't do a runner like Tom S. much good the following day. Thus a good part of the pasta meal is wasted, if the idea in the first place was to build glycogen.

The key to building glycogen is to maintain a strong level of blood glucose all the time. You do this by eating smaller, high-carbohydrate meals and snacks throughout the day. The following table gives an example of Tom's choice of foods and snacks for 1 day. His total food intake is 4,000 calories. The choice of foods are intended as a guide and would have to be adjusted for personal taste, level of activity, and body size. A corresponding female long-distance runner might expend, say, 3,000 calories.

TABLE 11.1: HIGH-CARBOHYDRATE MENU (1 DAY) FOR TOM S., A LONG-DISTANCE RUNNER. TOTAL CALORIES, 4,000

Breakfast	958 calories, 65 percent from carbohydrates
	orange and banana
	A bowl of cooked oatmeal (1½ cups dry), garnished with 3 T of raisins and 2 T walnuts
	A glass of skim milk
	2 slices of buttered whole-grain toast, lightly coated with jam
Lunch	864 calories, 57 percent from carbohydrates
	A large dish of whole-grain linguini (11 ounces, dry) with zucchini
	Green salad with olive oil and lime juice
	2 pieces of fruit mixed with 1 cup of low-fat yogurt
Dinner	1,105 calories, 63 percent from carbohydrates
	Medium chicken breast (7 ounces), roasted
	2 large baked potatoes, plain
	Mixed vegetables, lightly steamed; broccoli, carrots, beans, chard
	2 pieces of fruit
Snacks: eaten throughout the day	1,070 calories, 78 percent from carbohydrates
	4 pieces of fruit
	1 cup of low-fat yogurt
	4 fig cookies
	11/4 ounces mixed nuts
	2 glasses apple cider

Calories and percent carbohydrate calculated from USDA databases.
T = tablespoon

Bright Idea
Some people find it difficult to work up the incentive to take a walk. In that case, incorporate the walk into daily activity, like walking to work. If you drive a long distance, park a couple of miles from the job and walk the rest of the way.

Hydration is also a critical matter for an endurance sport. Because he exercises over a 2-hour period, Tom is careful to maintain fluid intake during his run. As part of the fluid, he sips apple cider diluted with water, 2:1 or 3:1, depending on the temperature—more water on hotter days.

Keep in mind the amount of food Tom eats is high compared to a person with normal activity. It's presented as an example of how to construct a high-carbohydrate diet from quality level 1 and 2 foods. He avoids refined sugar and foods made from refined flour. Thus, his diet is nutrient-dense, chock-full of vitamins, minerals, and phytochemicals.

On the other hand, the diet is not calorie-dense. It's bulky and requires a lot of chewing. How do you fit consumption of this amount of food into a busy day? Some athletes may find eating this much food a problem. One solution is to eat smaller meals more frequently, and to snack often. However you do it, you have to work out an eating schedule that fits your athletic activity and lifestyle. Your weight is an indicator. If you are eating adequately, your weight should not fluctuate.

In summary, endurance athletes should remember these tips:

- Eat a high-carbohydrate diet, 60 to 70 percent of calories.

- Eat upper-level foods: whole grains, fresh fruits and vegetables.

- Avoid foods and drinks that contain refined flour and refined sugar.

- Bracket your workout with before and after snacks.

Moneysaver
Apple cider is juice from apples that have been coarsely pressed. The juice is not made from concentrate and contains a lot of the fiber and other substances from the apples. Don't waste your money on canned apple juice that's highly purified and usually made from concentrate. This juice is little more than sugar and water.

- Maintain hydration. Water is sufficient, or include diluted fruit juice.

- To ensure glycogen rebuilding you must eat throughout your waking hours. Divide your snacks and meals accordingly.

Carbohydrate loading: Is it for you?

Carbohydrate loading is practiced by many athletes engaged in endurance sports. As mentioned, exhaustion of muscle glycogen limits any endurance activity. When glycogen is depleted, muscles stop working. With this fact in mind, athletes ask if there is a way of overloading muscles with glycogen—that is, forcing muscles to store a glycogen bonus. With extra glycogen packed into muscles at the start of an event, the athlete can go faster for a longer period.

Sports physiologists have worked out several ways of overloading muscles with glycogen. But keep in mind that carbohydrate loading is designed for a single endurance event, usually a competition. Carbohydrate loading is not intended for regular workouts.

The carbohydrate-loading regimen most often used is called the Sherman/Costill method. It's simple and the least stressful on the body. The regimen starts a week before the competition and combines a high-carbohydrate (60 to 70 percent) diet with gradually reduced exercise. The key to forcing muscles to build more glycogen than they normally would is halving exercise time every second day, as shown in the following table. The example in the table starts with an individual's normal workout time—in this case, 2 hours.

Watch Out!
Many athletes wait until after exercise before drinking water. Big mistake. Drinking water then helps, but you should sip water regularly during exercise. Remember, by the time you feel thirsty, you are already seriously dehydrated.

Bright Idea
All muscles in the body store glycogen, but each muscle stores its own glycogen. Glycogen in arm and shoulder muscles, for example, is unavailable for the leg muscles. Thus, when a runner glycogen loads, only the muscles being exercised (in this case, leg muscles) actually build up an excess of glycogen.

TABLE 11.2: CARBOHYDRATE LOADING BEFORE A COMPETITION—EXERCISE REGIMEN

Day	Exercise Time
1	120 minutes
2 and 3	60 minutes
4 and 5	30 minutes
6	Rest
7	Competition

(*Source: Sherman et al., International Journal Sports Medicine, 1981:2, 114–118.*)

Experience shows that this method of overloading muscles with carbohydrates can be done several times a year without any harm. However, to repeat, carbohydrate loading only makes sense for events lasting 1½ to 2 hours or more and involving intense exercise, such as marathons, bicycle time trials, cross-country skiing, triathlons, and mountain climbing. Team sports, downhill skiing, hiking, and weightlifting are not activities that benefit from carbohydrate loading.

Do dietary supplements enhance performance?

Smart nutrition is about supporting physical performance through sound, no-gimmicks nutrition. This book does not recommend any nutritional supplements taken to enhance performance. Nevertheless, many athletes hear about and take dietary supplements they believe enhance their performance. Therefore, the latter part of this chapter is devoted to a critique of some of the common supplements, giving reasons why they cannot aid, and in all likelihood diminish, performance.

The major sports bodies, incidentally, are silent on the issue of dietary supplements designed to enhance athletic performance. The Olympic

Committee, the National Football League, and several other sports federations ban performance-enhancing drugs, but they leave the issue of dietary supplements wide open.

Here are some of the dietary supplements athletes swear by.

Free amino acids

When you eat a food containing protein, the digestive system breaks the protein into the individual 20 amino acids. The digested amino acids then pass through the liver and are directed to muscles and other tissues, which use them to synthesize body proteins. In the early 1980s, manufacturers, having learned how to make individual amino acids, came up with the idea of marketing them as predigested protein—"better than a protein supplement," they advertised. "The amino acids save your body the work of digestion."

The idea of amino acids as a protein supplement is based on the false premise that "more is better." Let's say as an athlete you eat a normal meal of chicken, vegetables, and a fruit dessert. Now supposing the coach puts three or five such meals in front of you. Can you eat any more? No, you can only eat so much, and putting more food on the table doesn't increase your food consumption.

Muscles look at excess in the same way. They use a certain amount of amino acids to build protein, and that's all. The extra amino acids, as already mentioned, burden the body.

An athlete's normal diet, even the high-carbohydrate diets, provide more than enough protein. An athlete, whether a long-distance runner or weightlifter, doesn't need to supplement with protein powder or with amino acids.

Unofficially...
Athletes try all sorts of ways to enhance performance. In the 1988 Olympics at Seoul, Janet Evans, the American swimmer, won a gold medal wearing a slime swimsuit. This slippery garment, developed in secret, cut her time. While the Olympic committee banned dozens of drugs, they didn't ban slimy swimsuits!

Marketing strategy for amino acids, however, has evolved. Free amino acids are no longer just a predigested, protein supplement. They have become hormone enhancers. The body secretes a hormone, called growth hormone, which guides muscle growth. The marketing people reason that, if the body can be forced to secrete more growth hormone, that would boost muscle building. Certain amino acids were said to release extra growth hormone. Bodybuilders, in particular, embraced amino acids as a "natural steroid," not subject to official censure.

The idea that amino acids release growth hormone started with an experiment with two amino acids, arginine and ornithine. The researchers injected these amino acid into the subjects and found that their blood level of growth hormone increased. But note that the researchers *injected* the amino acids. Do you want your teenage son in his bedroom shooting up amino acids?

Nevertheless, the idea caught on, and arginine and ornithine were promoted not as something to put in a syringe but something to be taken by mouth. But here's the catch. An oral supplement behaves differently than the same substance when injected. The oral form enters the liver, which alters the amino acid. It is no longer the same.

This all may sound technical. But there's a practical point. An experiment done in the lab to prove a supplement works cannot easily be transferred to field experience. Yet the way such products are promoted, the athlete is tricked into believing the supplement will in some way enhance her or his performance. Keep in mind, as described in Chapter 8, "To Supplement or Not to Supplement Is No Longer the Question," that dietary supplements and their claims are not regulated by the government.

In any event, since that early study on arginine and ornithine, several more amino acids have been promoted as growth hormone releasers: cysteine, glycine, histidine, lysine, phenlyalanine, tryptophane, and tyrosine. Several studies report that they give a competitive edge. But for every study showing positive results, another study shows the amino acids don't work. In short, the idea of amino acid supplements enhancing performance remains controversial.

The bottom line for the athlete: Save your money, and leave amino acid supplements alone.

Creatine

Creatine is a normal muscle constituent that in the form of creatine phosphate stores energy for quick action. When your brain gives the signal to sprint out of the starting blocks, the message takes about one-fifth of a second to travel to the leg muscles. The muscles respond with an instant explosion of energy. That instant energy comes from creatine phosphate. This detail of body biochemistry led to another "more is better" idea. Even though the body makes all the creatine it needs, sprinters who took 20 grams of creatine a day were said to enhance their performance. But like the amino acid claims, these studies were done under laboratory conditions, not under the many pressures of actual competition. Moreover, other studies found creatine supplementation to be of no value.

There's a serious downside, too. Creatine is an amino acid, and 20 grams a day on top of one's normal protein intake represents a huge overload. All the disadvantages to the body of disposing extra amino acids apply in this case. (Mark McGuire, the home run champion, stopped taking creatine and didn't notice any drop in his performance.)

Watch Out!
Watch out for yellow urine. If your urine is bright yellow, it means the kidneys are conserving water and putting out a concentrated fluid. Your kidneys are warning you that you are dehydrated. Your urine should be a light yellow.

Moneysaver
It's easy to overindulge in high-sugar, high-calorie foods. A talented swimmer who ate regular meals ate two or three sports candy bars every workout, ending up 25 pounds over-weight. Save your money, snack on fruit.

Finally, creatine taken as a supplement suppresses the muscles' own synthesis of creatine. So what's the point of taking creatine as a supplement? Forget it. Enhance your performance through superior training and a superior diet.

Sports drinks

Are sports drinks all that helpful? Do they help maintain fluid balance and provide quick energy? Well, yes and no. Consider, first, your water balance. The body doesn't tolerate fluid loss, and even moderate exercise on a warm day causes loss of a quart or more of water as sweat. The problem is that you don't know you are becoming dehydrated because you don't feel thirsty. The sensation of thirst doesn't kick in until you've lost about 2 percent of body water. For an average-size woman this amount equals two 12-ounce bottles of water. Moreover, by the time you are down that much water, your body has already lost efficiency, and you are performing subpar.

Athletes can't afford to become dehydrated, waiting until they feel thirsty before drinking. Smart athletes drink water before a workout or event to ensure they are well hydrated at the start. They sip water at frequent intervals while exercising.

So, is water all you need, or should you take a sports drink? Proponents of sports drinks say they offer two advantages over pure water.

■ Sports drinks contain the electrolytes, sodium, and potassium, which you lose in sweat. Thus the drink provides instant replacement.

■ Sports drinks contain carbohydrates, either as simple sugars or glucose polymers, such as maltodextrin. The carbohydrate, easily digested, flows into the bloodstream and keeps blood glucose at an optimum level.

Neither of these features offers any advantage to the sweating athlete. Plain water is all you need. True, sodium and potassium are lost in sweat, but the losses are readily made up from the food of your next snack or meal. You don't need the extras from a sports drink.

As for the carbohydrate, a needed boost to blood glucose applies only to strenuous workouts or events lasting over 1 ½ hours. We are talking about events, such as long-distance running or cross-country skiing. Under those situations the athlete is better off sipping a fruit juice diluted with water.

A danger with sports drinks containing glucose, glucose polymers, or sucrose is that the individual can drink too much at one time. The muscles can't handle the amount immediately, and the excess provokes an insulin response. In 20 minutes or so, the blood glucose undergoes a precipitous drop. The athlete feels weak, light-headed, and loses fine control over muscles.

Some sports drinks try to get around the insulin problem by using fructose or high-fructose corn syrup as the carbohydrate. Fructose doesn't provoke an insulin response, but it carries its own baggage. Fructose eaten as part of a fibrous fruit or in a complex juice is not the same as eating pure fructose. The load on the liver is different. More work is necessary to digest it.

So here's a sports drink that is supposed to provide an easy source of nourishment. In fact, it creates work for the liver. The body has to divert blood to the liver—blood the athlete needs to keep his or her muscles well supplied with oxygen.

In sum, remember these hydration tips:

■ Drink water before a workout or event and at frequent intervals during the event. The goal

Unofficially...
One reason athletes of the former Soviet Union dominated Olympic gold was that they started young. The Soviet sports program identified talented 6-year-olds and put them in special schools. The kids were given a diet similar to that recommended in this chapter. The lips of the future gold-medal winners never touched soft drinks, fast foods, potato chips, or sugary sports drinks.

is to prevent dehydration. If you feel thirsty, you are already dehydrated.

■ Choose water as your beverage. Sports drinks are overrated gimmicks. For long-endurance sports, after about 1 $\frac{1}{2}$ hours start sipping diluted fruit juice for extra carbohydrates.

Nutrition and physical fitness: A wrap-up

Athletes and coaches get caught up in the training aspect of sports. They concentrate on developing the athlete's body and skills, while neglecting the foundation of superior performance—the athlete's nourishment. Remember these seven points.

1. Eat a high-carbohydrate diet, consisting of upper-level foods—that is, quality levels 1 and 2. One's muscles run mainly on glycogen, which is the muscle's store of pure carbohydrate. Muscles replenish glycogen from the carbohydrate you eat. The body cannot use fat to make glycogen, and it uses protein for that purpose only with difficulty. Thus high-protein, high-fat diets are not for anyone engaged in physical activity.

2. Bracket your workout or event with snacks. The pregame snack, preferably fruit, increases blood glucose. You begin with a body fully charged with fuel. The postgame snack caters to famished muscles, launching immediately glycogen recovery.

3. Eat enough. Sports consume a lot of energy, and the athlete has to eat a lot of food. In the typical high-carbohydrate diet, that means a large volume and a lot of chewing. There can be a tendency to shirk eating so much food.

The trick is to pace food intake; eat smaller meals more frequently and snack often. Be a nibbler if necessary.

4. Don't skip breakfast or eat only a muffin and coffee. Your body hasn't received food for 10 hours or so. If you don't eat at this point in the day, the body starts consuming itself. Notably, it tears down muscle to keep the number one priority organ—the brain—going.

5. Maintain body hydration. Don't wait until after the workout or event to drink water. Drink water at frequent intervals during the event to avoid dehydration. A dehydrated body is an inefficient body.

   Avoid sports drinks to replace lost body fluid. Plain water does the job. The sodium and potassium in the drink are unnecessary. Food supplies plenty of these two electrolytes. The carbohydrate in the sports drink is also unnecessary for most sports workouts or events. The extra carbohydrate becomes a burden because it has to be digested. The body diverts blood to the digestive system that would be better used delivering oxygen to muscles.

6. Avoid so-called performance-enhancing dietary supplements. Don't take amino acids or protein powders as a protein supplement. These supplements are totally unnecessary. One's regular meals and snacks provide all the needed protein. The excess in these supplements burdens the body with the job of disposing them.

7. Avoid so-called energy candy bars and liquid meals. Liquid meals are touted as providing balanced, high-carbohydrate nutrition. In fact, the carbohydrate comes from refined sugar—

Watch Out!
Forget androstenedione, the hormone reputed to increase muscle mass and athletic ability. A report in the *Journal of the American Medical Association* (June, 1999) says it does not boost testosterone (the male sex hormone). In fact, it boosts levels of the female sex hormone, estrogen—bad news for men, unless they want enlarged breasts and higher risk of heart disease.

for example, sucrose or high-fructose corn syrup. The meals provide some vitamins and minerals, but not the complete spectrum the body needs. The refined calories in a liquid meal come empty-handed. Such liquid meals on an empty stomach can provoke an insulin response. You experience a sugar high, followed 20 to 30 minutes later by a blood sugar crash.

Most energy bars are little better than a candy bar. They offer refined sugars and fat. This is not the right kind of snack your body needs. It needs high carbohydrate without the fat, and the carbohydrate should be either complex, as in a whole-grain product or a fruit. Energy bars, however, are a mixed bag. Read the labels. Some are well balanced, made of whole grains, seeds, and dried fruit. They are okay.

Just the facts

- Glycogen powers exercise. One hour of intense exercise depletes much of the muscle and liver stores. Avoid glycogen depletion by eating a preworkout high-carb snack, and promote glycogen replenishment immediately after workout with a postexercise snack.

- The best diet for general health and for supporting physical exercise is one high in carbohydrates. By constructing the diet from upper-level foods, the diet is relatively low in fat and adequate for protein.

- Maintain hydration by sipping water at frequent intervals, whether or not you're thirsty. Forget sports drinks. For long-duration sports, drink diluted fruit juice.

- Sports-minded children, whether preteen or teenage, need nutrition guidance. In their desire to reach a goal, kids make serous dietary errors.

- Avoid dietary supplements, promoted as performance enhancers. They don't work. Your best performance enhancer is an upper-level diet and proper training.

GET THE SCOOP ON...
Permanent weight adjustment ▪ Why diet/"lite"
foods promote weight gain ▪ Why dieters lose
muscle protein ▪ Pitfalls of the high-fat,
low-carbohydrate diet ▪ Pitfalls of the low-fat,
high-carbohydrate diet

Sensible Weight Loss Versus Fad Diets

Chapter 12

This book offers you a revolutionary new guide to weight control. What, you say, another revolutionary new way of losing weight? It seems every diet book you pick up promises a "revolutionary" way of shedding pounds. Well, revolutionary or not, the goal of this chapter might better be called not weight *loss* but weight *adjustment*.

Dieting to lose weight is a short-term dead end. Through sheer willpower, the dieter manages to follow a calorie-restricted diet. Then, having lost poundage, the individual slips into his or her old dietary habits, and weight creeps back. It's a lose-lose situation. Smart nutrition, by contrast, focuses on establishing a good eating pattern. By adjusting your eating pattern toward positive choices, your weight more naturally slides into its natural groove.

Human beings are not clones of each other. Each of us has a different bone structure and different size. Some of us are naturally stringy, others

Unofficially...
Maybe children
should fidget
more. The
President's
Council on
Physical Fitness
says children's
obesity is sky-
rocketing, regis-
tering a marked
percent increase
in the last
decade.
Children's cloth-
ing manufactur-
ers have taken
heed and include
in their lines
sizes for fat kids.

more compact. Some people fidget a lot, burning as much energy a day as someone who takes a 5-mile walk. Others can sit motionless, conserving energy. The point is that your weight has a natural groove, one that fits your body build and temperament. There is a body size that, while not excessively huge (or excessively skinny) is just right for you.

There's another "secret" to weight control. Don't add weight in the first place. It's easier to stop weight creepage now than to try to shed accumulated poundage. So, whether you'd like to shed excess weight or you are comfortable with your present weight and wish to avoid weight gain, the key to weight control is straightforward: It's not how much you eat, but what you eat.

This chapter profiles a smart nutrition strategy for weight adjustment and the health benefits that you gain. It avoids a count-the-calories strategy and instead focuses on the quality of the food you eat. It is hard, if not impossible, to overeat quality food.

This chapter contrasts a quality eating strategy with the calorie restrictions or bizarre food selection found in fad diets. Do such diets work? Yes, in the sense that you do lose weight. But more importantly, do they benefit your body and health in the long run? For many diets, the answer is a resounding *no*. We'll look at diet foods and why such foods can actually make you fat.

As food quality moves up, weight moves down

There's nothing gimmicky about the smart-nutrition strategy to weight control. The strategy is based on sound, well-established science. If there is a magic in some sense, it's because this strategy makes it easier for you to choose foods in the modern food market using the guides to food quality levels. Part II of this book describes these guides for all major food categories. The complete guides are collected for easy reference in one location in Appendix E. The following table summarizes the moves you should make.

TABLE 12.1: HOW TO MOVE YOUR FOOD SELECTIONS UP THE QUALITY SCALE

Food Group	Move From	Move To
Fruits	Dried and canned	Raw
Fruit juices	Juice drinks, made from concentrate	Premium, freshly squeezed
Vegetables	Canned and frozen	Green salads and fresh, lightly cooked vegetables
Potatoes	French fries	Baked or steamed
Vegetable oil	Blended oils, margarine with hydrogenated fat	Mechanically expressed, unrefined
Meat	Bacon, wieners, luncheon meats	Lean steaks and chops, grilled or broiled
Seafood	Fish sticks, canned fish	Wild (preferable) or farmed fish, fresh as possible
Fluid milk	Canned and ultra-pasteurized	Pasteurized, nonhomogenized, organic
Eggs	Egg substitutes	Free-range eggs
Poultry	Deep-fried chicken, rolled turkey breasts	Free-range chickens and turkeys, broiled or roasted
Breads	Commercial white breads made from frozen dough	Breads and baked goods made from whole-grain flours
Dried beans, peas, and lentils	Pork and beans and other canned beans	Organically grown, soaked, and freshly cooked

When you move your food selections up a quality level, your weight will move down with greater ease. And, if weight gain is your goal, a higher quality diet together with muscle-strengthening exercise can increase your weight.

Eat only until you are satisfied

Eat only until you are satisfied. The science behind this strategy is deceptively simple. Foods ranked at quality levels 3 and 4 are calorie dense; they deliver a lot of calories per mouthful. But such foods are also nutrient light; they fail to deliver the spectrum of vitamins and minerals needed to efficiently metabolize the ingested calories.

Foods ranked in the upper quality levels, 1 and 2, are the reverse—calorie light and nutrient rich. The calories of such foods are accompanied by the vitamins and minerals needed to convert them into energy and renewed body tissues. By eating foods ranked at quality levels 1 and 2, you experience two weight-control benefits:

- You become satiated more quickly with calorie-light foods. Good foods fill you to satisfaction without calorie overload. Moreover, you aren't tempted to overeat. Calorie-dense foods, on the other hand, with their high fat or sugar (or both), seduce you into overeating. We all have had the experience of feeling we "couldn't eat another bite" until a seductive sugar-loaded dessert arrived on the table. The sugar/fat duo has the power to cut off the brain's appetite control center, which is shouting, "You've eaten enough—stop!" You just keep on eating.

- Nutrient-rich foods stimulate your basal metabolic rate (BMR) (see Chapter 1, "The Basics of Smart Nutrition"). The flow of nutrients into the body causes cells to burn fuel faster. Your body operates more effectively at a higher energy level. Your brain sharpens, and you feel as if you have more energy, which indeed you do.

In short, eating quality level 1 and 2 foods helps control calorie intake. You eat the exact number of calories to match your energy expenditure for the day. You don't overeat; you don't undereat. And there's another benefit—peace of mind. You can:

- Forget about counting total calories. You're able to eat until full. Your appetite control mechanism works and you won't inadvertently overeat. You'll eat just the right amount of food to match your daily energy needs.

- Forget about counting fat calories. Level 1 and 2 foods are relatively low in fat, and the fats they do deliver are high in cell builders needed for the job of constant repair. You are in little danger of overloading your arteries with fat.

- Throw out your bathroom scales. Once your body adjusts to the size right for you—in the groove—your weight will not fluctuate. No more keeping several wardrobes of different-sized clothes.

The beauty of moving up the quality food scale is that you can eat a normal diet. You don't have to deprive yourself of food. You don't have to worry about weight gain. Instead of focusing on weight, you can focus on enjoying your food.

One diet does not fit all

The smart nutrition strategy is not a diet. It is a strategy for selecting and eating nutritionally high-quality foods. Within the strategy you can follow a vegetarian regimen, or a partial vegetarian plan, or

Bright Idea
Take a tip from wild animals. You don't find obese animals in the wild. The amount and kind of food an animal needs and the exercise to obtain the food are in perfect balance. The message for humans is don't overeat and exercise regularly.

you can be a hearty meat eater. The smart nutrition strategy accommodates personal dietary preferences. There is no need to change your preference.

The smart nutrition strategy also accommodates individuality. If you put on your friend's eyeglasses, would you expect to see perfectly? Hardly—we're all different. Similarly, our bodies respond to different foods in different ways. Some folks may do fine on a low-fat diet. Others don't do well and may wish to include more fat-containing foods, like quality cheeses and meats.

As we will see below, one problem with most highly publicized diets is that they are written as though everyone can benefit from that one diet. This belief defies human biology. Your body is a highly personalized biological instrument. You have to be able to adjust your style of eating to what works best for *you*. You can do this within the smart nutrition strategy for weight adjustment, emphasizing quality level 1 and 2 foods.

Remember that within the strategy of selecting level 1 and 2 foods, you must eat a balanced diet. Eat a variety of foods selected from the basic food categories:

- Fruits and vegetables

- Whole grains and legumes

- If you wish, meat and dairy

Finally, we mustn't forget exercise. You have to complement an upper-level diet with some form of physical exercise. Once you are reasonably fit, you should be able to sustain an hour workout or 5-mile walk three or four times a week.

Watch Out!
It's the era of mega-calories. A baked potato with cheese sauce contains 475 calories. A fast-food lunch of an ordinary hamburger, medium fries, and a shake with chocolate syrup adds up to 1,420 calories. This makes it all the more important to keep an eye on the kinds of foods you are eating.

As weight goes up, life shortens

According to the National Center for Health Statistics, one adult in two over age 20 is overweight. Worse, one adult in four is considered clinically obese. And this trend is increasing. The average American adult gained 11 pounds in the last decade. Carrying around excess weight increases the chances of some kind of breakdown within the body, leading to a disease or condition, including:

- High blood pressure
- Heart attack
- Stroke
- Adult-onset diabetes
- Apnea (a condition in which one stops breathing temporarily while asleep)
- Arthritis
- Cancer of the breast and endometrium
- Female infertility

All these diseases and conditions are life-threatening. The National Institutes of Health says that obesity is the second-leading cause of preventable death (after smoking).

How does body mass index (BMI) bear on health?

A new method of setting ideal weights, called the *body mass index (BMI)* calculates a ratio between weight and height. Unlike the height and weight charts, BMI is the same for both men and women.

You can find your BMI on the accompanying chart. A BMI of 25 is considered the cut-off point. Any number below 25 (excluding, of course, extreme underweight) is considered a

Bright Idea
The fat you eat turns directly into body fat at a small energy cost to the body. Conversion of carbohydrate to fat, in contrast, consumes one-quarter of ingested calories. This is one reason why people eating a high-carbohydrate diet can eat more without gaining weight: The body burns more of what they eat in the process of digesting and processing the food.

FIGURE 12.1: BMI BY HEIGHT AND WEIGHT

WEIGHT	100	105	110	115	120	125	130	135	140	145	150	155	160	165	170	175	180	185	190	195	200	205	210	215	220	225	230	235	240	245	250
HEIGHT																															
5'0"	20	21	21	22	23	24	**25**	26	27	28	29	30	31	32	33	34	35	36	37	38	39	40	41	42	43	44	45	46	47	48	49
5'1"	19	20	21	22	23	24	**25**	26	26	27	28	29	30	31	32	33	34	35	36	37	38	39	40	41	42	43	43	44	45	46	47
5'2"	18	19	20	21	22	23	24	**25**	26	27	27	28	29	30	31	32	33	34	35	36	37	37	38	39	40	41	42	43	44	45	46
5'3"	18	19	19	20	21	22	23	24	**25**	26	27	27	28	29	30	31	32	33	34	35	35	36	37	38	39	40	41	42	43	43	44
5'4"	17	18	19	20	21	21	22	23	24	**25**	26	27	27	28	29	30	31	32	33	33	34	35	36	37	38	39	39	40	41	42	43
5'5"	17	17	18	19	20	21	22	22	23	24	**25**	26	27	27	28	29	30	31	32	32	33	34	35	36	37	37	38	39	40	41	42
5'6"	16	17	18	19	19	20	21	22	23	23	24	**25**	26	27	27	28	29	30	31	31	32	33	34	35	36	36	37	38	39	40	40
5'7"	16	16	17	18	19	20	20	21	22	23	23	24	**25**	26	27	27	28	29	30	31	31	32	33	34	34	35	36	37	38	38	39
5'8"	15	16	17	17	18	19	20	21	21	22	23	24	24	**25**	26	27	27	28	29	30	30	31	32	33	33	34	35	36	36	37	38
5'9"	15	16	16	17	18	18	19	20	21	21	22	23	24	24	**25**	26	27	27	28	29	30	30	31	32	32	33	34	35	35	36	37
5'10"	14	15	16	16	17	18	19	19	20	21	22	22	23	24	24	**25**	26	27	27	28	29	29	30	31	32	32	33	34	34	35	36
5'11"	14	15	15	16	17	17	18	19	20	20	21	22	22	23	24	24	**25**	26	26	27	28	29	29	30	31	31	32	33	33	34	35
6'0"	14	14	15	16	16	17	18	18	19	20	20	21	22	22	23	24	24	**25**	26	26	27	28	28	29	30	31	31	32	33	33	34
6'1"	13	14	15	15	16	16	17	18	18	19	20	20	21	22	22	23	24	24	**25**	26	26	27	28	28	29	30	30	31	32	32	33
6'2"	13	13	14	15	15	16	17	17	18	19	19	20	21	21	22	22	23	24	24	**25**	26	26	27	28	28	29	30	30	31	31	32
6'3"	12	13	14	14	15	16	16	17	17	18	19	19	20	21	21	22	22	23	24	24	**25**	26	26	27	27	28	29	29	30	31	31
6'4"	12	13	13	14	15	15	16	16	17	18	18	19	19	20	21	21	22	23	23	24	24	**25**	26	26	27	27	28	29	29	30	30

The body mass index (BMI). A BMI of 25 is considered the dividing point between normal weight and overweight. Chart courtesy of Shape Up America 1997, 6707 Democracy Blvd., Ste. 306, Bethesda, MD 20817; www.shapeup.org/bmi/chart.htm/.

low-risk weight. Individuals with BMIs above 25 are considered overweight. Health risks go up as your BMI increases (see the following table).

TABLE 12.2: HEALTH RISKS BASED ON BODY MASS INDEX (BMI)

BMI Range	Health Risk
19–24	Minimal
25–26	Low
27–29	Moderate
30–34	High
35–39	Very High
40+	Extremely High

The BMI is designed to apply to the amount of body fat a person carries. It doesn't work for a well-conditioned, muscular athlete who is heavy yet carries relatively little body fat. Also, the BMI should not be applied to pregnant or lactating women or growing children.

For the average citizen—and that's most adults—BMI is a good measure of health risks. A 15-year study led by JoAnn Manson, an endocrinologist at Brigham Young and Woman's Hospital, Boston, of 115,000 young and middle-aged female nurses, showed a close correlation between BMI and deaths from all causes (*New England Journal Medicine*, 333, 677, 1995). The higher the BMI, the higher the number of deaths:

- Skinniest women, a BMI of 19 or less, had the lowest mortality.
- Women with BMI of 19 to 25, mortality 20 percent over the skinny women.
- Women with BMI of 27 to 29, mortality 25 percent over the skinny women.
- Women with BMI of 29+, mortality double that of skinny women.

Unofficially...
The BMI is only the start in assessing health risks. Doctors should take into account other risk factors, such as physical fitness, blood cholesterol, blood pressure, and disease history before recommending efforts to change weight.

For the record, the BMI of the average U.S. woman is 26. For a lot of women, shooting for a goal of BMI of 19 is unrealistic. A 5'6" woman with a BMI of 26 weighs 160 pounds. To achieve a BMI of 19 she would have to drop to a skinny 120 pounds. Does she really have to lose 40 pounds in order to win the health benefits? The good news is that other studies suggest a BMI under 25 is enough to win all the health benefits.

In any event, we shouldn't get carried away equating health with numbers. The BMI, while a useful tool, is not perfect. BMI, for example, doesn't apply to individuals over age 74. For older folks, overweight is not a factor in their health or longevity.

And then there's the issue of physical activity. A person with a higher BMI who exercises regularly and is in good physical shape has a better health outlook than a person with a lower BMI who leads a sedentary life.

Whatever your weight, this book does not recommend a weight-loss diet. More critical to your health and vitality is plain healthy living. If you adopt the smart nutrition strategy of eating upper-level foods, your weight in time will adjust to a value that fits your genes, body build, and lifestyle.

In sum, remember these tips for a healthy lifestyle:

- Eat a balanced diet chosen from upper-level foods (see the table earlier in this chapter about moving your food selections up the quality scale).

- Take regular exercise—1-hour workouts or 5-mile walks three or four times a week.

People who consume good quantities of whole grains, fruits, and vegetables are slimmer than average.

It is not because of any conscious effort to stay slim—their diet just encourages a trimmer profile. They have the peace of mind that comes from enjoying their food. They eat to satisfy their appetites, not to conform to some restrictive diet plan.

Fad diets: Do they work?

Unfortunately for many folks, following a restrictive diet plan is the norm. On any given day, one-third of American women and one-quarter of American men are trying to lose weight. They spend over $30 billion a year on diet programs, diet centers, books, and tapes. Although many lose weight, a large number gain more fat back within a year. Others manage to keep weight off only through heroic, restrictive effort.

Weight-loss programs "succeed" because people restrict the number of calories they eat. They are eating fewer calories than their daily energy expenditure, so the body draws upon its stores, thereby reducing weight. But restrictive diets have two major pitfalls:

- The smaller amounts of food in such diets don't provide enough of the full spectrum of vitamins, minerals, and other nutrients. The dieters undercut their body vitality.

- Dieters indeed lose weight, but that weight loss is due to more than fat. They also lose living protein, and that's not good. You have a working body consisting of organs, brain, bones, and muscle. Health depends on the vitality of this working body. You can't afford to lose any of it needlessly, but that can happen. Why? Your working body has a certain level of protein intake. It needs this amount of protein in the

Watch Out!
Be comfortable with your own body. Don't try to emulate fashion or magazine models. The average model is 5'10", weighs 120 pounds, wears a size 6 dress, and carries 18 percent body fat. The average American woman is 5'4", weighs 140 pounds, wears a size 12 dress, and carries 32 percent body fat.

diet each day, regardless of its level of activity. A restrictive weight-loss diet may fail to provide this base amount of protein. The body's alarm bells begin to ring. The protein deficit signals the working body that there is not enough food available. The working body hunkers down, keeping the metabolic fires stoked by consuming itself. Low-priority proteins in muscles and digestive enzymes are the first to go.

Individuals on such diets only watch the needle on the bathroom scales. They don't realize that they shed not only fat but also part of their working body, a loss the dieters will not likely recover. They sacrifice long-term vitality.

Restrictive diets—or fad diets, if you will—pop up continually. But although they are always proclaimed as new and revolutionary, they fall into a few basic types that have been practiced for centuries. We look here at two of the most common types—the high-fat/low-carbohydrate diet and the polar opposite, the low-fat/high-carbohydrate diet. Both extremes have their proponents and detractors.

Watch Out!
Fit is as important as thin. Researcher Chong Lee and colleagues at the University of Alabama, in a study of 21,000 men, found unfit men with a BMI of 25 or less had twice the mortality as fit men with a BMI of 27.8 or higher. (*Science*, May 29, 1998, p. 1366.)

Lose weight: Eat steak, eggs, and cheese

For lovers of dinner-plate-size steaks, barbecued spare ribs, eggs Benedict, and cheesecake topped with whipped cream, the high-fat diet is a dream. Eat your favorite foods and lose weight? Robert Atkins, in his 1970s book *Dr. Atkins' Diet Revolution*, did much to popularize this type of eating in America, recommending that dieters restrict carbohydrates to 20 grams a day. That amount of carbohydrate is equivalent to two slices of bread. The day's meals are mostly fat with some protein.

One reason for the diet's popular appeal is the fact that the diet *works*. People lose weight without denying themselves their favorite foods.

The high-fat diet, however, is not exactly new—it's been around since the 1860s. After a life of heavy eating, an Englishman, William Banting, at age 65 found his 5'5" frame supporting 202 pounds. He was so obese he couldn't tie his shoes and had to walk up staircases sideways. His doctor prescribed a diet devoid of starches and sugars. Banting lost 52 pounds eating lean meat, vegetables, dry toast, and soft-boiled eggs. Banting, to this point in life a casket maker, became Banting the author. He wrote a book, *Letter on Corpulence,* which became an instant best-seller. And so was born the high-fat, low-carbohydrate diet.

The diet works because the virtual absence of carbohydrates, as in the case of low protein, throws the body into starvation mode. The body is forced to cope with absent carbohydrates three ways:

1. The body switches into ketosis. Instead of burning fat completely, which generates a lot of energy, the body converts part of the fat into substances called ketone bodies. The ketone bodies are excreted in urine and also to some extent exhaled in one's breath. It's a case of eating fat without having to pay for all the calories it normally generates.

2. The diet drains the body of stored glycogen. The stored carbohydrate holds water, which is lost along with the glycogen. So an individual going on to this diet experiences an immediate water loss with a consequent gratifying weight loss. This is not a diet for active people.

Anyone engaged in sports activity cannot afford to lose glycogen. Nor can they afford to lose muscle protein, which can happen. A body deprived of dietary carbohydrate drains protein to make needed blood glucose.

3. Individuals lose appetite. This is one of the protective mechanisms of starvation. From the starving body's perspective, food is unavailable, so the individual loses interest in food. People on the high-fat, low-carbohydrate diet just don't feel hungry. They may even feel sick. As one dieter said, you soon get tired of eating hot dogs without the buns.

All these factors contribute to the diet's successful weight loss. But you can always lose weight by starving yourself. Critics of this diet say that's the problem with this diet. Throwing the body into starvation mode is okay for survival in an emergency, but not for the long term. Two critics, Mary Flynn, a nutritionist, and Kevin Vigilante, a public health specialist, both of Brown University, cowrote *Low-Fat Lies: High-Fat Frauds and the Healthiest Diet in the World* (Lifeline Press). In this book, they roundly condemn the high-fat diet as based on fraudulent and speculative science. They claim that over the long term the diet increases the risk of heart disease and cancer.

The diet consists almost entirely of fat and protein. The high-protein component of the diet places a heavy load on the kidneys, which must excrete the nitrogen produced by the metabolism of the protein. This high excretion washes out body calcium. Ironically, according to Johanna Dwyer of Tufts University and Paul Lachance of Rutgers University, the high-protein content of the diet also pulls protein out of muscle.

Unofficially...
At lunch in a New York restaurant with reporter Alex Witchel of the *New York Times,* Dr. Atkins ordered a bib salad and Gorgonzola and veal paillard— a high-fat, low-carbohydrate meal.

All in all, the diet places abnormal stresses on the body—not good for the long term. Finally, can someone live with such a restrictive diet? Dr. Atkins' version prohibits

- Bread and birthday cake.
- Ice cream.
- Candy and cookies.
- Potatoes and rice.
- Cereals and pastas.
- Milk and yogurt.
- Many fruits and vegetables.

Few animal foods contain carbohydrates, while plant foods are mostly carbohydrates. Thus, a diet that excludes carbohydrates excludes most plant foods with their rich store of vitamins and minerals, to say nothing of all those protective phytochemicals and fiber. It's impossible to construct a balanced, health-protecting diet by excluding foods from the plant world.

"The Zone," a junior version of the high-fat, low-carbohydrate diet

Another carbohydrate-bashing diet is trumpeted by Barry Sears, who puts a new spin on Atkins' diet in his book *The Zone*. Sears' diet, not as severe as the Dr. Atkins high-fat diet, recommends that 40 percent of calories come from carbohydrates, 30 percent from fat, and 30 percent from protein. By keeping amounts of carbohydrates, fat, and protein at these magic proportions, according to Sears, insulin is stabilized and you enter a euphoric zone—you feel energized.

Sears blames the epidemic of obesity on the high-carbohydrate diets that Americans eat. The cure, he

Watch Out!
The Zone diet claims it can reverse cancer, heart disease, and multiple sclerosis, even AIDS. *The University of California at Berkeley, Wellness Letter*, in a critique of The Zone diet (June 1998), says there is no evidence for this and that such claims raise false hopes for sick people.

claims, is to reduce the amount of carbohydrate and increase the amount of protein people eat. He centers his argument for those proportions of carbohydrate, fat, and protein on the hormone insulin. The body, Sears says, turns carbohydrate into fat, because carbohydrates provoke insulin release into the blood, which stimulates fat production.

This statement misleads because it lumps all carbohydrates into the same bag. Simple carbohydrates, such as refined sugar, a major part of the average American diet, provoke an insulin release into the blood. But the complex carbohydrates of whole grains, fruits, and vegetables do not. You can keep your insulin levels stable merely by avoiding sugary foods and drinks, including most fruit juices.

We covered this point in the previous chapter on nutrition and physical fitness. The high-carbohydrate diet described in that chapter, for example, consists of over 60 percent carbohydrates, most complex. Yet these complex foods do not provoke an insulin response. In other words, there is nothing magic about The Zone's carbohydrate, fat, and protein proportions. The smart choice of foods keeps your insulin level on an even keel, not some arbitrarily selected percentage of carbohydrate and protein.

The Zone pivots the diet on protein, that supposed-magic 30 percent. Sears recommends a person eat meat three times a day. At least a person is not thrown into ketosis, because the diet contains sufficient carbohydrate to prevent that from happening. But the high protein level suffers the same faults as the Dr. Atkins diet—excessive burden on the kidneys.

The main problem with both The Zone and the Dr. Atkins diet is that they focus on percentages of protein, fat, and carbohydrate; it's *not* the percentage of fat, protein, and carbohydrate that determine a diet's value to the body, it's the quality of the food. You can follow these diets to the letter and be eating nothing but low-level foods. The diets don't distinguish between nutritious, upper-level foods and highly processed foods. The Dr. Atkins diet ignores plant foods completely, and The Zone allows only a limited amount. These diets consequently are unbalanced, low in fiber, low in phytochemicals, and low in a broad spectrum of vitamins and minerals.

The effect on one's long-term health is not good. Following such diets attracts all the long-term health problems connected with poor eating habits.

Sugar-busting

Another weight-loss diet, Sugar Busters, like Dr. Atkins' Diet Revolution and The Zone, creates an unbalanced selection of foods. At first glance, the diet seems on the right track. It condemns refined table sugar (sucrose) and white flour. It advises you to eat whole-wheat pasta and whole-grain breads. So far, so good. But the diet falls apart because it's stuck on a single dietary issue, the glycemic index.

What's that? The *glycemic index* is a way of measuring how much a food provokes the body to releasing insulin into the blood. When insulin is released into the blood, it causes the body to convert blood sugar (glucose) into fat. Provoking a high level of insulin speeds up the conversion—too quickly. The level of sugar in the blood plummets. The individual loses energy and feels light-headed. (Chapter 11, "Don't Let Bad Food Habits Cancel Fitness Benefits," takes up this point. Drinking a sugary sports drink while involved in physical exercise can provoke this undesirable response.) In the interests of good health and a consistent energy level, the ideal is to avoid high blood levels of insulin.

The higher the glycemic index, the more the food provokes an insulin response. Foods like refined table sugar (sucrose) and corn syrup (glucose) have a high glycemic index and, surprisingly, so do foods containing complex carbohydrates, like carrots, parsnips, potatoes, and beets.

Sugar Busters, while telling dieters to cut out refined sucrose and glucose, also tells them to throw out these vegetables. The dieter is deprived of foods full of vitamins, minerals, phytochemicals, and fiber. This advice doesn't make any scientific sense. The authors fail to realize that the glycemic index has validity only when the food is eaten alone. But the laboratory is not the real world. People eat foods in combination. A meal with carrots mixed with other vegetables plus meat or meat substitute does not provoke an insulin response.

The rational for Sugar Busters is therefore false. In striving to meet a goal of avoiding foods with a high laboratory glycemic index, Sugar Busters pushes the dieter into the high-fat, low-carbohydrate diet of that English casket maker, Mr. Banting. It's another version of The Zone and Dr. Atkins' Diet Revolution.

A high-fat, high-cholesterol diet puts you at risk for heart disease, colon cancer, and other ills. Such diets are not associated with longevity. The Sugar Busters diet is not about healthy eating.

The lowdown on the low-fat Pritikin and Ornish diets

We've had a look at diets that claim you can gain a slim body, health, and longevity only through a

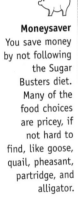

Moneysaver
You save money by not following the Sugar Busters diet. Many of the food choices are pricey, if not hard to find, like goose, quail, pheasant, partridge, and alligator.

high-fat diet. We now turn to a diet that makes the same claim, but you can win only through low fat. Nathan Pritikin, an engineer, was the first to popularize the diet. When he was in his 40s, Pritikin was overweight and suffered from heart disease and cancer. He concluded that he could salvage his health through exercise and a change of diet. Impressed by the fact that the hardiest and longest-living peoples of the world ate what might be termed primitive foods, he devised a diet consisting of:

- Carbohydrates, 80 percent.

- Protein, 10 percent.

- Fat, 10 percent.

The Pritikin diet features unrefined foods high in fiber-rich carbohydrates. It promotes food "as grown," eaten raw or cooked. According to Pritikin, the diet is in harmony with the digestive and metabolic machinery we've had for eons. The diet worked for him personally. He lost excess weight and overcame his heart disease.

The Pritikin low-fat diet rigorously excludes fats, whether animal or vegetable—it didn't seem to matter to Pritikin. For him, fat is fat. The problem with the fixation on a number—10 percent fat—is that this very low fat diet throws out foods containing essential fatty acids, especially the omega-3s. Another issue is the absorption of the fat-soluble vitamins A, D, E, and K. They dissolve in fat in the intestinal tract and in this way are absorbed along with the fat into the bloodstream. The low-fat diet risks a deficit of one or more of these vitamins.

Through several books on diet and health, Dean Ornish, a clinical professor at University of

Watch Out!
The American Heart Association recommends against population-wide adoption of very low-fat diets. The association says such diets could be harmful to certain subgroups. What's critical is not so much how much fat you eat, but the type of fat.

California at San Francisco, has also picked up on the 10 percent fat diet. Ornish calls his version the low-fat vegetarian diet. Unfortunately, it's not easy, even on a vegetarian regimen, to lower one's fat intake to 10 percent of calories. Recall that Chapter 9, "Vegetarianism: Should You Move Towards a Plant-Based Diet?," presents sample vegetarian diets. The foods in the diets were selected on the basis of wholesomeness and attractiveness, with no special attention paid to fat. The amount of fat in those diets turned out to be in the 25 to 30 percent range.

You have to work hard to move down to a 10 percent fat diet. Ornish lowers the fat content of his diet by saying no to:

- Oils in cooking and on salads.

- Avocados.

- Olives.

- Nuts.

- Seeds.

- Egg yolks.

- Dairy products containing fat.

The plus side of both the Pritikin and Ornish diets is that they emphasize whole foods—foods that are unprocessed or minimally processed. The diets include plenty of raw fruits and salads.

The minus side, as already mentioned, is the danger of poor absorption of the fat-soluble vitamins and shortchanging the body of the essential fatty acids. Ornish, in countering this problem, recommends taking 2 grams of fish oil and 2 grams of flaxseed every day, both sources of essential fatty acids.

Because of the rigorous exclusion of fat, the diets ban highly nutritious foods, like nuts, olive oil, and egg yolks. It's a case of being obsessed with a number, rather than looking at the total nutritional value of food.

On the practical side, diets limited to 10 percent fat are bland and, for many people, unappealing. After all, fat, whether vegetable or animal, gives food a certain taste and palatability. Both Pritikin and Ornish devised their diets for sick people, primarily individuals with heart conditions. A person faced with a life-threatening situation has more incentive to follow such a diet. It is not easy, on the other hand, to take such a diet and persuade healthy people to adopt it.

Both Pritikin and Ornish claim many successes, people who followed the 10 percent diet and overcame their heart conditions. But if you look closely at these claims, you see individuals who originally were overweight, eating a diet high in hamburger, hot dogs, french fries, sugar, and processed foods.

Patient improvement through the Pritikin and Ornish diets probably has as much or more to do with the whole grains, fruits, and vegetables than the fact the diet is 10 percent fat.

This book takes the position that the key to a balanced, wholesome, and weight-adjusting diet is the choice of food. You have to look at the total nutritional value of the food and how it fits into your total daily food pattern. The percentages of fat, protein, and carbohydrates should be kept in reason, but are not critical. We noted in Chapter 9, for example, that peoples in the Mediterranean following a traditional diet—which, in fact, is 30 to 40 percent fat—have a low incidence of heart disease. The reason for their healthy life has nothing to do with fat percentage. It is due to their food, which is nonprocessed and highly nutritious.

Unofficially...
According to Nathan Pritikin's son Robert, interviewed in the *New York Times* (July 28, 1993), the diet guru didn't concern himself with the palatability of food. He believed that if you told people about the health benefits of the diet, they would eat it.

The lowdown on diet/"lite," low-cal food and drink

People eat and drink diet/"lite" or low-cal products because they think such products will reduce or at least control an expanding waistline, but it doesn't happen. Studies find that people who buy "lite" foods are no more able to control their waistlines than people who eat regular foods.

What's going on? Are diet foods really "lite," or is there a deception at play here? More than likely, it's self-deception. People eating a diet cookie or dessert think, "Ah, fewer calories, so I can eat more," taking a second cookie or a bigger helping.

Beer companies, aware of this self-deception, heavily promote "lite" beer. The beer does indeed have fewer calories:

- Lite beer, 110 calories per 12-ounce bottle
- Regular beer, 150 calories per 12-ounce bottle

Unofficially...
Making a fat-free cookie is not easy. Marian Burros, a food critic of the *New York Times*, tasted 36 different nonfat cookies. She found only nine that really tasted good. Nineteen others deserved phrases like "bitter," "artificial taste and aroma," and "very dry." (*New York Times*, April 7, 1993)

Beer companies found that consumers who would normally drink one or two bottles of regular beer now would drink an extra bottle of the "lite" beer—presumably to reach the same level of satisfaction. The individual winds up consuming as many or more calories, and the beer companies wind up with increased sales.

The diet/"lite" industry targets two food components the public associates with dispensable calories: sugar and fat. The industry therefore manufactures

- Sugar-free soft drinks, pastries, candies, cookies, and dessert foods, all artificially sweetened.
- Reduced fat and fat-free foods in which fat is replaced with fake fat or a fat-mimicking ingredient.

What do consumers really get when they consume such products? We'll look at both categories.

Sugar-free foods and drinks

The diet/"lite" industry is full of paradoxes. As the sale of sugar-free foods and drinks has gone up, so has sugar consumption. In the last 25 years, per capita consumption of sugar has increased by 30 pounds a year. Every child and adult in the U.S. now consumes 83 pounds of sugar per year, or 3.6 ounces per day. It seems that artificially sweetened foods awaken a desire in people for the real thing.

At least with sugar in the food you know what you are getting. With sugar-free products, you don't. After all, the sugar-free products aren't exactly free—they bring to the consumer chemical additives and controversy.

First, the additives. From the food manufacturer's perspective, sugar does more than sweeten a product. Sugar adds body, which improves that all-important "mouthfeel," and sugar helps disperse other ingredients in the food product. Take out the sugar and the manufacturer has to add something else to bulk up the product. That something else is often another sugarlike product—a chemically treated starch called polydextrose. This nonsweet ingredient is poorly digested, so it contributes only a quarter as many calories as sugar. It means, however, that you have a synthetic substance, not a natural fiber, passing all the way through your intestinal tract.

Second, the diet/"lite" industry relies on two artificial sweeteners, both surrounded by controversy.

■ Saccharin (trade name Sweet 'N Low)

Watch Out!
Reduced fat doesn't mean reduced calories. Two tablespoons of Skippy Super Chunk Peanut Butter gives you 190 calories. The same amount of the reduced fat version gives you...190 calories.

- Aspartame, (trade names Nutrasweet and Equal)

Saccharin, 200 to 700 times sweeter than sucrose, has a century-long history of being banned and later reinstated. Harvey Wiley, head of the Board of the Food and Drug Inspection Agency (later the FDA) in 1907 banned it as a poisonous substance. The ban was lifted a few years later. FDA scientists in 1951 found that saccharin harmed the kidneys of rats. Later studies suggested that the artificial sweetener causes bladder tumors in rats. Since 1981, while permitting saccharin on the market, FDA has classified it as a suspected carcinogen. Both the United States and Canada require food products containing saccharin to carry a label warning consumers that the product may be hazardous to your health.

In 1998, an FDA panel of nine scientists voted six to three to remove saccharin from the FDA's list of suspected carcinogens. But keep in mind that the vote was not unanimous—three of the experts thought saccharin still presented a hazard to users.

So there the matter rests—a controversial substance that is still used to sweeten toothpaste, candies, chewing gum, mouthwashes, salad dressing, pastries, and many other items, including diet products.

Aspartame, 180 times sweeter than sucrose, has no less of a controversial history. It was approved for use in soft drinks, chewing gum, confections, and fruit spreads and fillings amid claims it triggers a variety of nervous disorders, including brain tumors (in laboratory animals). The FDA and the company that sells aspartame dispute such claims, saying there is no reason to doubt its safety.

Aspartame proves unstable in heat. When a diet drink is stored at room temperature in the summer, aspartame breaks down to a substance called dike-topiperazine, a chemical known to be toxic to humans. Unfortunately, when you buy a bottle of diet cola, you have no idea if it has been stored for any length of time at elevated temperature.

The bottom line for users of artificially sweetened foods and drinks is this: They don't save you calories, and you ingest chemicals bearing a baggage of questionable safety. So why use them?

Reduced-fat and nonfat foods

Here's another paradox. People look at reduced-fat or nonfat food items, thinking that they are low cal, drop their guard, and indulge. Surprise! The nonfat food is not necessarily much lighter in calories. A Nabisco regular Oreo cookie, for example, gives you 53 calories. The reduced-fat Oreo gives you 43 calories. If you're tempted to eat two, you take in 86 calories.

If you read labels, you won't make the mistake of believing no-fat foods are low cal. So what's the value of such products? Sales. From the food manufacturer's point of view, the terms "reduced fat," "nonfat," and "fat-free" sell food. That's the sole rationale for developing such products. Some nutritionists, on the other hand, see the advantage in that a person eats less fat. But if you're eating less fat, what else do you ingest when you eat these products?

Fat plays a big role in commercial food products. It tastes good, masks bad flavors, holds color and flavors, and gives foods that creamy texture. If the fat is taken away, the manufacturer has to scramble to duplicate the job fat did. Most fat replacements are some form of gelling or emulsifying agents. The idea is to incorporate more water and at the same time achieve the "mouthfeel" of the fat. Manufacturers, for example, use:

Watch Out!
The Canadian government requires the label of a food containing saccharin to state that the product should not be used by a pregnant woman except on the advice of a physician.

- Chemically modified starches.

- Modified prune or plum purees.

- Gums like carrageenan.

- Modified whey proteins, which are chemically shaped to impart a fatlike creaminess.

All these fat replacements add calories back to the product, accompanied by additives. So before you think of indulging freely, read the label.

Low-fat meat products present a different challenge. The meat contains fat to begin with, which the manufacturer removes by grinding up the meat and mechanically separating the fat. The missing fat is replaced with a chemical emulsifying agent. The products are indeed low in fat. But don't make the mistake of basing a nutritional judgment on that single factor. Because of the heavy processing, the nutritional value of low-fat meat products drops to level 4 (bottom level) on the quality meat scale. There are better nutritional meat products to choose. (See Chapter 5, "Meats, Fish, Poultry, and Eggs.")

Watch Out!
Both the high-fat and low-fat diets were created and promoted by overweight, sick men to solve their personal health problems. The idea that either type of diet should be applied to the general population defies common sense.

Sensible weight loss versus fad diets: A wrap-up

Fad diets share a common fundamental flaw—they focus on a single factor that bears on weight loss. This single-minded focus undermines a person's health in one or more ways:

- Long-term health is sacrificed for short-term gain (weight loss).

- A bizarre selection of foods destroys nutritional balance.

- The body loses vital proteins permanently.

- The dieter is denied the full spectrum of vitamins, minerals, phytochemicals, and fiber.

- Diets are hard to maintain; discouraged, dieters give up and lapse into old eating habits.

This book recommends avoiding any weight-loss diet, no matter how marvelous the claims. Instead, put the spotlight on your health and your daily eating pattern. Don't diet, just eat normally.

Remember to choose a balanced diet from upper-level foods—that is, nonprocessed or minimally processed foods. Eat a variety of fresh fruits (raw) and vegetables, including a daily salad. Don't forget exercise, an hour or so of vigorous exercise three of four times a week. Follow this program and you enjoy three benefits:

1. You can eat to satisfy your appetite—no holding back.

2. Your weight adjusts more naturally to fit your particular body type, age, and temperament.

3. You get all the long-term health benefits of sound nutrition.

Just the facts

- Sensible weight lost is better called sensible weight adjustment. This is not a diet but a way of eating quality foods all the time. Eat sensibly and your weight automatically adjusts to an optimum level for you.

- The high-fat, low-carbohydrate diet causes weight loss but unduly stresses the body.

- By eliminating plant foods, the high-fat, low-carbohydrate diet is woefully short of phytochemicals, fiber, and a full spectrum of vitamins and minerals.

- Low-fat, high-carbohydrate diets, while more nutritionally balanced, prove unsatisfying in the long run because they are overly restrictive for the normal eater.

- Diet/"lite" foods and drinks do not promote weight loss. In fact, they promote the opposite, because people let down their guard and overindulge.

- Reduced fat and fat-free foods are not necessarily low-cal. Such foods are highly processed in order to mimic their fat-containing counterparts.

GET THE SCOOP ON...
Symptoms of food poisoning ▪ Foods that invite
germs ▪ Chemicals in food that may make you
sick ▪ Food safety at home

Food Safety: Avoiding Foodborne Illness

Chapter 13

Food is your most intimate contact with nature. Food plugs you into the rhythms of living plants and animals, which through their life give you life. You become part of those rhythms and, if you grow your own food, you see, touch, and smell those cycles of renewal and growth. You know exactly what happens between soil and dinner plate. That's the ideal.

For most people, however, contact with nature's rhythms is remote. A long train of hands, machines, and chemicals intervenes between field and plate. At every stage opportunity abounds for mishandling food products, turning them into more than substance for life—instead, they become vehicles for sickness. What's worse, agents of sickness, whether microbes or chemicals, are often invisible and tasteless. You have no way of knowing whether or not the food you eat today will make you sick tomorrow.

Food-safety issues fall into two broad categories:

- **Bacteria and viruses.** If food is contaminated, you fall ill, but despite your suffering, you generally recover. Nevertheless, a small percentage of episodes of foodborne illness prove fatal. In addition, although individuals recover from an illness, aftereffects may linger for years or even a lifetime.

- **Chemical contaminants.** Chemicals play a major role in modern food production, from pesticides and fertilizer in the field to food additives and chemicals used in food processing. In addition, industrial waste chemicals enter the food system, contaminating food products and adding to the consumer's chemical burden. Chemical contaminants don't make one sick in the short term, but exposure day after day weakens immune defenses, increases risk of cancer, and can cause birth defects.

This chapter brings you information to make you more savvy about these issues. It gives you facts so you can take steps in your own home to minimize risks of illness, whether short-term sickness or the long-term specter of cancer and other debilitating diseases.

Foodborne illness: Bacteria and viruses

Two hundred and sixty guests at an evening wedding banquet feasted on barbecued chicken. The chicken pieces looked good and tasted good. Unknown to the guests, the caterer that morning had partially cooked the chicken pieces, then put them in a large container which was refrigerated. That evening a second set of cooks, assuming the chicken had been completely cooked, brushed the pieces with barbecue sauce and warmed them. Seven out of ten guests became violently ill.

Why? The chicken was probably contaminated to begin with. The initial cooking did not heat the pieces to the centers, so the bacteria remained. That evening the warm chicken proved a marvelous incubation medium for the contaminating bacteria. Such bacteria double in number every 20 minutes, and it doesn't take long for the numbers to build sufficiently to cause illness.

This is just one of all too many horror stories collected by the government's Centers For Disease Control and Prevention in Atlanta, GA. According to this agency, foodborne illness is on the rise. The agency cites six main reasons.

Changing agricultural practices

Normal soil organisms, such as botulinum and listeria, enter the food chain and cause illness. Salmonella and *E. Coli* 0157:H7, both deadly microorganisms, reside in farm animals. The bacteria do not make the animals sick but are capable of sickening humans. Several episodes have been recorded in which *E. Coli* 0157:H7 contaminated undercooked hamburger and caused the death of small children. Children are more vulnerable because their still-developing immune systems make them less able than adults to survive the illness.

Food workers

Workers who handle food in its long chain of processing, packaging, and retailing are, on average, low paid. There is tremendous turnover and notable lack of knowledge of hygiene as it relates to food safety. Workers who are infected or carriers of diseases are a major source of food contamination.

Unofficially...
At the 1998 World Figure Skating Championship in Minneapolis, MN, Arturs Dmitriev, an Olympic gold pairs champion and the favorite to take the gold medal, was unable to skate in his competition. The night before, he had eaten raw fish at a sushi bar and became violently ill.

Food safety at home

With growing affluence and rising disinterest in home cooking, people are eating more prepared or partially prepared meals. Relying on other peoples' cooking increases the risk of illness. Moreover, attention to food safety in many homes is nonexistent. A survey by the American Meat Institute found that one person in two has no grasp of safe-food practices in the home.

Imported food

Food has become a worldwide commodity. Americans eat a vast amount of imported food. Food-safety surveillance in many countries is minimal compared to that in the United States. This fact has become an issue, particularly with fresh produce, because so much is imported during winter months. Raspberries imported in 1996 from Guatemala, for example, caused an epidemic. Apparently, the berries were sprayed before harvest with a fungicide mixed with contaminated water.

Unofficially...
When a group of adults was asked if they washed their hands after using a public washroom, 94 percent replied yes. However, when observed, 74 percent of the women and only 61 percent of the men actually washed.

Antibiotic resistance

The microbial world fights antibiotics by becoming resistant. But they only become resistant when exposed, and indiscriminate exposure, particularly in agriculture, has become a serious issue. Some 2 dozen antibiotics, including the common ones used in human medicine, are added to animal feed for two reasons.

First, because farm animals are raised in confined quarters, the threat of infectious disease is ever present. The antibiotics minimize infectious outbreaks. Second, the antibiotics stimulate the animals to grow a little faster, imparting a slight economic advantage. Antibiotics in animal feed have been used in this way since the 1950s.

Bacteria continually exposed to low levels of an antibiotic mutate and become resistant to that antibiotic. During the 50 years antibiotics have been used in agriculture, many of the bacteria that make people ill have become resistant. For example, a salmonella strain sweeping Europe and North America in 1999 was resistant to the following antibiotics used in human medicine: ampicillin, chloramphenicol, streptomycin, sulfonamides, and tetracycline. For individuals infected with this salmonella strain, which causes a life-threatening bloody diarrhea, treatment is difficult.

Emergence of new types of infection

The Centers for Disease Control and Prevention finds new types of infection one of the more troubling issues. *E. Coli*, for example, is a common type of bacteria found in the human intestinal tract as well as the intestinal tracts of all other animals. Most strains of *E. Coli* are harmless. But in the 1990s, as already noted, a new strain appeared and was given the laboratory designation *E. Coli* 0157:H7. This strain, which can cause devastating illnesses in children, is so widespread in the population of farm animals that you are wise to assume that all meat is contaminated.

Mad cow disease, otherwise known by the scientific name *bovine spongiform encephalopathy (BSE)*, causes a fatal disease in cattle. In the 1990s, a serious outbreak of BSE in Great Britain led to the discovery that BSE appears to cause a similar disease in humans called Creutzfeldt-Jacob disease. Victims of this disease lose coordination, suffer personality

Bright Idea
If you buy hot takeout foods, make sure they are hot when you receive them. Take them home and eat within 2 hours. If you plan to eat later, transfer food to shallow dishes, cover loosely and immediately refrigerate. If contaminants are present and food is not kept hot, the level of contamination can rise quickly.

changes, and eventually lose their minds as their solid brain turns into a spongelike mass.

BSE can only be transmitted by eating meat from an infected animal. Cows don't naturally eat meat, but in the high-pressure business of milk production, cows are fed high-protein meal made from the blood, organs, and other body parts of dead cows and sheep. Defenders of this practice say the best nutrition for a cow is another cow. Humans can get the disease from eating meat taken from infected animals that are slaughtered before the infection has caused the animal to go mad.

BSE has not crossed the Atlantic. Nevertheless, BSE and its human version, Creutzfeldt-Jacob disease, have emerged on the scene as another foodborne disease, one which is 100 percent fatal.

While the human population is subject to a large number of potential foodborne illnesses, most illnesses are caused by one of the following bacteria:

- *Campylobacter jejuni*
- Salmonella
- *Listeria monocytogenes*
- Shigella
- *Escherichia coli* O157:H7
- Hepatitis A (a virus)

We now examine each of these disease-causing microbes in more detail.

Campylobacter jejuni

Within 2 to 11 days after ingesting *Campylobacter jejuni,* the victim experiences diarrhea, abdominal cramping, fever, chills, headache, and general malaise. These symptoms last 1 to 2 weeks. Deaths are rare, and if they do occur it is usually among young children or the elderly. Adding to the short-term misery, however, is the possibility of lingering conditions, such as arthritis and Guillian-Barré syndrome. This syndrome, which occurs in one out every thousand infections, leads to acute neuromuscular paralysis.

A main source of infection is poultry. Other food sources are unpasteurized milk, barbecued pork, and contaminated drinking water. Handling young pets with diarrhea is another source.

Campylobacter jejuni is the most commonly reported bacterial cause of foodborne infection in the United States—as many as 8 million cases a year. Mishandling of raw poultry and consumption of undercooked poultry are the major reasons people get sick from this bacteria.

Disturbingly, an increasing proportion of campylobacter infections are resistant to antibiotics such as ciprofloxacin and fluoroquinolone.

A campylobacter victim becomes dehydrated because of diarrhea and vomiting. Replacement fluids are essential. Antibiotics in general are unnecessary, and the patient should definitely avoid antidiarrheal medication, such as loperamide (Imodium) or diphenoxylate with atropine (Lomotil).

Salmonella

Individuals infected with salmonella develop diarrhea, fever, and abdominal cramps 12 to 72 hours after infection. The illness usually lasts 4 to 7 days, and most persons recover without treatment. In some cases, however, the diarrhea may be so severe that the patient needs to be hospitalized. In these patients, the salmonella infection may spread from the intestines to the bloodstream and then to other body sites, and can cause death unless the person is

Watch Out!
In one study, 98 percent of chicken samples in a supermarket were contaminated with *Campylobacter jejuni*.

treated promptly with antibiotics. The elderly, infants, and those with impaired immune systems are susceptible to the severe form of the illness.

Foods contaminated with animal or human feces are the major sources of infection. Raw foods can become contaminated, for example, from the unwashed hands of a food handler. Salmonella can infect the ovaries of chickens with the result that salmonella resides inside the egg. Undercooked eggs thus are a possible source. In some cases, salmonella have been known to survive the making of an omelet.

Salmonella is the second-most common cause of foodborne illness. Many different kinds of salmonella bacteria have been identified, *Salmonella typhimurium* and *Salmonella enteritidis* being the most common in the U.S. (The name "salmonella," by the way, has nothing to do with the fish. The microorganism was discovered by an American scientist named Salmon.)

Salmonella infections usually resolve themselves in five to seven days and often do not require treatment unless the patient becomes severely dehydrated or the infection spreads from the intestines. Persons with severe diarrhea may require rehydration, often with intravenous fluids. Antibiotics are not usually necessary unless the infection spreads from the intestines. Then it can be treated with ampicillin, gentamicin, trimethoprim/sulfamethoxazole, or ciprofloxacin.

Some salmonella bacteria have become resistant to antibiotics, largely as a result of the use of antibiotics to promote the growth of food animals.

Listeria monocytogenes

The symptoms of *Listeria monocytogenes* appear almost immediately. An infected person usually has

> 66
> If you come down with diarrhea, stomach cramps, and other symptoms of food poisoning after eating in a restaurant, there is a 60 percent chance the culprit is salmonella. Six out of ten foodborne illnesses from eating restaurant food are caused by salmonella.
> —Centers for Disease Control and Prevention
> 99

fever, muscle aches, and sometimes gastrointestinal symptoms such as nausea or diarrhea. If infection spreads to the nervous system, symptoms such as headache, stiff neck, confusion, loss of balance, or convulsions can occur. Infected pregnant women may experience only a mild, flu-like illness; however, infection during pregnancy can lead to miscarriage, infection of the newborn, or even stillbirth.

Healthy adults and children are rarely infected. The disease primarily affects pregnant women, newborns, and adults with weakened immune systems. In the U.S., an estimated 1,850 persons become seriously ill with this bacteria each year. Of these, 425 die.

Precooked meats like wieners and deli meats are the main sources of contamination. The chance of infection is relatively low. Nevertheless, pregnant women and immunosuppressed persons might wish to avoid these foods or thoroughly reheat the meat before eating. Other possible sources are contaminated cottage cheese, milk, and soft-surface, ripened cheeses, such as Brie, Camembert, feta, blue-veined cheeses, and Mexican-style cheese.

According to the Centers for Disease Control and Prevention, you need not avoid hard cheese, processed cheese, cream cheese, cottage cheese, or yogurt.

When infection occurs during pregnancy, antibiotics (trimethoprim/sulfamethoxazole, ampicillin, or penicillin G) given promptly to the pregnant woman can often prevent infection of the fetus or newborn. Babies with a listeria infection receive the same antibiotics as adults, although a combination of antibiotics is often used until physicians are certain of the diagnosis. Even with prompt treatment,

Watch Out!
Instruct your children on how to handle food safely. Seventy percent of women are in the workforce, and three-quarters of them work full-time. The result: More children are home alone and prepare food for themselves.

some infections result in death. This is particularly likely in the elderly and in persons with other serious medical problems.

Shigella

The symptoms of shigella appear within 1 to 7 days: diarrhea, fever, vomiting, abdominal cramps, and bloody mucus in the stool. These last 4 to 7 days, although it may take several months for bowel habits to return to normal.

Shigella is a family of microorganisms discovered a hundred years ago by the Japanese scientist, Shiga, for whom they are named. Interestingly, once a person recovers from an infection of one strain of shigella, the person acquires an immunity to that strain lasting for years. The immunity, unfortunately, doesn't carry over to the other strains of shigella.

Shigella bacteria pass from one infected person to the next. The bacteria are present in the diarrheal stools of infected persons while they are sick and for a week or two afterwards. Most shigella infections result from the bacterium passing from stools or soiled fingers of one person to the mouth of another person. This happens when basic hygiene and handwashing habits are inadequate. It is particularly likely to occur among toddlers who are not fully toilet-trained.

Food becomes contaminated by infected food handlers who neglect to wash their hands with soap after using the bathroom. Vegetables become contaminated if they are harvested from a field with sewage in it. Flies can breed in infected feces and then contaminate food. Shigella infections can also be acquired by drinking or swimming in contaminated water. Water may become contaminated if sewage runs into it or if someone infected with shigella swims in it.

About 18,000 cases are reported every year in the United States. The actual number of cases is probably 20 times higher, because most individuals do not have their disease diagnosed.

Shigella infections can usually be treated with antibiotics, such as ampicillin, trimethoprim/ sulfamethoxazole, nalidixic acid, or ciprofloxacin. Appropriate treatment kills the shigella bacteria that might be present in the patient's stools and shortens the illness. Persons with mild infections will usually recover quickly without antibiotic treatment. Therefore, when many persons in a community are infected by shigella, as a rule antibiotics are used to treat only the more severe cases.

Antidiarrheal agents are likely to make the illness worse and should be avoided.

Unfortunately, some shigella strains have become resistant to antibiotics, and using antibiotics to treat an infection can actually make the germs more resistant in the future.

Escherichia Coli O157:H7

The symptoms of *Escherichia coli* O157:H7 appear within 1 to 8 days after exposure. These include bloody diarrhea (a sign the intestinal wall is being destroyed) and abdominal cramps. Usually little or no fever is present. The illness lasts 5 to 8 days.

In about 5 percent of cases in children under five years of age, a complication arises—hemolytic uremia. In this disorder, red blood cells are destroyed and the kidneys fail. This is the principal cause of kidney failure and death in young children.

Watch Out!
Don't get poisoned by *Clostridium botulinum*. This bacteria, the cause of botulism, can grow in canned food and precooked meat like wieners. It produces a deadly toxin that causes the disease. Fortunately, the toxin is destroyed by heat. Heat your wieners to the boiling point for 10 minutes before eating them.

E. coli O157:H7 is just one of hundreds of strains of *E. coli*. Most are harmless, but this particular strain produces a toxin that causes the illness. The major source of human infection comes from eating undercooked hamburger. The meat becomes contaminated in the slaughterhouse from the animals' feces, and the bacteria is thoroughly mixed into the meat when it is ground into hamburger. Solid meat, like steaks and roasts, are less of a problem. The bacteria remain on the surface and are killed by the heat, even though the center of the meat remains rare.

Most individuals recover without antibiotics within 5 to 7 days. Because the disease is caused by the toxin released by the bacteria, antibiotics do not help and may cause complications with the kidneys. As with the other bacterial infections that cause diarrhea, the patient needs plenty of replacement fluids and should avoid antidiarrheal drugs.

Hepatitis A (a virus)

Persons infected with the hepatitis A virus may not have any symptoms. When they do occur, they are more likely present in older persons and occur abruptly. They include fever, tiredness, loss of appetite, nausea, abdominal discomfort, dark urine, and jaundice (yellowing of skin and eyes). Symptoms may persist 2 months, and sometimes as long as 6 months. The average incubation period after exposure is 28 days (occasionally as much as 50 days).

The method of transmission of hepatitis A is what could be called feces to mouth. In the most common mode, a food worker who is a carrier or is sick from the virus does not wash his hands thoroughly after using the bathroom. Consequently, fecal contamination is passed to the food. The disease can also be transmitted when water contaminated with infected feces is used to spray or wash food.

Unofficially...
According to the American Medical Association, half the visitors to Mexico come down with traveler's diarrhea. Most visitors eat at resort hotels. To minimize your risk, don't drink tap water or use it to brush teeth. Don't use ice cubes. Be wary of salads, undercooked eggs, and all dairy products. Skip shellfish, and don't buy food from street vendors.

Because hepatitis A is a virus, antibiotics or other drugs are ineffective treatments. Treatment includes making sure the individual remains hydrated. Individuals can be vaccinated against the disease, but the vaccine has to be given at least 4 weeks before potential exposure.

Hepatitis A is not a sufficient health risk in the United States or Canada to warrant general vaccination of the population. The Centers for Disease Control and Prevention does, however, recommend vaccination for tourists traveling to developing countries, even if staying in a luxury tourist hotel.

Chronic disease resulting from foodborne illness

The majority of food poisoning cases, 97 to 98 percent, resolve themselves, and the individual is none the worse for wear. The remaining 2 to 3 percent of cases, however, suffer long-term effects, which can be much more serious than the original foodborne sickness.

Chronic disease arises for two reasons. The original infection provides a route for another and more deadly microorganism to invade the body, or the original infection evokes an immune response that overreacts, leading to an autoimmune problem like acute arthritis. Whether or not a foodborne illness leads to an autoimmmune response involves genes. Some individuals are genetically predisposed to be more susceptible.

Here is a list of some of the chronic diseases that can result from an initial episode of a foodborne illness:

- Ankylosing spondylitis—a stiffening and immobilizing of the spinal column as the vertebrae disintegrate

- Reactive arthritis—an acute inflammation of joints
- Kidney disease
- Cardiac disease
- Neurologic disorders, including Guillian-Barré syndrome and personality changes
- Inflammatory bowel disease—inflammation of the gut lining, causing nutritional deficiencies because of poor absorption

The fact that only 2 to 3 percent of foodborne illness leads to chronic disorders may seem a small number, but consider that in the United States 80 million cases of foodborne illness occur every year. Thus, we are looking at some 2 million people a year who develop a chronic disease because of a food poisoning episode. In terms of human suffering, healthcare costs, and lost time, the chronic disorders are more of a national burden than the original foodborne illnesses.

The four cardinal rules of food safety

You have no information on the history of food products you see in the supermarket. You have no control over the safety of the food except by judging the integrity of the company and the store selling the products. In short, you can't do anything about the food before it arrives on the store shelf. But there is much you can do to protect yourself and your family and not be one of those 80 million food poisoning cases a year. Here are the FDA's four cardinal rules of personal food safety:

Rule Number 1: Food safety starts with shopping

Organize your trip at the supermarket by following these tips:

- Pick up packaged and canned foods first. Don't buy food in cans that are bulging or dented or in jars that are cracked or have loose or bulging lids.

- Check "use by" or "sell by" dates on dairy products such as cottage cheese, cream cheese, yogurt, and sour cream, and pick the ones with the latest date.

- Choose eggs that are refrigerated in the store. Open the carton and make sure that none are cracked or leaking.

- Save for last frozen foods and perishables such as meat, poultry, or fish. Always put these products in separate plastic bags so that drippings don't contaminate other foods in your shopping cart. Don't buy frozen seafood if the packages are open, torn, or crushed on the edges. Avoid packages that are above the frost line in the store's freezer. If the package cover is transparent, look for signs of frost or ice crystals. This could mean that the fish has either been stored for a long time or thawed and refrozen.

- Check for cleanliness at the meat or fish counter and the salad bar. For instance, cooked shrimp lying on the same bed of ice as raw fish could become contaminated.

- When shopping for shellfish, buy from markets that get their supplies from state-approved sources. Stay clear of vendors who sell shellfish from roadside stands or the back of a truck.

Bright Idea
When grocery shopping, take an ice chest in your car to keep frozen and perishable foods cold if it takes more than an hour to get your groceries home.

Rule Number 2: Store food safely
Treat all food as perishable and store each item in an appropriate way:

- Refrigerate or freeze perishables right away. Refrigerator temperature should be 40°F (4°C) and the freezer should be 0°F (18°C). Buy a good refrigerator thermometer.

- Poultry and meat heading for the refrigerator may be stored as purchased in the plastic wrap for a day or two. If only part of the meat or poultry is going to be used right away, it can be wrapped loosely for refrigerator storage. Put a plate under the meat or poultry to prevent leaking juices from contaminating other foods.

- Tightly wrap foods destined for the freezer in a good-quality freezer paper or plastic bag. Mark the date.

- Store eggs in their carton on a refrigerator shelf rather than on the door. The temperature is warmer on the door, and the eggs are jarred by the opening and closing of the door.

- Keep seafood in the refrigerator or freezer until preparation time.

- Practice good housekeeping in the refrigerator. Don't crowd the items so that air can't circulate. On a daily basis, check the leftovers in covered dishes and storage bags and other foods for spoilage. Throw out anything that looks or smells suspicious.

- A sure sign of spoilage is the presence of mold, which can grow even under refrigeration. Mold itself is not a major health threat, however. You can often save a part of the food, such as opened jars of jam or jelly, by cutting off and discarding the visible mold along with a large section of the food around it.

Moneysaver
Always check the labels on cans or jars to determine how the contents should be stored. Once the bottle or can is opened, the contents are exposed to air and can become contaminated. If you've neglected to refrigerate items, be safe—throw them out.

- Many items besides fresh meats, vegetables, and dairy products need to be kept cold. For instance, mayonnaise and ketchup should go in the refrigerator after opening. Ground spices, too, keep best when refrigerated.

- Many foods store best at room temperature. Nevertheless, take some precautions. Potatoes and onions should not be stored under the sink, because leakage from the pipes can damage the food. Potatoes don't belong in the refrigerator, either. Store them in a cool, dry place. Don't store foods near household cleaning products and chemicals.

- When putting canned goods away, move the older ones to the front of the shelf and put the new cans in the back row. Check cans to see if any are sticky on the outside. This may indicate a leak.

Rule Number 3: Keep your kitchen clean

The cleanliness rule applies to the areas where food is prepared and, most importantly, to the cook. It's common sense to wash hands with warm water and soap for at least 20 seconds before starting to prepare a meal and after handling raw meat or poultry. Cover long hair with a net or scarf, and be sure that any open sores or cuts on the hands are completely covered. If the sore or cut is infected, stay out of the kitchen. Here are more tips:

- Keep the work area clean and uncluttered. Wash countertops with a solution of one teaspoon of chlorine bleach to about one quart of water, or use a commercial kitchen-cleaning agent diluted according to product directions. They're the most effective at getting rid of bacteria.

Watch Out!
Bacteria love moisture and room temperature. Sponges and dishcloths are perfect breeding places. Sanitize dishcloths and sponges every day by immersing in boiling water. Wash frequently in the clothes washer (hot water cycle).

- Sanitize the kitchen sink drain periodically by pouring down the sink the bleach solution or a commercial cleaning agent. Food particles get trapped in the drain and disposal and, along with moistness, create an ideal environment for bacterial growth.

- Use smooth cutting boards made of hard maple or plastic that are free of cracks and crevices. Avoid boards made of soft, porous materials. Wash cutting boards with hot water, soap, and a scrub brush. Then sanitize them in an automatic dishwasher or by rinsing with a bleach solution.

- Keep separate cutting boards for raw meat/fish and for fresh produce and bread.

- Be careful of cross-contamination from utensils—for example, using a knife to cut raw meat, then using the same knife without careful cleaning to cut fresh produce.

- Wash the lids of canned foods before opening to keep dirt from getting into the food. Also, clean the blade of the can opener after each use.

- Food processors and meat grinders should be taken apart and cleaned as soon as possible after they are used.

- Do not put cooked meat on an unwashed plate or platter that has held raw meat.

- Wash fresh fruits and vegetables thoroughly, rinsing in warm water. Don't use soap or other detergents. If necessary and appropriate, use a small scrub brush to remove surface dirt.

Rule Number 4: Cook it thoroughly

Assume that raw meat, poultry, and fish are contaminated with one or all of the microorganisms mentioned earlier. Cooking temperature must be sufficient to kill germs. Fortunately, the germs that cause illness are sensitive to heat. Follow these steps to ensure that bacteria are destroyed:

- Use a thermometer to determine whether meats are completely cooked. Insert the thermometer 1 to 2 inches into the center of the food and wait 30 seconds to ensure an accurate measurement. Beef, lamb, and pork should be cooked to at least 160°F (71°C); whole poultry and thighs to 180°F (82°C); poultry breasts to 170°F (77°C); and ground chicken or turkey to 165°F (74°C). Don't eat poultry that's pink inside.

- Eggs should be cooked until the white is firm and the yolk begins to harden. Avoid foods containing raw eggs, such as homemade ice cream, cookie dough, cake batter, mayonnaise, and eggnog, because they carry a salmonella risk. Their commercial counterparts are made with pasteurized eggs. Cooking an egg-containing product to an internal temperature of at least 145°F (63°C) will kill the bacteria.

- Seafood should be thoroughly cooked. The FDA's 1997 Food Code recommends cooking most seafood to an internal temperature of 145°F (63°C) for 15 seconds. If you don't have a meat thermometer, look for other signs of doneness. Fish is done when the thickest part becomes opaque and the fish flakes easily when poked with a fork. Shrimp can be simmered

Bright Idea
Don't thaw meat and other frozen foods by leaving them on the kitchen counter. Instead, move them from the freezer to the refrigerator a day or two in advance of using, defrost by submerging in flowing cold water, or put the frozen item directly in a microwave oven and cook it, using the defrost setting.

3 to 5 minutes or until the shells turn red. Clams and mussels are steamed over boiling water until the shells open (5 to 10 minutes), then boil 3 to 5 minutes longer. Oysters should be sautéed, baked, or boiled until plump—about 5 minutes.

Eat cooked foods promptly. Apart from the safety issue, once a food, whether vegetable or meat, is cooked, nutritional value deteriorates quickly.

Cooked foods should not be left standing on the table or kitchen counter for more than 2 hours. Disease-causing bacteria grow at temperatures between 40° and 140°F (4° and 40°C). Cooked foods that have been in this temperature range for more than 2 hours should not be eaten.

If a dish is to be served hot, get it from the stove to the table as quickly as possible. Reheated foods should be brought to a temperature of at least 165°F (74°C). Keep cold foods in the refrigerator or on a bed of ice until serving. This rule is particularly important to remember in the summer months. After the meal, leftovers should be refrigerated as soon as possible.

If all this seems like a lot to keep in mind, at least remember these food safety musts:

- Wash hands before handling food.
- Put perishable foods into the refrigerator as soon as possible.
- Wash raw fruits and vegetables.
- Keep kitchen and food preparation areas clean and uncluttered.
- Keep hot foods hot and cold foods cold.
- Cook meats and fish thoroughly.

Foodborne illness: Chemical contamination

Chemical contaminants in foods raise safety issues more difficult to resolve than issues of germs in foods. With germs you are either sick or not sick; there is no middle ground. Not so with chemical contaminants.

Chemicals in foods don't normally cause immediate illness. Their danger comes from long-term exposure leading to cancer or other devastating disease later in life. Or, exposure may lead to a subtle degradation of one's life outlook. For example, some pesticide residues are linked to diminished intelligence in children.

Chemical contamination of food arises from four sources—two of them deliberate, two of them unintentional:

Chemicals deliberately added to food:

- Chemical pesticides are sprayed on crops to kill insects, fungi, and weeds. Pesticide residues remain in and on food products.

- Food additives are chemicals not used in home cooking and baking, but on the industrial scale of commercial manufacturing.

Chemicals that unintentionally enter food products:

- Packaging materials. Chemicals leach from plastic wraps or are rubbed off package lining and mix with the packaged food.

- Industrial waste chemicals, such as dioxin and PCBs, contaminate waterways and the air. This general pollution contaminates land in agricultural areas and enters the food supply.

Watch Out!
Maine lobsters carry a high concentration of the industrial toxic chemical polychlorinated biphenyls (PCBs), particularly in the tomalley (that green stuff in the body—actually the animal's liver). If you eat lobster rarely, don't worry about it. If you eat lobster frequently, shun the tomalley.

Bright Idea
Plastics contain chemicals called plasticizers, which can leach into stored food, particularly fatty foods. Consumers Union says that plastic containers marked with recyclable numbers 1, 2, and 5 are best for storage. Look for the number on the bottom of the container. Note: These containers cannot be microwaved.

Chemicals from all four sources contaminate foods—not necessarily every item, but in enough items so that you can't avoid exposure. The issue then becomes, are the chemical residues to which you are exposed in foods a health hazard? It would be nice if we could answer that question in clear, unambiguous terms. Unfortunately, we can't, because of a dearth of information.

This dearth of information is particularly acute when it comes to the safety of children. Take pesticides as an example. The EPA sets a tolerance for each pesticide in each food—that is, the maximum amount of a pesticide residue allowed in the food. This tolerance is based on the EPA's estimate of what a human can tolerate without becoming ill. Who is this "human"? The government human is a male in his 30s of medium height and weight and in robust health. Having established what this robust male can tolerate, the government agency then reduces the legally permitted amount of pesticide by a factor of 10. It does this to accommodate the greater sensitivity of subpopulations.

The problem with this reasoning is that the factor of 10 is not enough to protect infants and children. They are especially sensitive to health risks posed by pesticides for several reasons:

- Their internal organs are still developing and maturing.

- In relation to their body weight, infants and children eat and drink more than adults, possibly increasing their exposure to pesticides in food and water.

- Certain behaviors—such as playing on floors or lawns or putting objects in their mouths—increase children's exposure to pesticides used in homes and yards.

■ Pesticides may harm a developing child by blocking the absorption of important food nutrients necessary for normal healthy growth.

■ A child's detoxifying mechanisms are not fully developed. The child's body may not fully remove pesticides.

■ There are critical periods in fetal and child development when exposure to a toxic chemical can damage an individual for life.

There is real reason for concern that legal tolerances for pesticide residues set for a robust adult male don't protect kids. This issue took on more urgency in 1993 when the National Research Council of the National Academy of Sciences issued a report, "Pesticides in the Diets of Infants and Children." The report found that levels of pesticide residues set for adults could cause permanent loss of brain function in fetuses and children.

This conclusion is supported by other studies. University of Arizona anthropologist Elizabeth Guillette has found a link between pesticide ingestion by children and lower intelligence and reduced motor skills. Based on a study of the effects of pesticides on the learning abilities of young rats, Warren Potter of the University of Wisconsin has concluded that pesticide exposure may be part of the reason for rising rates of learning disabilities and hyper aggression in children.

The fact that toxic chemicals, such as pesticides, could damage the developing brain of children opened up a new area of concern. Prior to such findings, the safety testing of chemical residues in

> **"**
> Pesticides and other contaminants in food pose particular threats to our children's health. Children eat more (by weight) of fewer foods than adults and are more vulnerable to toxic pesticides and potentially deadly foodborne bacteria. Roughly half of the food kids eat includes detectable residues of one or more pesticides, almost none of which have been fully tested for their effects on children.
> —Physicians for Social Responsibility
> **"**

food had focused on whether the chemicals caused serious disease like cancer. Brain function was not covered. Yet isn't intelligence a health issue? A child whose brain capacity is diminished may not be sick per se, but the child is denied full use of his or her genetic endowment.

The growing evidence that the bodies and brains of children are not adequately protected by the present system of setting pesticide tolerance levels led Congress in 1996 to pass the Food Quality Protection Act. This act includes three features designed to give the public, especially children, better protection from the dangers of pesticide residues in food.

1. The act requires the agricultural industry to lower pesticide use, seeking alternative ways of growing crops.
2. The act requires the Environmental Protection Agency to reevaluate all existing pesticide tolerance levels, not from the standpoint of a robust adult male, but from the point of view of little kids.
3. The act requires the total danger from pesticides to be assessed. A child, for example, can ingest a dozen different pesticides in apple juice, plus the same pesticides in raisins and other foods. The accumulated toxicity of all the pesticides in all the foods the child might eat has to be taken into account.

This latter point is a new direction in pesticide regulation. Currently, tolerance levels are set for a single pesticide in a single food. The tolerance level is set as if the food contained no other pesticide residues and the person ate no other foods containing pesticides.

Clearly, this approach does not represent the real world. The new act is trying to make pesticide regulation more consistent with the real-life experience of people eating a variety of food, all conveying into the body a variety of pesticide residues.

It will take the EPA some time to reduce the hazards of pesticides in foods. Over 9,700 separate legal tolerances for pesticide residues in foods exist, and the EPA must review each in detail. The agency estimates it will take a minimum of 10 years to work through these tolerances. It may take much longer to bring about the necessary changes in agricultural practice so that the accumulative risk of pesticides is indeed lower than it is today.

So far we have talked only of pesticides. Of the four sources of chemicals in foods—pesticides, food additives, chemical contamination from packaging, and industrial waste chemicals—we have the best handle on the pesticides. Yet, as we have seen, in the case of pesticides serious unanswered questions about safety remain. Our understanding about the safety of the rest of the chemical contaminants is even cloudier. It's fair to say that our use of chemicals and permissible tolerances in foods has overreached government and industry ability to assess the danger.

The food-safety issue remains fluid. Evidence of new dangers from chemical contamination of food come to light all the time. In the 1990s, for example, endocrine disrupters emerged as a hitherto unknown threat. *Endocrine disrupters* are chemicals that mimic the sex hormones—mostly the female hormone, estrogen. Scientists discovered that a number of common pesticides, such as the herbicides 2, 4-D (used on lawns) and atrazine (used on corn),

Unofficially...
The Consumers Union estimates that if the EPA eliminated or tightly restricted the worst 40 insecticide-food combinations, the risk to infants and children from chemical poisons found on nine of the foods children eat most— apples, pears, peaches, grapes, oranges, green beans, peas, potatoes, and tomatoes—would decrease by 95 percent.

as well as industrial wastes like PCBs and dioxin (universal food contaminates), mimic estrogen.

These substances have the potential of interfering with the wiring of the human brain during the fetal stage of life, leading to lowered intelligence and behavioral abnormalities in the affected child. The fetus is exposed through the mother. In adult women, endocrine disrupters may add to the incidence of breast cancer and endometriosis. The latter is a painful disease in which bits of the uterine lining migrate to other pelvic organs, causing infertility, internal bleeding, and other serious problems.

Because of this new threat, the EPA and the chemical industry have established programs to assess more specifically the dangers from endocrine disrupters. Again, it will take years for these programs to move ahead and result in a reduction of the public's exposure to chemical contaminants in foods that are endocrine disrupters.

Risk reduction

So where does this leave the consumer? What practical options are available to reduce your exposure to chemical contaminants in foods? Here are five tips:

- Choose organically grown fruits and vegetables. This produce has not been sprayed or dusted with chemical pesticides.

- Thoroughly wash fresh fruits and vegetables. Scrub and peel as needed. Remove outer lettuce and cabbage leaves. Doing this removes up to 90 percent of surface pesticide residues.

- Eat fewer foods that are highly processed. Read the ingredient list and choose foods that limit the number of chemical additives.

Unofficially...
According to the *Toronto Globe and Mail* (April 11, 1998), Allan Graff is an Alberta farmer who switched from chemical farming to organic farming. Graff says his soil is better, his grain is denser, and yields are better. What few problems there are, he adds, are minor.

- Eat lower on the food chain—that is, eat fewer animal foods. The industrial wastes—like dioxin and PCBs—that blanket the country contaminate grass and all crops. Animals eat the grass and crops and concentrate the waste chemicals in their body fat. Thus, meat can have a 200-fold higher concentration of these chemicals than vegetables or grains.

- Eat a diverse diet. Contamination of fruits and vegetables and animal products varies from item to item. This week, the supermarket carrots may be contaminated with pesticides while the cauliflower is not. The next week it's the reverse—contaminated cauliflower and pesticide-free carrots. You don't know, so minimize the risk by broadening your selection of foods.

Genetic engineering, a new safety issue

Yet a new challenge to food safety has emerged—genetic engineering. This new technology, which also goes by the names of *genetic modification* (GM) and *transgenic,* enables scientists to insert foreign genes into plants and animals.

How is this really new? After all, agriculturists since the beginning of civilization have bred plants and animals. Our current selection of fruits and vegetables, for example, is the result of centuries of plant breeding and selection. The difference is this: Plant and animal breeding hitherto required that the breeder cross different varieties within the same species. Plant breeders crossed one variety of carrot with another variety of carrot. Or they crossed two varieties of wheat with each other. But the breeders could never cross a carrot with wheat.

Genetic engineering, however, allows scientist to insert a carrot gene into wheat, or the reverse. For

> ❝
> . . . There is a danger especially in the areas as sensitive as food, health, and the long-term future of our environment, in putting all our efforts into establishing what is technically possible [genetic engineering] without first stopping to ask whether this is something we *should* be doing.
> —Charles, Prince of Wales (*The Ecologist,* Sept./Oct. 1998)
> ❞

that matter, they can insert a human gene into carrots or wheat. Moreover, they can create artificial genes and insert those. The possibilities are unlimited.

This new technology is changing the genetic makeup of crops and farm animals. Already, two-thirds of the soybean and corn crops consist of genetically engineered varieties. Although the engineered crops don't seem to pose short-term health threats, the technology is still new. We have no idea of what it means to the long-term health of children who will live their entire lives eating genetically engineered foods.

For the consumer, the safety issues of genetically engineered foods are impossible to address in an informed way. The technology is going ahead with little public comment. Foods containing genetically engineered crops are not labeled as such. You therefore have no way of knowing whether or not the food product contains genetically engineered material.

Gordon Conway, president of the Rockefeller Foundation, which has given $100 million in support of genetic engineering, believes the issues of public safety deserve more open debate. He favors labeling genetically engineered foods so that people who wish to avoid them can do so. He also feels we need to be more alert to health hazards. He says, for example, that the increasing allergic reactions to soy products could be an outgrowth of genetic alteration.

Food safety: A wrap-up

The issues and challenges involving food safety are constantly changing. New foodborne diseases such as *E. Coli* O157:H7 and mad cow disease (BSE), unheard of before 1990, have suddenly appeared as new disease threats. Strains of common foodborne bacteria, like salmonella and shigella, have developed resistance to antibiotics, making treatment difficult.

As for exposure to toxic chemicals in food, new dangers are being revealed. In the mid 1990s, for example, it became apparent that many chemical contaminants are endocrine disrupters, mimicking the female sex hormone estrogen. They have the potential of causing a wide range of health problems, from cancer to interference with the mental development of kids.

What's being done to protect the consumer? Consumers are certainly responsible for the safe handling and preparation of food, once purchased. Yet the greatest opportunity for bacterial and chemical contamination of food products occurs before the point of sale. It is here that the U.S. government must provide the oversight.

Although the government is reasonably successful in ensuring that food is free of disease-causing microbes, it has been less successful in protecting the public from toxic chemical contamination. The variety of toxic chemicals from pesticides to industrial wastes, and the ease with which they enter food products, has outstripped the government's ability to regulate safety. The 1996 Food Quality Protection Act is an attempt to catch up. The act gives priority to protecting children from overexposure to toxic chemicals in their food. However, it may be years—even decades—before the act is fully effective.

Just the facts

- Most foodborne illness is caused by about half a dozen bacteria and one virus (hepatitis A).

Salmonella accounts for half of all foodborne cases resulting from eating restaurant food.

■ The most common route for food contamination is feces to mouth. Infected food workers fail to practice good personal hygiene and contaminate the food.

■ Practice food safety at home. Keep the kitchen—and the cook—clean. Keep hot foods hot and cold foods cold. Remember that microbes multiply fast in food that is warm or at room temperature.

■ Chemical contamination of food comes from pesticide residues, industrial waste chemicals, chemicals used in food manufacturing, and from packaging material. Exposure to toxic chemicals in food is not likely to cause immediate illness, but chronic exposure may lead to cancer, neurological effects, birth defects, and other serious disorders.

Medical Issues

PART V

GET THE SCOOP ON...
How to avoid the five dietary traps ▪ Heart
disease and diet ▪ Cancer ▪ Adult-onset
diabetes ▪ Osteoporosis

Chapter 14

Holistic Nutrition Against Cancer, Heart Disease, and Other Degenerative Diseases

The disease pattern of the United States and Canada has undergone a remarkable shift since the beginning of the 20th century. The shift has gone from diseases of poverty to diseases of affluence. A population, generally poor (as it was in the last century) and unable to afford sufficient food and adequate public health services, is vulnerable to infectious disease. At the beginning of the 20th century, the major public health issues in this country were tuberculosis, pneumonia, diphtheria, measles, and other infectious diseases. For example, entire hospitals were filled with people suffering from tuberculosis.

With rising affluence, people's nourishment improved, public health services were upgraded, and medical attention become generally available.

One result: Infectious disease faded as a serious public health issue. All those tuberculosis hospitals have long been closed. And how often do you hear about diphtheria today?

As infectious disease vanished, however, a new disease pattern emerged—diseases of affluence. From a cell's-eye view, this pattern can best be described as premature degeneration of one or another body system. The degeneration leads to a clinically defined and often disabling disease. What are the diseases of affluence of our times? They are painfully familiar to all, just as a century ago everyone had friends and relatives who suffered from or had died of tuberculosis or diphtheria. The modern diseases are:

- Cancer
- Heart disease
- Atherosclerosis
- Stroke
- Adult-onset diabetes
- Osteoporosis
- Obesity

If you search for causes of these diseases of affluence, you find that poor nutrition is at the root of most of them. Other factors may be involved—a genetic predisposition, environmental contaminants—but for each of these modern diseases, nutrition is a major component. Diseases of affluence are not rooted in a lack of food, but rather in too much and in the wrong kinds of food.

Diseases of affluence become a health issue in every country that rises out of general poverty into material wealth. The Chinese population is now undergoing that transition, experiencing the same change in disease pattern that we have experienced in North America. A huge study done by nutrition scientists of Cornell University in collaboration with Chinese scientists demonstrated this.

The study started in 1983, when most Chinese ate a traditional plant-based diet. The study team found no obesity, in spite of the fact the Chinese consumed 20 percent more calories than Americans do. It wasn't so much a case of how much the Chinese ate, but what they ate. The Chinese ate a third as much fat as Americans, and twice the carbohydrates.

But as the Chinese have gained a more affluent lifestyle, according to the Cornell study director, Colin Campbell, their diet has been changing—more meat, less plant fiber. Cancer, heart disease, and adult-onset diabetes, hitherto rare, are now commonplace in affluent sections of the country.

The Cornell study is part of a large body of evidence linking diet and the degenerative diseases of affluence. But must we pay for affluence by accepting a high risk of developing a degenerative disease? No. You can enjoy nutritious, sensual food and at the same time enjoy a low risk of these diseases. The problem is that as the standard of living rises, people lower their standard of discrimination in food choice. They go for the sensual and forget the nutrition.

This book takes a cell's-eye view of the link between diet and the prevention of degenerative disease. Poor food choice stresses your body's biochemistry. Inner workings lose efficiency, and over time the stress causes a breakdown. Outwardly, the manifestation is a heart condition, or adult-onset diabetes, or cancer.

Watch Out!
Beware of narrowly based diets tied to a single degenerative disease. Promoted in books and articles are diets that prevent heart disease, or control adult-onset diabetes, or claim to prevent cancer. Unfortunately, you can't possibly follow different diets simultaneously. This puts you in the odd position of choosing the disease you wish to avoid.

This way of looking at degenerative diseases differs from conventional wisdom, which sees specific dietary indiscretions linked to specific diseases. The idea here is to focus on the nutritional needs of the whole body, rather than focus on diet and a specific disease.

We can use smart nutrition to avoid inner stress and keep body cells working at top efficiency. The reward? You minimize the risk of not just one but all degenerative disease.

Okay, enough theory. What do you do in practical terms? We come back to the question: Just because we have an affluent diet, do we have to accept those degenerative diseases? Certainly not. This chapter asks what it is about modern foods that leads to body breakdown and degenerative diseases.

The answer is straightforward. Modern foods lay five traps that lure you into making poor food choices and consequently stressing your body biochemistry. The longer you remain trapped, the higher your risk of developing one or more degenerative diseases.

This chapter explains the five traps and how to avoid them. In addition, because diet and disease figure so prominently in books and articles, the chapter examines four of the current controversies over the links between diet and degenerative diseases: heart disease, cancer, adult-onset diabetes, and osteoporosis.

Five dietary traps linked to degenerative diseases

Imagine you were a medical student in the early years of the 20th century. Your professors wouldn't spend time teaching about sudden heart attacks—because they were almost unheard of. Doctors spent entire careers never having seen a heart attack victim. That situation rapidly changed as heart attacks and other forms of heart disease became the number one cause of death. Today, according to the American Heart Association, although deaths from heart attacks have dropped due to improved medical care, in absolute terms the overall incidence of heart disease continues to rise. And this is in spite of 40 years of telling the public to avoid saturated fat and cholesterol.

All the evidence points to nutrition as a major link to heart disease. Yet the advice about cholesterol and saturated fat clearly is not working. Why? The advice isolates one component of food—in this case, fat—and makes it the sole dietary focus. The advice to lower saturated fat and cholesterol in the diet and therefore lower the risk of heart disease, by itself, clearly falls short.

You see the same tired, one-note approach in dealing with osteoporosis. Individuals are told to drink milk or take a calcium supplement. The goal is simply to get more calcium into the body. Such an approach doesn't work either, as we will see in a moment. There's much more to stemming osteoporosis than taking in more calcium.

Excessively narrow approaches to dealing with degenerative diseases are doomed to failure. Cancer, heart disease, adult-onset diabetes, and the other degenerative diseases are like a flood threatening to inundate a town. A one-note approach is equivalent to building a section of a dike—it doesn't work. The flood sweeps around it. You have to build a total dike—in other words, a solid nutritional base.

A higher percentage of women today contract breast cancer. Without suggesting that changes in the nature of food are the sole reason for this

Unofficially...
Affluence doesn't have to lead to disease. The Japanese have a high standard of living but still have a life expectancy greater than that of Americans. A Japanese woman's chance of contracting breast cancer is one-quarter of the rate of a woman living in the United States or Canada.

disheartening increase, such changes are certainly part of the story.

From a cell's-eye view, five changes in the American diet during the 20th century have encouraged the rising incidence of degenerative diseases. Each change represents a dietary trap. If you are aware of the traps, they're easy to avoid.

The five dietary traps are:

1. Refined sugars.

2. Refined and bleached wheat flour.

3. Refined vegetable oils.

4. Chemical burden—pesticide and industrial waste residues, food additives, and chemicals from manufacturer processes and from packaging.

5. Shrunken food diversity—the bulk of the American diet is created from soybeans, wheat, corn, and sugar.

If you look at each of these traps in isolation, you might be tempted to ask, "How can sugar or refined flour be a cause of cancer or heart disease?" But don't look at each trap in isolation; think of all five together. Avoiding all five builds a formidable defense against disease.

Trap 1—refined sugars

People love sugar, or to be more exact, they love sweetness. And sugar provides plenty of that. In the United States, the average person consumes per day 4 to 5 ounces of refined sugars, the equivalent of about 25 of those sugar packets restaurants provide for sweetening tea and coffee. When you translate that into daily calories, adults are getting 16 to 20 percent of their calories from refined sugar. This amount is in addition to the natural sugars contained in fruits and vegetables.

People eat more sugar than they realize. It's hidden in canned vegetables, tomato ketchup, salad dressing, pickles, crackers, breads, frozen vegetables, spaghetti sauce, and toothpaste. Then consider all the foods where you expect to find sugar, like jams, sweet cakes, candy, ice cream, and soft drinks.

Why this fondness for sweetness? Thank our caveman ancestors for this heritage. Primitive people foraging for food instinctively felt that sweet-tasting food was safe. They were right. Few sweet foods existing in nature are known to be poisonous. From a cell's-eye view, sweetness also marks the presence of carbohydrates, and that signals nourishment. So when you munch on sweet vegetables, fruits, or grains, the roughly 10,000 taste buds on your tongue register sweetness in the brain.

You may hear the claim that refined sugar is just another carbohydrate, like the starch in potatoes or grains. This is a half-truth. Sugar indeed is a carbohydrate, delivering the same number of calories as other carbohydrates—four per gram. But the truth ends there. Exuberant use of refined sugars in foods subverts the natural connection between sweetness and safety plus nutrition.

Here are three reasons:

■ Refined sugar, as the name implies, is pure sugar extracted from sugar cane, sugar beets, and corn. Sucrose, or table sugar, accounts for 44 percent of the refined sugar consumed in United States and Canada. The remaining 56 percent is refined from corn into either corn syrup (pure glucose) or high fructose corn syrup (HFCS), a mixture of fructose and glucose. These are pure calories. Most of the vitamins, minerals, fiber, and phytochemicals

Unofficially...
Linda Bartoshuk, a researcher in taste perception at Yale University, claims that some people are super-tasters. They need only half the amount of sugar of most people to perceive the same level of sweetness.

of the original cane, beets, or corn have been stripped away. Consider the impact on the body. Refined sugar arrives in the body without any nutrients the body requires to metabolize sugar into energy.

▪ You eat only so much food. Refined sugars replace more nutritious choices and squeeze out foods that promote inner body vitality.

▪ Much of the refined sugar people eat is combined with fat—a seductive combination. We all love the smooth, pleasant "mouthfeel" and taste of the sugar/fat duo in ice cream, cookies, cakes, pies, and pastries. It's all too easy to overindulge, however, because this combination does not trigger the normal signal to the brain that you've eaten enough. It's a sure way to become overweight.

There are ways to avoid the sugar trap. This may take some adjustment in diet, but it would be worth it in terms of weight control, health, and energy. You can avoid the sugar trap by heeding these tips:

▪ Avoid soft drinks. Soft drinks are the biggest single source of refined sugar in the diet. On average, people drink more gallons of soft drinks than they do water. Don't be an average person on this one. In place of soda, try a carbonated water with a twist of lime or lemon.

▪ Control your urge to eat the sugar/fat combo in candy, pastries, and so forth. Consider them as a fun food saved for rare treats. Make fresh fruit your regular dinner dessert.

▪ You can educate your taste buds to less sweet. If you put sugar in your coffee, try putting a little less for a few days, then cut down a bit

Bright Idea
The ultimate way to avoid eating refined sugar is not to buy it or keep it around the house. Instead, keep a jar of honey handy. Honey is much sweeter on a weight basis than table sugar, so you are inclined to use less of it.

more, or add milk. You'll find the coffee taste
just as enjoyable.

- Cut down on low-level foods (quality levels 3
  and 4) that are packaged or highly processed.
  Such products often have added sugar. Check
  the labels.

- If you enjoy ready-to-eat breakfast cereal, read
  the labels. Many, like corn flakes, are loaded
  with sugar.

- When you do add sweetness, use honey. Unlike
  refined sugar, honey brings a roster of nutrients: vitamins E and C, phytochemicals, and
  active enzymes (when not pasteurized).

- Remember the trick that food manufacturers
  use to disguise the amount of sugar in foods.
  By using several different sugars in a food
  product, manufacturers avoid listing the first-
  named ingredient as sugar. They also use a
  variety of substitute terms for sugar.

Trap 2—refined and bleached flours

Refined and bleached flours, of which wheat flour is
the most common, are almost pure carbohydrate.
Like refined sugar, refined and bleached flour
delivers pure calories. Thus, all the nutritional sins
associated with sugar also can be hung on refined
flour. The refined flour doesn't bring with it the
fiber, phytochemicals, vitamins, and minerals the
natural grain once had, components the body
needs. It drains living tissues of their vitamins and
minerals in order for the body to metabolize the
carbohydrate into energy and body tissues.

North Americans eat a lot of refined and
bleached wheat flour: in breads, bagels, cakes,
muffins, pastries, breakfast cereals, and pizza crusts.

Moneysaver
Whole grains satisfy hunger faster than comparable products made from so-called enriched flour. You eat less, yet benefit because you get fiber, phytochemicals, vitamins, and minerals, all packed into fewer calories. You weigh less, feel better, and you save cash.

All the pasta shapes are made from refined and bleached semolina flour. Semolina is made from durum wheat, one of many varieties of wheat. Regardless of variety, nearly all the flours are refined and bleached.

On average, Americans consume $8\frac{1}{3}$ ounces a day of this nutritionally naked carbohydrate, equivalent to $1\frac{1}{2}$ cups of flour—enough flour to fill an empty soft-drink can.

Consider one fallout from eating refined and bleached flours—slow bowel transit time. A person eating whole grains and plenty of fruits and vegetables consumes a lot of fiber; this speeds up the flow of food through the intestinal tract. Transit time for such people is 24 to 48 hours. In contrast, transit time for the average American is 48 to 96 hours. The stop-and-go traffic through the bowel leads to:

- **Constipation.** Fiber absorbs water, making looser, easily passed stools. A compact, dense mass is simply harder to push through.

- **Increased risk of diverticulitis.** The heavy, muscular contractions of the colon necessary to force hard stools along cause the lining of the colon to bulge outwards, creating pockets. These pockets fill with stagnant feces, and in due course the pockets (diverticuli) become inflamed.

- **Increased risk of colon cancer.** Various cancer-causing substances either formed in the bowel or from the diet have a longer time to irritate the bowel lining and initiate a cancer.

- **Increased risk of heart disease.** The only mechanism the body has to eliminate excess cholesterol is to sweep it out the bowel with dietary fiber. Cholesterol clings to the fiber like a magnet, and out it goes. If cholesterol is not eliminated in this way, it is reabsorbed, creating a body overload.

As mentioned in Chapter 3, "Grains, Legumes, and Nuts," a wheat berry consists of three parts: an outer coat that contains fiber and the B vitamins; the germ or embryo that contains essential fatty acids and vitamin E; and the starchy endosperm. The endosperm, containing pure starch, is the berry's food store that feeds the embryo when it germinates.

Modern flour milling discards the bran coat along with B vitamins and the germ, altogether 30 percent of the wheat berry. On top of the refining, flour is treated with chemical bleaching agents which react with fats in the flour, forming unnatural fats such as dichlorostearic acid. This substance, according to the government, is not dangerous. Nevertheless, the chlorinated fat represents another burden imposed on the body, which must detoxify it.

Back around World War II, nutritionists, embarrassed by the nutritional poverty of refined and bleached flour, persuaded the government to restore some of the lost vitamins. Three vitamins—niacin, riboflavin, and thiamin—and one mineral—iron—were added. In the late 1990s one more B vitamin was added—folic acid. This flour is called *enriched* flour, and that is the term you see on the labels of food packages. But don't be misled by the term. Adding the four vitamins and iron doesn't in any way restore the full spectrum of vitamins and minerals, plus essential fatty acids, phytochemicals, and fiber lost in the 30 percent of the wheat berry that is discarded.

Unofficially...
Government nutritionists recognize that enriched flour has lost the full spectrum of vitamins and minerals as well as fiber and phytochemicals. The official nutrition guidelines issued by the USDA say, "Eat several servings of whole-grain breads and cereals every day."

Trap 3—refined vegetable oils

A hundred years ago, added dietary fats (as opposed to fat in meat and milk) came from three animal sources: butter, lard (pigs), and tallow (cattle). That all changed, as described in Chapter 4, "Extracted Fats and Oils," with an almost total shift to fat from plant sources. Say what you will about animal fats— at least they aren't refined. They are consumed as they come from the animal. Vegetable fats, in contrast, are highly refined products.

As a result, the public consumes more:

- **Polyunsaturated fat.** The body stores most of its fat as saturated fat. Thus in dealing with a large dietary intake of polyunsaturated fat, the body, in order to store it, must first convert it—the process is added stress.

  Perhaps more serious is the fact that polyunsaturated fats are vulnerable to oxidation in blood and in cells, creating cancer-causing breakdown products. The body defends with its antioxidants, but a large influx of polyunsaturated fat can overwhelm these defenses. Vegetable fats in their natural unrefined state contain vitamin E, an antioxidant. Refining, however, largely eliminates the vitamin.

- **Trans fats.** During the refining of vegetable oils, the product is partially hydrogenated, an industrial process that creates the unnatural trans fats. (See Chapter 4.) Hydrogenated vegetable oils with their trans fats are widely used in margarine, vegetable shortening, cooking oils, deep frying oils, and retail products from baked goods to peanut butter.

Bright Idea
The major source of the unnatural trans fats in the American diet is potato chips and french fries. Replacing these two items with better choices, like baked chips or a baked potato, eliminates most of the trans fats you encounter.

What happens to the trans fats in the body?
Some of them are metabolized like saturated fat,
Trans fats in effect add to the body's total intake of
saturated fat. Perhaps worse, trans fats mimic essential fatty acids.

These unnatural fats crowd out the essential
fatty acids that normally are built into delicate nerve
structures of the brain and into heart and muscle
tissue. These tissues just don't function as well and
over the years are more vulnerable to breakdown.

Having mentioned these two health negatives,
we should keep in mind the positive features you get
from the unrefined versions of vegetable oils. Olive
oil is an important component of the Mediterranean diet, which has been established to be very
healthful. Several vegetable oils provide omega-6
and omega-3 fatty acids, essential for health and life.

To avoid the trap of refined vegetable oils,
remember to:

- Buy mechanically expressed (pressed), unrefined vegetable oils.

- Avoid any product that contains hydrogenated
  or partially hydrogenated oil.

- Use butter instead of margarine. Margarines
  are highly processed and most are loaded with
  trans fats. However, smart eating mandates butter be used in moderation.

Trap 4—chemical burden

The chemical burden, as outlined in Chapter 13,
"Food Safety: Avoiding Foodborne Illnesses," consists of chemicals that add nothing to the nutritional
value of the food while forcing the body to devote

resources to detoxifying them. In the last 100 years, the chemical burden has skyrocketed with more food additives, and with people eating more foods that contain these food additives. In addition, modern foods contain pesticide residues, industrial waste chemicals, and contaminants from manufacturing and packaging materials.

There also has been an increase in unnatural food ingredients that fall into the category of a chemical burden. An example is modified food starch, a chemically altered starch that has no counterpart in nature. The human digestive system has not evolved the mechanisms to digest it properly. The ingredient also appears on food labels as polydextrose.

Other examples are the chlorinated fatty acids (the dichlorostearic acid produced during the bleaching of flour) and a series of brominated contaminants. Where does bromine come from? Millers treat refined and bleached flour with bromine to make it stiffer so that the baked bread loaf made from it stands rigid. The brominated substances are side-products. None of these ingredients of the refined flour are mentioned on the products label because they result from the manufacturing process. Yet they are present, and your body is forced to detoxify them.

Why does the FDA allow all these chemicals in foods, you might ask, if there is a danger? The answer is that neither the FDA nor the food industry knows if the total burden of the chemicals is hazardous.

The FDA looks at the possible danger of each chemical by itself, as if all the rest didn't exist. For instance, they don't study the entire group of chemical contaminants that you eat in refined and

Unofficially...
In 1999 the EPA carried out its first action under the 1996 Food Quality and Protection Act, banning two organophosphate pesticides—methyl parathion and azinphos methyl. The first is used on fruits and vegetables, the second on sugar cane. The EPA says the ban will make foods safer for kids.

bleached flour. A single chemical contaminant may present a limited danger, but in real life, a person on a standard American diet eats a collection of pesticide residues, industrial contaminants, chemical food additives, and assorted unnatural food ingredients. Neither the government nor industry has ever looked at the long-term effects of that total chemical burden. We do know in general that long-term exposure to such a burden just wears the body down, leaving it vulnerable to degenerative breakdown.

Why take the risk? To avoid this trap, check the unofficial guides to quality levels (Appendix E). Choose foods listed at levels 1 and 2. They are foods carrying the smallest burden of nonnutritional substances.

Trap 5—shrunken diversity

The trap of "shrunken diversity" may seem odd considering that shoppers have access to 30,000 items in the supermarket. Choices galore are offered by restaurants and delis. But despite the number of items available, people have limited themselves to a much smaller number of preferred foods. Let's set aside the dairy and meat cases of the supermarket and look at processed foods, which make up the bulk of people's diets.

When you look at what goes into processed foods from a cell's-eye perspective, the thousands of such foods shrink to four main ingredients.

How is that possible? Food technology takes four agricultural crops and, through chemical extraction and refining, creates raw materials from which all processed foods are made. The following table shows the four basic crops and the derived raw materials used in food manufacturing.

Bright Idea
One way to
increase the
amount of raw
vegetables in
your diet is to
get a juicer. You
can juice most
vegetables
except potatoes
and heavy leafy
vegetables. Just
don't make this
the sole source
of raw vegeta-
bles, because
you lose fiber
and some of the
phytochemicals.
And drink
the juice
immediately—
the juice starts
to oxidize
the instant it is
produced.

TABLE 14.1: THE FOUR BASIC CROPS USED IN FOOD MANUFACTURING

Crop	Raw materials made from the crop
Wheat	Refined and bleached flour, modified food starch
Corn	Corn flour, modified food starch, corn syrup, high-fructose corn syrup, and hydrogenated corn oil
Soybeans	Soy protein isolate, textured vegetable protein, hydrogenated soy oil
Sugar—beet and cane	Refined sugar

This book—as well as the USDA food guide—recommends eating a diversity of foods. Why? No single food provides a full spectrum of vitamins, minerals, fiber, and phytochemicals, plus a balance of protein, fat, and carbohydrates. No one food meets the body's full nutritional needs.

Moreover, agricultural crops are subject to the whims of nature. The nutritional content of crops can vary from farm to farm and from season to season. Carrots you buy this week have slightly different nutritional qualities from those you bought last week. For these reasons, eating a diversity of foods smoothes out inconsistencies, ensuring you higher-level, complete nutrition.

One might argue that a person obtains diversity through fruits and vegetables. Just look at the variety of fresh fruits and vegetables in the produce section of a supermarket. But only 1 person in 10 eats the recommended five servings of vegetables. And for nearly half the population, potatoes (in fact, french fries) are the sole vegetable they eat. Processed foods are the mainstay of the American diet.

For anyone eating mainly processed foods, diversity collapses into the highly processed raw materials of the four crops. Nutritional value shrinks along with diversity.

Avoiding the shrunken-diversity trap is easy. Minimize the amount of processed food in your diet. Increase the diversity of foods you eat by eating a variety of whole grains and patronizing the fresh produce section of your local supermarket.

The five traps: A summary

It's well established that the degenerative diseases listed at the start of this chapter are diet-related. Epidemiological and laboratory studies provide ample evidence of this. But the idea of approaching the diet issues from an integrated perspective is a departure from normal nutritional thinking.

Ask, for instance, what's in the diet that increases risk of heart disease, and you come up with a narrow answer: cholesterol and saturated fat. As already mentioned, telling people to cut down on cholesterol and saturated fat clearly has not worked.

But by integrating heart disease into the common pattern of degenerative disease, you can ask a more effective question: What is it in the way people eat that increases the risk of all the degenerative diseases, including heart disease? The answer: the five dietary traps.

So, having looked at the five traps, we turn to four of the major dietary-linked degenerative diseases. For each disease, a stream of articles and books appears that offer narrow dietary advice for that disease alone. Such advice raises questions about that disease and the diet connection. This next section of the chapter answers frequently asked questions (FAQs) about each of the four diseases within the context of the five dietary traps. We begin with diet and heart disease.

Unofficially...
Many dietary factors influence the onset of heart disease, but nuts seem to be a standout. In one study people who ate nuts five or more times a week had half the number of fatal heart attacks as non-nut eaters. Nuts are no magic panacea, however—they should be part of your all-around healthy diet and lifestyle.

FAQs about heart and diet

If one degenerative disease related to diet seizes the public's attention, it is heart disease. As noted in Chapter 7, "Reading Between the Lines of Nutrition Labels," nutrition labeling of all food packages is geared to heart disease and the theory that saturated fat and cholesterol are major risk factors. You see on every package the amount of cholesterol and saturated fat. Yet, surprisingly, the cholesterol/saturated fat theory is not proven. Moreover, if all you worry about is the amount of cholesterol and saturated fat in food, you can wind up making low-quality food choices. There is more to the heart disease/diet connection than cholesterol and saturated fat.

Here are the FAQs:

1. **Question:** What exactly is heart disease (and stroke)?

   Answer: Ironically, while the heart pumps the entire volume of the body's blood though its chambers, it can't use any of that blood for its own nourishment. The heart needs a constant supply of oxygen and nutrients, which it gets through a separate network of arteries. These arteries, called coronary arteries, thread through the heart muscle. Over the years, plaques consisting of cholesterol and fatty material build up on the inner arterial wall and obstruct the flow of blood. This process is called atherosclerosis. The buildup is gradual, and as a coronary artery narrows the individual experiences pain called angina. A completely blocked artery cuts off the blood supply from a region of the heart muscle. That is a heart attack.

The same buildup of plaques may also occur in arteries of the brain. A blockage of a brain artery causes a stroke.

2. **Question:** What is the cholesterol/saturated fat theory of heart disease?

   Answer: Simply put, the theory states that an excess of cholesterol and saturated fat in the diet causes an excess of cholesterol and fats (triglycerides) to circulate in the blood, causing formation and buildup of those plaques.

   The theory also states that cholesterol and saturated fat in the diet raises blood cholesterol levels. William Castelli, director of the Framingham, MA, Heart Study, sponsored by the National Heart, Lung, and Blood Institute, points out that this is true in a controlled experiment. When patients in a hospital are fed such a diet, their blood cholesterol is indeed elevated. But in the real world of jobs, kids, social life, and exercise, the correlation disappears.

3. **Question:** Does cholesterol have a function in the body?

   Answer: Yes. Every cell in the body needs cholesterol. Cholesterol is a critical part of the membranes that surround each cell. Nerve cells are particularly rich in cholesterol. Without cholesterol, you couldn't think, your muscles would be paralyzed, and your heart would stop. In addition, the body uses cholesterol to make bile acids, needed to digest fat. And your sexual performance depends on the sex hormones made from cholesterol.

   The body makes about 1½ grams of cholesterol a day. If you eat cholesterol in your diet,

> **❝**
> The more saturated fat one ate, the more cholesterol one ate, the more calories one ate, the lower people's serum cholesterol. We found that the people who ate the most cholesterol ate the most saturated fat, ate the most calories, weighed the least, and were the most physically active.
> —William Castelli, director of a lifelong study of some 5,000 residents of Framingham, MA
> **❞**

the body makes less. Only animal foods contain cholesterol; the substance doesn't exist in the plant world.

4. **Question:** What is meant by cholesterol balance in the body?

   Answer: There is a constant flow of cholesterol through body tissues. While the body makes about a gram and a half of new cholesterol every day, it has to get rid of a gram and a half of old cholesterol. The body has only one route to dispose of cholesterol, and that is dumping it into the intestine. The problem is that if the cholesterol is not swept out, it is reabsorbed. It takes dietary fiber—from fruits, vegetables, and whole grains—to prevent reabsorption. So if removal doesn't keep up with body synthesis and whatever cholesterol one might eat, cholesterol builds up in the body.

5. **Question:** Can a lack of balance between intake and outgo of cholesterol contribute to heart disease?

   Answer: The lack of fruits and vegetables in the diet is often cited as contributing to a higher risk of heart disease. The Scots, for instance, have one of the highest rates of heart disease in the world. The high rate has been blamed on the meat and animal fat in their diet. But a closer examination of dietary habits reveals that the Scots also eat few vegetables and fresh fruits. Their main vegetable is french fries, which they call chippies. Rather than blame the cholesterol and saturated fat in their diet for the high rate of heart disease, blame the total diet.

6. **Question:** How critical is cholesterol in the diet?

   Answer: The cholesterol/saturated fat theory says that you should limit the amount of cholesterol you eat. But this advice takes cholesterol out of the context of the food. Eggs, for instance, contain cholesterol, and for this reason people are warned to eat no more than three a week. Yet healthy people can eat two eggs a day, and this does not increase the risk of heart disease. On the other hand, consider margarine, which contains no cholesterol. Many brands contain trans fats, however, and a study from Harvard School of Public Health links the eating of margarine to an increased risk of heart disease. (Whether or not the link is due to the trans fat content is uncertain. All that can be concluded is that there is a correlation between eating margarine and increased risk of heart disease.)

   Practice smart nutrition and look at the merits of the total food rather than making a decision based on one component, like cholesterol.

7. **Question:** How is blood cholesterol linked to the risk of heart disease?

   Answer: This question remains controversial. Some authorities say that at the level of blood cholesterol above 200 milligrams per deciliter of blood, the risk of heart disease increases; other studies question this link.

8. **Question:** Will a low-fat diet save a person from heart disease?

Unofficially...
Frank Sacks, a nutrition professor at Harvard Medical School, wanted to set up a study to check the benefits of the 10 percent fat diet of Dean Ornish. Sachs had to abandon the experiment because he couldn't recruit enough individuals willing to follow the diet.

Answer: As described in Chapter 12, "Sensible Weight Loss Versus Fad Diets," a diet containing 10 percent fat was first promoted by Nathan Pritikin. Pritikin, adhering to the diet, was successful in reversing the course of his own heart disease. The diet has also been promoted by Dean Ornish. The diet is nutritionally sound, but it has one serious problem: With its low fat, the diet is devilishly hard to stick to.

Proponents of the low-fat route make a major mistake. They promote the diet as the only salvation for avoiding heart disease. Not true. The key to avoiding heart disease is to construct a sound diet that suits your temperament and preferred style of eating. If you construct a diet of upper-level foods (quality levels 1 and 2) that skirts the five dietary traps, you minimize the risk not only of heart disease but of the other degenerative diseases.

9. **Question:** Does soy protein help ward off heart disease?

Answer: Studies suggest that about 25 grams (1 ounce) of soy protein a day eaten in a diet already low in cholesterol and saturated fat may help reduce blood cholesterol levels. But soy may present hazards not yet fully explored, like its high content of isoflavones. Moreover, soy protein isolate and textured vegetable protein (a soy product) are highly processed foods that wrap in many food additives and rank at a quality level 4. Tofu, a relatively unprocessed soy protein, is a better choice. If you want legume protein, other dried beans are a healthy choice.

10. **Question:** The Inuit (Eskimos) eat a traditional diet with very little vegetables and fruits,
yet have a low rate of heart disease. How so?

Answer: The advice to eat your fruits and vegetables is given for people living the modern,
urban America. No one here would find the
traditional Inuit diet of raw seal blubber, fresh
blood, raw walrus organs, and raw fish appetizing. Yet, from the Inuit point of view, the diet
was highly satisfying and nutritious. You'd have
to grow up in that culture, however, to accept
this diet.

Nevertheless, we can learn from their traditional diet, which is high in protein and fat
and rich in cholesterol. One concern about
eating a high-protein diet is the ability of the
body to dispose of the large amount of the
sulfur-containing amino acid, methionine. To
handle methionine, the body needs plenty of
vitamin B_6 (pyridoxine). Otherwise a breakdown product of methionine, homosysteine,
builds up. Excess homocysteine has been
linked to heart disease. This is no problem for
the Inuit, because raw meat contains a large
amount of vitamin B_6.

Move south to urban America, however, and most meat is cooked; this destroys
about half the vitamin B_6. So urban peoples
have to rely on other sources for vitamin B_6—
vegetables and whole grains. Refined and
bleached flour has lost 90 percent of its original vitamin B_6. This vitamin is not one of the
vitamins added back to "enriched" white flour.

The relation between methionine, vitamin
B_6, homocysteine, and a possible link to heart

Watch Out!
Women who eat
little cereal fiber
but a lot of
white bread,
pasta made from
enriched
semolina, white
rice, potatoes,
and sugary soft
drinks greatly
increase their
risk of develop-
ing adult-onset
diabetes.

disease is only part of the picture. But the relation demonstrates the complex linkages between different components of the diet and degenerative disease. The practical lesson is not to think about a single link, like cholesterol and heart disease, but about your total diet and lifestyle. Avoid the five dietary traps, and get plenty of exercise.

FAQs about cancer and diet

Cancer is an all-pervasive disease in our modern society. Yet most cancers are caused by environmental factors under one's control. Environmental contaminants form part of those factors. Smoking accounts for a third of all cancers. Diet accounts for a large fraction of cancer deaths.

You can really cut down the risk of cancer in your life by avoiding the five dietary traps. Take fruits and vegetables, for instance. A study conducted by Gladys Brock at the University of California, Berkeley, School of Public Health found that people who ate generous portions of fruits and vegetables had half as much cancer as those who ate few of these foods. Just think: If everyone in the country started eating more fruits and vegetables, the cancer rate could fall by half!

Fortunately, we have a lot of answers to how diet relates to cancer. The fruit-and-vegetable connection is one. Here are other FAQs about cancer and diet:

1. **Question:** Why does avoiding the five traps reduce one's risk of cancer?

   Answer: Here's why:
   - By avoiding refined sugar, you eliminate naked calories devoid of the vitamins and

minerals the body needs. Dropping
refined sugar from your diet puts less
stress on the body, improves overall metabolism, and toughens immune defenses.

■ Avoid refined and bleached flour. By eating whole grains, you obtain vitamins, minerals, fiber, and phytochemicals. Your body
metabolism works more effectively, and the
antioxidant action of the fiber and phytochemicals blocks initiation of cancers.

■ Avoid refined vegetable oils. These oils
with their high polyunsaturated fat content
drain the body's antioxidant reserves. You
need antioxidants to stop cancer from
starting.

■ Avoid a high chemical burden.
Combinations of chemicals such as pesticide residues and waste industrial chemicals wear down the body's defenses against
cancer. You reduce exposure to chemicals
in your foods by choosing level 1 and 2
foods. Buy organically grown produce and
other foods to reduce the pesticide burden
your body has to deal with.

■ Pursue food diversity. Minimize processed
foods in your diet. Eat whole grains,
legumes, nuts, and a variety of fruits and
vegetables. This way you ensure getting a
full spectrum of all the nutrients the body
needs. Your pumped-up immune defenses
work at top efficiency and block cancers
before they start.

2. **Question:** Does alcohol increase the risk of
cancer?

Unofficially...
Classical nutri-
tion has focused
on vitamins,
minerals, pro-
tein, fats, and
carbohydrates.
We now realize
this is only a
partial view of
the complex rela-
tion between
diet and health.
Phytochemicals,
fiber, and other
components of
whole foods we
are just now
becoming aware
of are proving
important in pre-
venting chronic
diseases such as
cancer.

Answer: The American Cancer Society says that risk of cancer goes up with alcohol consumption. The higher risk may start with as little as two drinks a day: 24 ounces of beer, 10 ounces of wine, or 3 ounces of 80-proof distilled liquor. The Society notes that women who are at unusually high risk for breast cancer should consider abstaining from alcohol.

3. **Question:** In avoiding the five dietary traps, are there particular foods that help lower the risk of cancer?

   Answer: When choosing a variety of whole grains, fruits, and vegetables, include these:

   - Dried beans (except soybeans)
   - Sweet peppers
   - Green tea
   - Flaxseed (freshly ground)
   - Broccoli and the other cruciferous vegetables (cabbage, brussels sprouts, cauliflower, kale)
   - Tomatoes (canned when higher-quality fresh ones are unavailable)
   - Dark leafy vegetables
   - Olive oil
   - Garlic
   - Apples
   - Grapes
   - Oranges
   - Strawberries

4. **Question:** Does being overweight increase the risk of cancer?

   Answer: Yes, overweight people have a higher incidence of several cancers, including colon,

Bright Idea
To lower your risk of cancer, replace white rice with brown. Instead of eating an ordinary muffin, choose a whole-wheat muffin. Instead of eating white bread, choose whole grain. Instead of eating corn flakes for breakfast, choose oatmeal or shredded wheat. Instead of eating a regular cracker, choose a whole-grain cracker. In every choice you eat more fiber, more vitamins and minerals, and more phyto-chemicals.

breast, and endometrium. But you have to ask: Does cancer result from the mere fact that the person is overweight or from the cause of his or her overweight condition? People become overweight and obese generally because they eat a high proportion of calorie-dense foods, those high in fat and refined sugar (cakes, pies, cookies, ice cream, french fries), plus low-quality level meats and dairy quality levels 3 and 4. These are the foods that bait the dietary traps and, moreover, these folks generally aren't eating much fruits and vegetables. Overall, their nutrition is poor.

A study of some 4,000 individuals of England and Scotland who grew up in the 1930s found that persons who ate more fruits and vegetables as kids had less cancer as middle-age adults. Stephen Frankel, an epidemiologist at the University of Bristol, England, who conducted the study, points out that the fruit-and-vegetable-eating kids ate fewer cakes and cookies and were more slender than kids who eventually succumbed to cancer.

5. **Question:** Does red meat increase the risk of cancer?

Answer: A team led by Walter Willett of the Harvard School of Public Health studied 89,000 nurses in their mid years. Those nurses who ate beef, pork, or lamb daily had two-and-a-half times the rate of colon cancer as women who ate red meat less than once a month. Colon cancer ranks second as the cause of cancer deaths.

However, we need to be cautious about interpreting such a finding. The study doesn't go into detail, like hamburger versus steak or cured ham versus fresh ham, or whether or not red-meat eaters eat fewer fruits and vegetables. There may be something to the red-meat connection. But in your own meal planning, place this information in the overall context of avoiding the five dietary traps. If you eat red meat, do so in moderation and, above all, choose cuts in the quality levels 1 and 2. (See Chapter 5, "Meats, Fish, Poultry, and Eggs.")

FAQs about adult-onset diabetes

The American Diabetes Association warns of a near epidemic of Type II diabetes, also called adult-onset diabetes, as the baby boomer generation slides into their mid-50s and 60s. This disease generally occurs in older and overweight persons. But for the first time, diabetes clinics are seeing teenagers who have always been overweight being diagnosed with adult-onset diabetes. In fact, about 90 percent of those with adult-onset diabetes are overweight. Some 15 million persons in the United States have been diagnosed with diabetes, 90 percent with adult-onset diabetes.

Individuals with diabetes have a heightened risk of:

- Heart disease.

- Stroke.

- Kidney disease.

- Blockage of blood flow in limbs, leading to amputation.

- Blindness.

The following are FAQs about adult-onset diabetes and how it can be prevented or controlled through what you eat:

1. **Question:** What is diabetes?

   Answer: The disease centers on the hormone insulin. When you eat food, the carbohydrate portion enters the blood as glucose (blood sugar). The issue is the speed at which the carbohydrate enters the blood. Foods with refined sugar and flour are digested and enter the blood more quickly. The blood glucose level starts to rise, and in response, the pancreas secretes insulin into the blood. The insulin release signals the liver and other tissues to absorb glucose and convert it to fat. The important point: The blood is cleared of excess glucose.

   In some forms of diabetes, the insulin signal doesn't work and the glucose blood level rises dangerously high.

2. **Question:** What is the difference between Type I (juvenile) and Type II (adult-onset) diabetes?

   Answer: Juvenile diabetes, as the name implies, strikes before an individual becomes an adult. It is an autoimmune disease in which the body's own immune system attacks and destroys the islet cells in the pancreas, which produce insulin. These individuals no longer produce insulin, so every day they must take insulin shots to control blood glucose level. Juvenile diabetes has a hereditary component and appears to be unrelated to diet.

   A person with adult-onset diabetes, in contrast to the juvenile form, produces insulin, but the body tissues that normally absorb glucose are unable to respond. The cells of these tissues have receptors that bind the insulin and in this way receive the signal to get busy and absorb blood glucose. The receptors don't work. We say the person is insulin resistant.

More recently, some researchers prefer to use the distinction between insulin-dependent and noninsulin-dependent types of diabetes.

3. **Question:** How is adult-onset diabetes connected to diet?

Answer: Individuals who contract adult-onset diabetes are invariably, although not necessarily, overweight. Researchers find that persons who consume white bread, pasta made from enriched flour, sugary soft drinks, and other high sugar foods are at high risk. The high sugar snacks and soft drinks over the years provoke excessive insulin swings that gradually wear down the receptors in the liver and other tissues that respond to insulin. The individual thus gradually becomes insulin resistant. Furthermore, the general stress on the body's metabolic systems imposed by excess weight makes the body insulin resistant.

4. **Question:** What is the glycemic index?

Answer: This index measures the speed with which a carbohydrate enters the blood. The faster the entry, the higher the index. Fast entry of glucose into the blood provokes a strong insulin release from the pancreas. This is what happens when a person eats a candy bar or drinks a soft drink on an empty stomach. The insulin causes the blood sugar to drop to abnormally low levels. The individual feels listless, irritable, and often irrational.

But the glycemic index only works for single foods. The index is valuable to investigators in a laboratory but has no value in the real world of people eating mixed meals. As mentioned in Chapter 12, some diet advisers, misunderstanding this limitation of the glycemic index, mistakenly use it to construct diets.

5. **Question:** What changes in the diet are necessary to control adult-onset diabetes?

   Answer: First, avoid the five dietary traps. Second, eat level 1 and 2 foods. You still have much latitude in choice of foods that satisfy the way you like to eat. Remember overall to eat a balanced diet of fruits, vegetables, whole grains, and quality meats and dairy or legumes. Third, exercise vigorously for an hour or so every day, or at least three to four times a week. Regarding weight, it isn't necessary to embark on a special weight-loss program. Follow the first three recommendations and weight will automatically adjust to a lower level.

FAQs about osteoporosis and diet

Osteoporosis is a degenerative disease in which the inner structure of the bone literally dissolves away. The bones become less dense and less able to support weight or the normal physical movements of the body. The result: The bones fracture.

One's skeleton is set by age 30, and from then on there is gradual loss of bone density. For women, the loss accelerates after menopause. This is the normal life course but, for individuals with osteoporosis, the loss of bone mass is excessive. Once osteoporosis sets in, there is no effective treatment.

The answer to osteoporosis, then, is prevention. What can diet do? Here are the FAQs:

Watch Out!
A stress fracture in an athletic teenage girl may be a sign of osteoporosis. Girls who participate in dance, figure skating, and gymnastics where a lithe figure is held desirable are most likely to suffer this problem.

1. **Question:** Why don't big doses of calcium correct osteoporosis?

   Answer: The hard mass of a bone is composed of a complex mineral structure based on calcium. But this structure is not static. Although we talk about the skeleton being "fixed" by age 30, don't think of the skeleton as a fixed structure, like a set of steel girders.

   Bones are living, like all other parts of the body. Bones are constantly breaking down and being rebuilt. Biochemists call this process *remodeling*. At any one time, 10 percent of your bone mass is being remodeled. Calcium enters bones and calcium leaves. In the healthy person, calcium's entry and departure remains in perfect balance. The bones don't get bigger, and they don't get smaller, except for minute, yearly decreases due to normal aging.

   In the individual with osteoporosis, calcium departs faster than it enters. Consequently, there is a net loss of bone mass. The reason for the imbalance in calcium's entry and departure is rooted in some deep-seated biochemical problem. Thus, taking big doses of calcium doesn't solve the fact that more calcium leaves the bones than is normal. The best way to correct the problem of excess calcium loss is to adjust the whole diet. Avoid the five dietary traps and raise your dietary sights to foods that rank at levels 1 and 2.

2. **Question:** Is milk a good source of calcium?

   Answer: Yes, milk is a good source, but so are green leafy vegetables and other vegetables. There is nothing magic about milk as a source of calcium. The important thing in preserving one's bones is to maintain a steady intake of calcium.

3. **Question:** Are calcium supplements helpful?

   Answer: Nutrition authorities recommend that a healthy person get about 1,200 milligrams of calcium a day. The problem is that many individuals don't eat foods containing calcium. Teenagers in particular drink soft drinks rather than milk. They eat snack foods and hamburgers and shun vegetables. The government estimates that the average American gets about 450 milligrams of calcium a day.

   Under these circumstances, a calcium supplement may be helpful, but a better solution is to improve the diet. There is more to bone structure than calcium. Magnesium is just as important. Vitamin D (sunlight) is important. A calcium supplement is a one-note approach to a complex disorder. That's why the superior route is to fix your diet. Avoid those five dietary traps.

4. **Question:** Can you consume too much calcium?

   Answer: Yes. Too much calcium is just as undesirable as too little. Your total intake, food plus supplement, should not exceed 2,000 milligrams. Too much calcium leads to

   ■ Kidney stones (if you are predisposed).

   ■ An abnormal heartbeat.

   ■ Diminished kidney function.

5. **Question:** When does prevention of osteoporosis start?

   Answer: From conception on. One's bone structures are laid down during childhood until early adulthood. A good set of solid,

Unofficially...
According to the Osteoporosis and Related Bone Diseases National Resource Center, osteoporosis threatens 28 million Americans, eight out of ten of whom are women.

high-density bones at this stage of life mini-mizes the risk of osteoporosis later in life. In particular, teenage girls falling into the dietary traps and getting little exercise undermine the future of their skeletons.

The five dietary traps: A wrap-up

66

Human life is the outcome of…man's ability to choose between alterna-tives and to decide upon a course of action. —René Dubos, Bacterologist, formerly at Rockefeller University

99

The anticancer diet, if you will, is the same as the anti-heart-disease diet, the anti-osteoporosis diet, and so on. This is the beauty of looking at the total bundle of degenerative diseases. One diet resists the whole bundle. You go to the root problem and tune up your body biochemistry, beef up immune defenses, and slow the aging process. Do this, and you lower your risk not only of one but of all of the degenerative diseases.

Construct a diet that avoids the five dietary traps by doing the following:

- Choose quality foods ranking at levels 1 and 2 .
- Choose whole-grain breads, pastas, crackers, and other baked goods.
- Don't eat foods with refined sugar and refined white flour.
- Double the recommended servings of fruits and vegetables. The USDA dietary guidelines suggests five a day of vegetables. Eat 10, includ-ing raw vegetables like a salad. Eat two or three pieces of fresh fruit every day.
- Diversify the foods you eat. This means actual foods, not different packaged foods made from the same ingredients.
- If you eat meat and dairy, eat in moderation and choose quality level 1 and 2 products.

- If you follow a vegetarian regimen, include legumes, but vary them over the course of the week.

- Follow a prudent balance of protein, fat, and carbohydrates.

- Don't forget regular exercise—an hour or so a day, or at least three or four times a week.

A diet based on these recommendations avoids the five dietary traps. The diet is nutritionally sound and automatically sheds excess pounds. The diet is relatively high in carbohydrates, moderate to low in fat, and provides a recommended amount of protein.

Finally, some practical advice: We live in a real world. The foods you might like to buy may not be available all the time. Family schedules may make food shopping erratic at times. To stretch your budget, you may want to stock up on specials. One has to be realistic and make educated choices. The purpose of this book is to provide you with the information so you can indeed make those educated choices.

Just the facts

- Several degenerative disease are diet related, including cancer, heart disease, atherosclerosis, stroke, adult-onset diabetes, osteoporosis, and obesity. All these diseases are a manifestation of some deep-seated biochemical breakdown in the body.

- The nutritional goal is to construct a diet that goes to the root of the problem and reduces the risk of the whole bundle of degenerative diseases.

- Five dietary traps increase the risk of all these degenerative diseases. The traps include refined sugar, refined and bleached flour, refined vegetable oils, excess chemical contaminants, and a lack of diversity in diet.

- Avoid these five dietary traps by choosing quality level 1 and 2 foods in all categories. Eat a variety of whole grains, and fresh fruits and vegetables. Diversify your food choices, and eat a prudent balance of protein, fat, and carbohydrates.

GET THE SCOOP ON...
Symptoms of allergies ▪ Testing for allergies ▪
Recognizing allergens in processed foods ▪
Emerging problems for allergic people ▪ Why
organic foods minimize the problems

Dealing with Food Allergies

A food allergy is caused by the body's immune system reacting to a food or food component. We call the substance that triggers an allergic reaction an *allergen*. The body's immune system recognizes the allergen as foreign and produces antibodies to halt what it considers an invasion. The reaction to an allergen is more like an overreaction, because as the battle rages to fight the allergen, immune cells release powerful chemicals, including histamine. It is these chemicals circulating in the blood that cause the allergic symptoms. The most common are:

- Rhinitis (runny nose)
- Swelling of the lips
- Stomach cramps
- Vomiting
- Diarrhea
- Hives

■ Eczema

■ Swelling of the airways, causing wheezing and coughing

Most allergic reactions to foods occur within a few minutes to a few hours and are relatively mild. A small percentage of individuals with food allergies, however, suffer a severe reaction called *anaphylaxis*. This is a life-threatening situation. When anaphylaxis happens, several symptoms in different parts of the body occur simultaneously. The throat swells and the individual has difficulty in breathing. The condition may lead to cardiorespiratory arrest and shock.

In most cases of anaphylaxis, symptoms go away or are reversed by treatment with epinephrine (adrenaline)—the so-called "epi" shot.

The National Institutes of Health estimate that about 2 percent of the adult population suffers food allergies. About 5 percent of young children suffer some type of food allergy, although many outgrow allergies to common allergens, such as milk and eggs, by age 5.

Almost any food can cause an allergic reaction in someone, somewhere. About 80 percent of all food allergies, however, are triggered by eight foods:

■ Eggs

■ Fish

■ Milk

■ Peanuts

■ Crustaceans (lobsters, crabs, shrimp, other shellfish)

■ Soy products

■ Wheat

■ Tree nuts, such as walnuts

Bright Idea
Individuals who are allergic and parents with an allergic child should get online. The Internet has several sites with valuable information and support groups. You can have your name put on an e-mail list for receiving product alerts. (See Appendix B for resources.)

Children do not outgrow allergies to nuts, legumes, fish, and shellfish. Fruits and vegetables also can cause allergic reactions, but not as commonly as these eight. When kiwi fruit was introduced to the United States some years ago, many reported allergic reactions to it.

No medicine, vaccine, or treatment exists that can prevent an allergic reaction. The only recourse an individual has is to avoid the allergen.

In this chapter, we look at food allergies from the practical side, dealing with allergies in the midst of the rapidly changing ways foods are manufactured and marketed.

How do you know if you have a food allergy?

Knowing whether or not you have a food allergy requires intelligent sleuthing. Many people try to self-diagnose, believing they have allergic reactions to certain foods or food ingredients.

Regrettably, self-diagnosis can easily be made in error and lead individuals to restrict foods they mistakenly think are causing an allergy. In fact, in some cases the symptoms the person believes to be due to a food allergy are due to some other condition. If you have persistent symptoms you believe are related to food, see a qualified healthcare professional for proper diagnosis.

Many reactions to foods are not true allergies but food poisoning or food intolerance. Some people, for instance, are intolerant to the milk sugar lactose. The problem is caused by lack of the enzyme, lactase, in the gut, and has nothing to do with the immune system. We say these individuals are lactose intolerant.

Watch Out!
Food ingredients masquerade under often vague names. What does "modified food starch" mean? In fact, the starch can come from wheat, corn, tapioca, potato, or other starchy crops. You can't tell from the label.

True food allergies may be diagnosed by a simple skin-prick test. The suspected food is placed on the skin and the skin is pricked to allow the food to mix with blood. Or the food may be injected directly under the skin. A bump (wheal) that develops within 20 minutes indicates a positive response.

The skin test is often not very helpful in detecting an allergen. A more elaborate and reliable test is called the double-blind test. This test avoids the possibility that the patient or the healthcare professional conducting the test anticipates a positive reaction and records a false positive.

In the double-blind test, a third person puts the suspected food or substance in a capsule or hides it in a food. The third person may also give the patient a capsule with a placebo, an inert substance. The test is called double-blind because neither the healthcare professional nor the patient know which capsule or which test food contains the suspected allergen. After tests are completed, the "code" is broken, and the patient and healthcare professional can decide if symptoms are correctly related to the allergen.

FAQs about food allergies

The following are frequently asked questions about food allergies:

1. **Question:** As an adult, will I outgrow a food allergy?

   Answer: Although young children may outgrow egg and milk allergies, adults are not likely to. You should assume that as an adult you will not outgrow the allergy. Immune systems have long memories and, although by avoidance you are not exposed to the allergen for

Timesaver
Food ingredients appear on different product labels under different names. The Food Allergy Network (www. foodallergy.org) provides small laminated cards listing all the names of food ingredients for common allergens.

decades, a chance exposure can set off the allergic reaction.

2. **Question:** Will I get more allergies?

   Answer: It's possible. Sometimes when a principle allergen is removed from the diet, other allergens previously masked become apparent.

3. **Question:** Will my children inherit my allergies?

   Answer: There is a genetic component to allergies. Not all your children will inherit your allergies. When one parent is allergic, the child has a 50 percent chance of becoming allergic. However, if both parents suffer from allergies, the chance may be 100 percent. There is a practical issue. If a parent is allergic to certain foods, then the family meals may never include that food. The children, whether or not they have the allergies, grow up eating the same restricted diet of their parents and therefore are never exposed to the allergen.

4. **Question:** Do food additives cause allergic reactions?

   Answer: Many additives such as aspartame, monosodium glutamate (MSG), and food dyes have been studied. People may suffer adverse reactions to these chemicals, but their "bad" reactions do not appear to involve the immune system. For someone who reacts to such additives, of course, whether the reactions are allergic or not doesn't make any difference. The experience is equally unpleasant. (We'll discuss adverse reactions to food additives later in the chapter.)

5. **Question:** Is someone allergic to peanuts allergic to peanut oil?

Bright Idea
While it may be impractical to ban allergens from schools, the International Food Information Council Foundation has a couple of suggestions. The school can establish allergy-free tables in the cafeteria and prohibit lunch swapping.

Answer: The actual allergen in peanuts is most likely to be a protein. Most commercial peanut oil is extracted from peanuts using industrial solvents. The oil is refined, bleached, and deodorized—processes that leave virtually no protein in the oil. Research shows that individuals allergic to peanuts usually can use the refined peanut oil without experiencing a reaction. Thus they can eat processed food cooked with or containing the oil. The allergic individual, however, should avoid the less-processed gourmet brands of oil. These less-refined products contain some of the peanut proteins.

The same can be said for individuals allergic to soy. They probably can manage with the highly refined brands of soy oil.

The downside of this situation is that the nutritional value of highly refined vegetable oils ranks at the bottom of the quality levels scale, level 4. The less-refined oils rank at level 1 or 2.

You can use unrefined olive oil, which is not likely to be allergenic, and thus take advantage of its higher nutritional quality.

6. **Question:** Should allergenic foods, like peanuts, be banned from school?

Answer: Allergy authorities feel that banning an allergen from schools is not practical, because it is difficult to enforce. What's more, trying to render the school cafeteria safe for allergic children has its downside—the children have less incentive to learn how to take care of themselves. No environment can be rendered 100 percent safe, and the best defense against exposure is a child who understands the allergy and knows how to avoid exposure.

7. **Question:** Are corn or chocolate allergies really allergies?

Answer: True allergies to corn or chocolate are rare. Although many people claim to be allergic to corn or chocolate, allergy specialists are unable to prove an allergy using double-blind tests. There are probably several explanations for adverse reaction to corn or chocolate. An allergic reaction to corn may, for example, be due to a reaction to soy. Corn products are often carried and handled in the same equipment as soy products and thus become contaminated. Minute residues of soy may be enough to set off the allergic reaction.

An allergic reaction to chocolate may be due to some ingredient added to the chocolate or a substance carried over from the manufacturing process, rather than the chocolate itself.

8. **Question:** What is asthma?

Answer: Asthma is a chronic condition in which an irritant triggers a swelling of tissues in the air passages to the lungs, making breathing difficult. Irritants include dust, pollen, animal dander, and cigarette smoke. In about 8 percent of children and 2 percent of adults with asthma, foods trigger an attack.

Dairy intolerance: Lactase deficiency or allergy?

Milk can cause awkward and uncomfortable symptoms for one of two reasons: an allergy to a milk protein, usually casein, or an intolerance to the milk sugar, lactose. A true milk allergy generally shows up in infants,

Watch Out! Although cooking or canning renders fruits and vegetables nonallergenic, this is not true for the "big eight" allergenic foods. They remain allergic after heating and other forms of food processing.

and many infants outgrow the allergy by age 3. Lactose intolerance, on the other hand, doesn't usually appear until after age 3 and lasts a lifetime.

Lactose intolerance due to lactase deficiency

The human gut is unable to absorb lactose. Since all humans start out life drinking milk, nature provides the gut with an enzyme called *lactase*. Lactase splits lactose into two simple sugars, glucose and galactose, both of which are absorbed into the bloodstream.

In most cultures of the world, the need for lactase soon disappears. Older children and adults do not drink milk. Certainly in prehistoric times, milk drinking beyond infancy was unlikely. Thus, in terms of genetic heritage and in the interests of body efficiency, the gut stops making lactase after age 3. It is a question of body resources. Why devote energy to making an enzyme which is a protein and which is no longer needed?

Human beings, however, are a diverse lot. Those humans who settled in northern Europe and successfully developed a culture based on raising cows retain lactase throughout their adult lives.

North Americans who have a genetic heritage stemming from northern Europe retain their lactase. Native Americans and people whose heritage stems from Asia, Africa, and southern Europe are less likely to retain lactase into adulthood and thus become lactose intolerant.

This is just a general pattern; there are no absolutes. Moreover, lactose intolerance depends on the amount of milk ingested. Lactose-intolerant individuals may be able to handle small amounts of fluid milk without incurring symptoms.

Symptoms of lactose intolerance begin a half hour to two hours after eating or drinking foods that contain milk. The person experiences bloating, gas, abdominal cramps, nausea, and often diarrhea.

The reason for these symptoms is a matter of intestinal chemistry. The undigested lactose passes down the small intestine and into the large intestine (colon). There, bacteria convert lactose to short-chain fatty acids and two gases, carbon dioxide and hydrogen. The gases cause the colon to bulge, creating a feeling of bloating. The short-chain fatty acids cause water to flow into the large intestine, which leads to diarrhea.

How do you know symptoms are due to lactose intolerance?

Not everyone who claims to have lactose intolerance is a true sufferer. Other problems may cause similar symptoms. A simple test exists, however, to determine if the individual is lactose intolerant. A person experiencing difficulty in digesting lactose has hydrogen on the breath: Some of that hydrogen produced in the colon is absorbed into the blood and exhaled through the lungs.

If you suspect you might be lactose intolerant, you can have the test done at a health clinic. You ingest a known amount of lactose and afterwards exhale into a device that collects your breath and measures the amount of hydrogen. The test shows to what degree you are intolerant. The more hydrogen on the breath, the more intolerant you are.

Milk allergy is not intolerance

An individual allergic to milk experiences the same intestinal distress as that of a person with lactose intolerance. In addition, the allergic person may suffer rhinitis—an inflammation of the nasal passages—as well as dermatitis.

Unofficially...
Persons who normally digest milk without difficulty may become lactose intolerant due to disease. Some illnesses and intestinal infections create a temporary intolerance to lactose. The intolerance disappears when the individual gets better.

The allergens in milk are the proteins, casein, and whey protein. *Casein* is the protein that curdles and ends up in all the cheeses. *Whey protein,* as the name implies, remains in the whey, the fluid left over after milk curdles.

Both casein and whey are major food ingredients, used in a large variety of different food products, including breads, cakes, rolls, candies, cookies, cream fillings for snacks and confections, potato products, gravies, cream pies, and sausages. Whey is used as a fat replacer in some foods. If you're trying to avoid these milk products, you'll have to read labels.

Cooking does not diminish the allergenic potential of milk proteins, and may, in fact, increase their activity.

Timesaver
If in doubt about a food product, contact the food's manufacturer. The product label carries a phone number or an address.

Dealing with wheat allergies

Individuals allergic to wheat can still enjoy traditional breads and other baked goods using a variety of substitute flours. The following table lists some of the flours you can use.

Some people are allergic to specific proteins in wheat other than gluten. Thus, they can eat gluten-continuing grains. Other people are unable to tolerate the gluten well and so must avoid all grains that contain gluten. *Gluten* is the protein that gives bread dough its elasticity, providing the cell structure that allows the carbon dioxide from yeast to make the dough rise.

Gluten is also an issue for individuals with Celiac Sprue. The lining of their small intestine reacts to gluten and other components of grain including carbohydrates, and sloughs off. Without this lining, the intestine is unable to absorb nutrients. Celiac Sprue can occur in people from infants to older folk.

TABLE 15.1: FLOURS THAT CAN SUBSTITUTE FOR WHEAT FLOUR

Almond	Sorghum
Amaranth	Poi
Buckwheat	Potato
Cassava (tapioca)	Quinoa
Chestnut	Rice
Chickpea	Soy
Flaxseed	Teff
Hazelnut	Water chestnut
Jerusalem artichoke	Sweet potato
Kuzu (Kudzu)	Wild rice
Legumes, like peas, lentils, beans	Yam
Malanga	Lotus
Millet	

Note that barley, kamut, oat, rye, and spelt contain gluten. Individuals not allergic to gluten can use these grains as wheat substitutes.

(Source: Marjorie Hurt Jones, R.N., Mast Enterprises, Inc.)

Tracking your allergens can be a problem

Once foods that cause you an allergic reaction have been identified, the next task is to learn where the foods occur and how to avoid these foods. This is not an easy task, and it is only getting harder. Severe allergic reactions are becoming more common.

Keep in mind that the merest trace or whiff an allergen can set off an allergic reaction in some people. The foods they eat must be scrupulously clean of the offending allergen.

The obvious tactic in avoiding allergens is to check product labels. But labels are not infallible. Here are four reasons why:

Watch Out!
Allergies in some people are so severe that even minute amounts of the allergen triggers an allergic reaction. Some individuals allergic to wheat cannot tolerate wheat particles floating in the air, let alone eat any wheat-containing product. Other individuals allergic to shrimp become sick from just taking a few breaths of steam coming from a pot in which shrimp are cooking.

1. The manufacturer unintentionally leaves off the label an allergy-producing food used as an ingredient. According to Steve Taylor, codirector of the Food Allergy Research and Resource Program at the University of Nebraska, undeclared allergenic foods are the major cause of products recalls.

2. Manufacturers change formulations of products using different ingredients or different sources of the ingredients. You may know from experience that a certain product is safe to you, but without warning, the same product can suddenly cause an allergic reaction because of an ingredient change.

3. Shared equipment is another issue over which allergic individuals have no control. Manufacturers produce products in batches using the same equipment. A pasta maker, for instance, makes a batch of egg-containing pasta. The equipment is not adequately cleaned before making a run of no-egg pasta. The product is labeled and sold as "egg-free." Yet traces of egg remain in the product sufficient enough to cause an allergic reaction in susceptible individuals.

The following industries are among those that frequently use the same equipment to make several different product lines:

- Ice cream
- Cereal
- Confectionery
- Baked goods
- Soups
- Potato chips

Unofficially... Persons sensitive to one food often are sensitive to similar foods. Persons allergic to soy products, for example, often are allergic to other legumes.

4. Allergens pop up in unexpected places. You wouldn't expect a blueberry muffin to be a problem for someone allergic to soy. But those "blueberries" you see in the muffin have never been near a blueberry bush. They are, in fact, manufactured from dyed soy protein isolate to give the texture of genuine blueberries.

The fake soy "fruits" include cherry, apple, orange, and the spice cinnamon. You find them in bagels, nut breads, pound cakes, muffins, pancakes, waffles, cookies, ice cream, candies, cereals, donuts, trail mix, salad garnishes, and frozen desserts.

Soy products appear in many processed foods, and their presence is not always noted on the label. They might, for example, be hidden in that catchall phrase "natural flavors."

Persons allergic to wheat might be surprised to find wheat as an ingredient of crunchy, fake nuts, such as almonds, cashews, pecans, and walnuts. The fake nuts are used as toppings for nut logs, sundaes, pralines, and chocolates. They may appear in candy bars, popcorn, candies, brownies, fruit cakes, nut pies, sticky buns, and donuts.

Dining out

Trusting food preparation to others is always a risk. Even when assured that the ingredients of a dish are accurately described, the danger of cross-contamination in the kitchen remains. For example, restaurants often fry different foods in the same deep-fry oil. An order of french fries might contain traces of fish—a disaster to someone allergic to seafood. Or an ordered hamburger patty might be lifted with a spatula used previously to lift a cheeseburger—bad news for the milk-allergic individual.

Still, a person with allergies should not be denied the pleasures of dining out. Here are five tips that may make the evening out safer:

Bright Idea
If you are peanut sensitive, avoid Southeast Asian restaurants. If you are corn sensitive, avoid Mexican restaurants. And if you are wheat sensitive, avoid Italian restaurants.

1. Dine locally: You may be able to find a trustworthy restaurant. If the staff gets to know you, they'll be happy to meet your needs.

2. For a new restaurant, call in advance, preferably at a nonrush hour, and speak to the manager, owner, or chef to explain your problem. Ask them to suggest something they can prepare that suits your needs.

3. If dining out with a group on a social occasion, bring your own meal. Have the kitchen staff heat it and serve it along with the others. This way you can enjoy the occasion without fuss.

4. Most chain restaurants, including fast-food chains, on request provide a list of ingredients of the foods they serve. You can check for allergens. These chains generally have central factories where the food is prepared and then shipped to individual restaurants. You are eating factory-produced food with the possibility of inadvertent cross-contamination. On the other hand, the same food is shipped to all restaurants in the chain. If you find a chain that is reliable, you can patronize the chain in different towns with some assurance of safety.

5. Patronize an upscale restaurant. It may be pricey, but the restaurant has a live chef who prepares dishes from scratch. You can ask to have your meal prepared in a clean pan or on a clean grill.

Food additives that cause adverse reactions

As already mentioned, some substances cause a set of symptoms that can be similar to allergic reactions and just as devastating. Because these reactions to an ingested substance don't involve the immune system, they are categorized under the general term *adverse reactions*. Chemicals used in paint, perfumes, toiletries, cleaners, plastics, and food can cause these adverse reactions. Individuals who react to such chemicals are said to be chemical sensitive.

Some 3,000 chemicals are used as food additives, but of this number only a handful have been identified as causing adverse reactions in sensitive people. According to the American Academy of Allergy, Asthma, and Immunology, only nine chemical additives have been reported to cause adverse reactions in sensitive people; these are listed in the following table.

TABLE 15.2: FOOD ADDITIVES THAT MAY CAUSE ADVERSE REACTIONS

Additive	Purpose
Aspartame	Sweetener
Benzoates	Preservatives
BHA, BHT	Antioxidants
FD&C Dyes	Colorants
MSG	Flavor enhancer
Nitrates/Nitrites	Preservatives
Parabens	Preservatives
Sulfites	Preservatives

(Source: American Academy of Allergy, Asthma, and Immunology)

Let's take a closer look at these chemical additives, including where they are found and the types of adverse reactions you might expect. In listing the reactions, it should be noted that this is an ongoing area of research and that the link between chemical and adverse reaction is not always clear-cut.

- **Aspartame.** This substance is an artificial sweetener known under its brand name, Nutrasweet. Adverse reactions to aspartame, which is used in diet soft drinks and foods, are rare and reported to involve swelling of the eyelids, lips, hands, or feet.

- **Benzoates.** Benzoates, either as sodium benzoate or potassium benzoate, are a common preservative used in foods including baked goods, cereal, chocolate, dressings, fats, licorice, margarine, mayonnaise, powdered milk, oils, powdered potatoes, and dry yeast. True allergic reactions are rare.

- **BHA/BHT.** BHA (butylated hydroxyanisole) and BHT (butylated hydroxytoluene) are antioxidants widely used in processed foods that contain a fat or oil. You find these chemical additives in margarine, breakfast cereals, and salad dressings. People sensitive to BHA and BHT suffer hives and other skin reactions. True allergic reactions are rare.

- **FD&C Dyes.** The Food, Drug, and Cosmetic Act of 1938 approved a variety of dyes used in foods and beverages. They are identified on products labels by the phrase FD&C followed by a color and number. Sometimes the name of the dye is included on the food label. The permitted dyes include: Red #2, Amaranth; Red #3, Erythrosine; Red #40, Allura red; Yellow #5, Tartrazine; Yellow #6, Sunset yellow; Blue #1, Brilliant blue; Blue #2, Indigotine;

Green #3, Fast green. These chemical dyes manufactured from coal tar are used either singly or in combination to produce every color and hue imaginable. They are found in practically all types of processed foods. For example, Sunset yellow (Yellow #6) is permitted in bread, butter, ice cream, milk, jams, jellies, pickles, relishes, icing sugar, liqueurs, sherbet, smoked fish, lobster paste, caviar, tomato catsup, deli meats, anchovies, and shrimp.

Although the FD&C dyes are not allergens, they can cause similar symptoms in sensitive individuals. Of the dyes, FD&C Yellow #5 (tartrazine) seems to be the most prominent cause of symptoms.

■ **MSG (Monosodium glutamate).** MSG itself doesn't have much flavor, but like salt it intensifies other flavors. Asian cooking is well known for its liberal use of MSG, and reactions to MSG are often associated with this type of cooking. However, this association is misleading, because food manufacturers and restaurants also use it widely. You'll find it, for instance, in breaded, deep-fried chicken. MSG has a bad image in many people's minds, so manufacturers hide its presence under label terms such as "hydrolyzed vegetable protein." People sensitive to MSG report headaches, nausea, diarrhea, sweating, chest tightness, and a burning sensation along the back of the neck. Asthmatic reactions to MSG are rare.

■ **Parabens.** Parabens are a class of preservatives that include methyl, ethyl, propyl, and butyl parabens. They are used as preservatives.

Watch Out!
Nitrates and nitrites are widely used as preservatives in processed meats such as hot dogs, bologna, and salami. These chemicals may cause headaches and possibly hives in some individuals.

Sensitive individuals can suffer severe contact dermatitis or redness, swelling, itching, and pain of the skin.

▪ **Sulfites.** Sulfites go under a variety of names, including sulfur dioxide (SO_2), sodium or potassium sulfite, bisulfite, and metabisulfite. These chemicals are used to preserve foods, stabilize natural colors in dried fruit, and sterilize bottles used in wine making. Sulfites can be found in many foods, including baked goods, teas, condiments and relishes, processed seafood products, jams and jellies, dried fruit, fruit juices, canned and dehydrated vegetables, frozen and dehydrated potatoes, and soup mixes. They are also found in alcoholic beverages such as beer, wine, wine coolers, and hard cider.

Sulfites may cause reactions such as breathing difficulty, chest tightness, hives, abdominal cramps, diarrhea and vomiting, lowered blood pressure, light-headedness, weakness, and a rapid pulse. Sulfites also may trigger asthma attacks in sensitive asthmatics.

At one time restaurants sprayed a sulfite solution on the fresh items in their salad bars. The FDA received so many reports of adverse reactions from people dining in restaurants that in 1986 it banned the practice. Diners often have a glass of wine, and the sulfite both in the salad and in the wine was enough to set off an adverse reaction.

The problem of ingesting sulfite from several sources still exists. Sulfites appear in many foods, and eating two or three foods with sulfites might be enough to cause an adverse reaction. Check labels. The FDA requires that all foods containing more than 10 parts per million of any sulfite have to be labeled.

Transgenic foods (genetic engineering)

Industrial agriculture has taken a giant leap with the new technology of genetic engineering. Technologists introduce genes across species barriers. These genetically engineered plants and animals are called *transgenic.*

A gene from the Brazil nut, for example, has been inserted into a variety of soybeans. Brazil nuts contain many different proteins, only some of which are allergens. It turns out that the transgenic gene in this case includes Brazil nut allergens. If this variety of soybeans becomes widely used, persons allergic to Brazil nuts will have to guard against eating any soy product. As mentioned earlier, because product labels provide no information about ingredients that are transgenic, the consumer has no way of knowing whether or not the Brazil nut soy ingredient is present.

Here is a partial list of other transgenic crops and animals now on the market in the United States:

- Catfish, farmed
- Canola (rapeseed)
- Cheese-making enzymes
- Corn
- Cottonseed oil
- Potatoes
- Prawns, farmed
- Salmon, farmed
- Soybeans
- Tomatoes

Unofficially...
The FDA maintains a list of foods that contain allergenic substances. Food products that contain these allergenic ingredients must declare them on the label. In addition, chemicals, such as FD&C Yellow #5 (tartrazine) and sulfites, are on the list. If these substances are present in a food product but not listed on the label, the product is subject to recall.

"
The growth of agricultural biotechnology products [transgenic] is anticipated to continue at a tremendous pace, even accelerate with new products.
—*Chemical and Engineering News* (April 19, 1999)
"

Practically every commercial crop, fruit, and vegetable is being genetically engineered, and the transgenic varieties will soon make their way into products in your local supermarket.

Companies in the business of developing transgenic varieties are well aware of the issue of transfer and creation of new allergens. But it is impossible to identify or to predict in advance all the possible allergens that might be created.

Individuals with allergies should be aware of this trend. The genetically engineered crops taking over American agriculture present a new set of hurdles.

How to upgrade nutrition and avoid allergens

For a person with allergies, the number one priority is avoiding allergens. This goal has to take precedence. But interestingly, as you move up the quality nutrition scale, avoiding allergens becomes easier. The reason is straightforward. Difficulties in allergens arise mainly from processed foods. There are problems with unlabeled ingredients that are allergens, problems of cross-contamination, and problems of ever-changing manufacturing processes.

Foods ranked at level 1 and 2 on the quality nutrition scale either are unprocessed or minimally processed. These foods are "in the open," with no hidden ingredients. You know what you're getting.

If you buy a solid piece of meat—a steak or roast, for example—it ranks on level 1 or 2 (see Chapter 5) and you have a piece of meat, nothing more. Buy hamburger (level 3) or sausage (level 4), however, and you have meats with added ingredients that you can't be sure of. Restaurants, for example, often mix in cheaper soy-based textured vegetable protein (TVP) with the hamburger. You get inferior nutrition and a greater risk of unknown exposure to an allergen.

The same problem exists with deli meats, which are mostly made from chunked and reformed meat. They contain chemical binders, emulsifiers, and often meats from other animals. Chicken meat, for example, winds up in pork sausage.

The same can be said for all categories of foods. The lower they rank on the quality nutrition scale, the greater the risk of an unpleasant surprise.

One direction you ought to consider is going organic. Organically grown produce is free of chemical pesticide residues. Organically raised meats come from animals not injected with hormones or fed antibiotics to accelerate growth. In short, you have foods containing fewer chemicals, so there is less chance of invoking chemical sensitivities.

Organic farmers and manufacturers of organic products avoid using transgenic varieties. Products such as cereals, soups, sauces, and canned goods are made without chemical additives. You won't find artificial preservatives, artificial colors or flavors, refined sugars, or MSG. This reduces the chance of unexpected exposure to an allergen.

Organic produce and goods are slightly more expensive, but in terms of high nutritional quality and low risk of an allergic reaction, they offer a bargain. Mainstream supermarkets now carry such products, and most towns and cities have a natural food store or co-op.

Bright Idea
When traveling by air, take a prepared meal with you in an ovenproof container. Aircraft do not carry microwave ovens, but do use convection ovens. The flight attendants are usually happy to heat the meal for you.

Just the facts

- A food allergy occurs when the body's immune system reacts to a food or food component. The substance triggering an allergic reaction is an *allergen*.

- The "big eight" foods that provoke 80 percent of all allergic reactions are eggs, fish, milk, peanuts, crustaceans (lobsters, crabs, shrimp, other shellfish), soy products, wheat, and tree nuts, such as walnuts.

- About 2 percent of adults and about 5 percent of children suffer food allergies. Many children outgrow allergies to milk and eggs by age 5. Allergies to peanuts, fish, legumes, and nuts are for life.

- Some people develop adverse reactions to chemicals in food products. These reactions are not true allergies but are equally devastating.

- For individuals with allergies, the only recourse is avoidance of the food. But the allergenic ingredient is not always listed on the product label, and can enter the product through cross-contamination.

- Eating foods ranked at levels 1 and 2 of the quality nutrition sale reduces the chance of unexpected exposure to an allergen.

The Art of Smart Nutrition

PART VI

GET THE SCOOP ON...
Why kids don't like the taste of fruits and
vegetables ▪ The key nutrient for brain development in the fetus ▪ Why breast-feeding is best
for baby ▪ Why fast foods drag down the
immune defenses

Teen Health Starts in the Womb

Chapter 16

You are a child only once—and a fetus only once. One's nutritional experiences through the fetal stage and through childhood are cast in the adult body. For better or worse, much of your adult health pattern can be traced back to nutrition during these early years.

It behooves parents, therefore, to give their children nutrition that builds not only physically strong bodies but robust health. Parents prepare their children for life by encouraging a well-rounded personality, supplying them with a good education, and possibly saving up an inheritance. But while material advantages are showered on their children, nutritional development receives less attention than it deserves.

The reasons for this neglect are diverse and have been touched on in previous chapters. Lifestyles are changing—there is less time spent in the kitchen while access to finger foods of minimal nutritional merit, fast foods, and take-out foods are growing. Overall, the trend is to let others do the cooking, and in effect others decide our nutrition. Even though children don't go hungry in these times, their nutrition often simply falls through the cracks.

Your child deserves a superior nutritional inheritance. This chapter provides tips and ideas on how to upgrade your child's nutrition.

A fetus deserves mom's nutrition

Bright Idea
Think of pregnancy as extending back in time, months before conception. Prepare your body and make food choices accordingly.

Nutrition of a fetus begins long before conception. Nutritional preparation of the body before pregnancy is as important as nutrition during pregnancy. It's like training to be good at a sport. You whip your body and skills into shape in advance of competition. Likewise, the inner body, through nutrition, has to be nurtured to a high standard of readiness for the most complex of all biological processes, the creation of a life.

Individuals already eating a high-quality diet, including fruits and vegetables, are already prepared. Others, for whom pregnancy becomes an incentive to upgrade nutrition, need to start upgrading months or even years ahead.

Eat upper-level foods

The key to satisfying the fetus's nutritional needs is to eat a balanced diet selected from upper-level foods. Upper-level foods are those ranked at quality levels 1 and 2. In Part II, quality levels were described in detail. The following table summarizes the quality levels of the different food categories.

The concept behind choosing upper-level foods listed in the table above is really very simple. As we've discussed, each choice gives you maximum nutrition for that particular food category. The choices provide ample flexibility in constructing a

TABLE 16.1: UPPER-LEVEL FOODS
(QUALITY LEVELS 1 AND 2)

Food Category	Level 1	Level 2
Vegetables	Fresh, raw (preferably organic)	Fresh, lightly cooked (some vegetables, such as potatoes, need to be cooked)
Fruits	Fresh, raw (preferably organic)	Frozen
Fruit juices	Freshly squeezed	Premium juice in dated carton or bottle
Breads	Whole wheat, whole wheat with other whole grains (preferably organic)	Whole wheat mixed with unbleached, white flour
Pasta	Fresh, whole grain	Dry, whole grain
Corn and corn flours	Sweet corn on the cob, fresh	Whole-corn flour (unbolted), masa, blue-corn flour
Dried beans	Organic dried beans, lentils, peas, soaked and home cooked	Nonorganic beans, lentils, peas, soaked and home cooked
Nuts	Nuts in the shell, raw	Nuts, preshelled, raw
Peanut butter	Peanuts, freshly ground	Peanuts, ground (nothing added) and packed in their own oil
Olive oil	Extra virgin, mechanically expressed, low temperature	Virgin, or extra virgin blended with solvent-extracted olive oil
Vegetable oils	Mechanically expressed (cold) and unrefined	Cold pressed, unrefined
Meat	Meat from free-range, organically raised animals	Lean steaks, pork chops, broiled or grilled; beef and pork roasts, baked
Poultry	Free-range, organically raised chickens and turkeys, grilled, broiled, or roasted	Fresh chicken and turkey, grilled, broiled, or roasted
Eggs	Fresh eggs, free-range, organic hens	Commercial eggs (look for those rich in the omega-3 fatty acids)
Fish	Wild sea fish, fresh, broiled, grilled, baked	Farm fish, fresh, broiled, grilled, baked
Fluid milk	Milk from organically raised cows	Pasteurized, nonhomogenized milk

balanced diet that suits your personal preference. You can lean toward meat and dairy, vegetarian, Mediterranean diet, or some other style.

If you aren't sure about constructing a balanced diet, the USDA Food Guide Pyramid is a good place to start. This guide makes the grain group the foundation, with the fruit-and-vegetable group the second tier. Preferably the tiers should be reversed, with fruits and vegetables as the foundation. Why? Although upper-level choices within the grain group provide an excellent spectrum of nutrients, the fruit and vegetable groups provide an even more varied spectrum, particularly those all-important phytochemicals. With this in mind, a balanced diet would look like the one in the following table.

TABLE 16.2: A SUGGESTED BALANCED DIET, FEATURING FRUITS AND VEGETABLES

Food Group	Serving Size
Vegetables (excluding potatoes)	6–10 servings. Vegetables with main meal, for example, should cover $1/3$–$1/2$ of the dinner plate.
Fruits	2–4 pieces a day
Grains, pasta (including potatoes)	4–8 servings (1 slice of bread, $1/2$ cup cooked brown rice or pasta, $1/2$ cup of potatoes all equal 1 serving)
Meat or legumes and nuts	2–3 servings (Meat the size of 2–3 packs of cards, 1–$1^1/2$ cups cooked dry beans, the amount of nuts you can hold in one hand— about $1/3$ cup all equal 1 serving)
Dairy: milk, yogurt, cheese	2–3 servings (1 cup of milk or yogurt, $1^1/2$ ounces of quality cheese equal 1 serving)
Sweets and added fats or oils	Sweets: Avoid or use sparingly. Use small amounts of added fats like salad oil or butter.

Individuals sensitive to dairy products can adjust the size of the other groups accordingly.

Eating for two

The growing fetus has a demanding list of nutrients it must have in order to develop. The nutrients come both from the mother's diet and from her bones and tissues. This is one reason why the mother-to-be should be nutritionally prepared for pregnancy long before conception. Here's something else you might not normally think of. During pregnancy, in addition to baby, you are creating a brand-new organ, the placenta. Mother's and baby's bloods do not mix. The placenta (which weighs about a pound) transfers nutrients from mother's blood into the baby's blood, and in the reverse direction transfers waste products from baby to the mother's blood. This exacting process works wonderfully well when the mother is properly nourished. So to have a super pregnancy and create that super baby, keep these additional tips in mind:

- A weight gain of 25 to 30 pounds is considered normal. The gain should be slow during the first trimester, accelerating in the second and third trimesters. Along with weight gain comes increased appetite. The pregnant woman can eat additional food above normal diet equivalent to 150 calories during the first trimester and 350 calories during the next two trimesters.

- Nausea in the first trimester may be minimized by eating smaller meals more frequently.

- Don't drink any alcohol whatsoever. Also avoid tea, coffee, and cola drinks (discussed below).

- Nature, anticipating the increased calcium and iron needs of baby and mother, causes the intestinal tract of the pregnant woman to absorb these minerals more efficiently. A

Bright Idea
Take a tip from wild monkeys. Katherine Milton, a professor of environment policy and management at the U.C. Berkeley, studied the eating habits of Panamanian wild monkeys. The animals selected fruits and other foods rich in vitamin C, calcium, and omega-3 fatty acid. The latter nutrient is almost absent in American diets, yet is absolutely essential to the growth of the brain.

nonpregnant woman, for instance, absorbs about 10 percent of the iron she eats. During pregnancy, absorption doubles. Individuals eating a balanced diet of upper-level foods will get plenty of both minerals in their foods.

■ Follow the guidelines outlined in Chapter 8, "To Supplement or Not to Supplement Is No Longer the Question," for taking antioxidant vitamins and other supplements. Vegetarians should be sure to include a vitamin B_{12} sublingual supplement.

■ Persons eating a balanced diet of upper-level foods will get more than enough protein. Incidentally, the extra protein needs of pregnancy (about 14 grams) are met by 2 large eggs, 2 ounces of cheddar cheese, 2 8-ounce glasses of milk, 2 ounces of meat, 2 ounces of walnut or other nuts (a small handful), or 1 cup of cooked, dry beans.

The fetus creates a brain

The fetus does a superb job of creating the wonderfully intricate nervous system and brain. All the neurons an individual has for life are created during the third trimester of fetal development and the first 6 months of life. In fact, by the time of birth, the baby's brain consumes 60 percent of its energy. Of all the organs, the brain takes top priority. This fact has special significance in the mother's nutrition, because the principle building blocks of the brain are the essential fatty acids, the omega-6 and omega-3 fatty acids described in Chapter 4, "Extracted Fats and Oils."

Of the two classes of essential fatty acids that build neurons, the omega-3s are the critical ones,

Watch Out!
If for any reason a healthcare provider recommends calcium supplements, avoid bone meal and dolomite. Both these sources contain lead, a poison that decreases the mental acuity of the baby.

and the scarcest in the average diet. Small amounts are found in eggs and meat. Fish contain more. Plants make only one member of the omega-3 class, linolenic acid. The baby's brain, however, uses two other omega-3s, EPA (eicosopentaenoic acid) and DHA (docosohexaenoic acid).

DHA, especially, is one of the most prominent fatty acids in the brain and in the eye's retina. What does all this mean in terms what you should eat? Do the following:

- Avoid sunflower, safflower, and corn oils. Also minimize use of or avoid canola, grape, cottonseed, corn, and soy oils. All these oils contain a high percentage of omega-6 fatty acid. While this substance is an essential fatty acid, the diet already provides plenty of it. The problem is that excess amounts of the omega-6 fatty acid restricts the baby's body from converting linolenic acid into EPA and DHA. Your best bet is olive oil for salads and cooking or peanut oil for cooking.

- Eat 2 to 3 tablespoons of freshly ground flaxseed every day. A coffee grinder works well. Sprinkle on cereal. Most plant foods contain small amounts of omega-3 fatty acid, but flaxseed is the richest source.

Bright Idea
If you eat eggs, look for special brands that contain a high level of omega-3 fatty acids. The chickens are fed flaxseed. The eggs have various trade names but the word "omega" or "three" generally appears in the name.

If you eat a balanced diet of upper-level foods, stick to olive and peanut oils, and supplement with flaxseed. If it could talk, the fetus would thank you for giving it the omega-3 building block for a superior brain.

While we are on the subject of diet and brain, what about other sources of the omega-3 fatty acids? There are two obvious sources, but both present problems for the mother-to-be:

- EPA and DHA supplements are sold, but these two substances are unstable and vulnerable to oxidation, which creates toxic by-products. So not only can't you be sure that the material in the capsule offers any benefit, but the toxic by-products may in fact harm the fetus.

- Fish are a rich source of all the omega-3 fatty acids, including generous amounts of EPA and DHA. You might think that all you need do is eat fish a few times a week. But fish present a dilemma. Fish are at the end of industrial waste pipes. Many species, especially freshwater and inshore species, are badly contaminated with toxic chemicals; this offsets the benefits of the fishes' omega-3 fatty acids. Government advisories, in fact, suggest pregnant women steer clear of fish, or at the most eat one fish meal per month. (See Chapter 5, "Meats, Fish, Poultry, and Eggs," for a fuller discussion of this issue.) So use discretion in buying fish.

What about the old standby, canned tuna? Canned fish has about the same amount of the omega-3s as the fresh fish. Canned tuna, for instance, is a source of DHA, but the amount is not large. You'd have to eat $6^1/2$ 6-ounce cans of tuna to get an amount of DHA equivalent to the omega-3 fatty acid (linolenic) in 2 tablespoons of flaxseed.

The fetus detoxifies contaminants poorly

The developing brain takes top priority during the fetal stage of life. Other organs and body systems don't fully develop until later. One system that waits until later—later in childhood, to be exact—is the body's ability to deal with substances that are poisonous (toxic).

Human adults have body systems that destroy toxic substances or transport them to the urine, where they are excreted. The fetal systems are still in a rudimentary stage. The fetus, to put it bluntly, is wide open to chemical assault.

The most feared result of such an assault is a birth defect. But toxic chemicals inflict other types of less obvious damage. For instance, they can interfere with the wiring (neural network) of the brain, interfere with sexual development, and possibly create a hidden vulnerability to cancer later in life.

For all these reasons, the mother should protect her fetus as much as possible. Consider the following steps:

- Eat as many foods as possible that are certified organic. Eating such foods cuts down the pesticide residues you ingest, sparing the fetus. Keep in mind that the Environmental Protection Agency, alarmed by the pesticide load babies and young children currently bear, is reviewing all pesticides used in agriculture.

- Give up tea, coffee, and cola for the duration of the pregnancy. Caffeine is a drug, a possible agent for birth defects.

- Be aware that many drugs, both prescribed and over-the-counter, may cause birth defects. Consult your healthcare provider.

- By eating upper-level foods, you avoid processed foods and their chemical additives. None of these additives has been studied for harmful effects on children and fetuses.

The overall objective is to minimize the fetus's total exposure to toxic substances. Think of it as providing a clean environment in the womb.

Unofficially... David M. Ferguson and L. John Horwood of Christchurch School of Medicine studied the academic achievement of 1,000 New Zealand school children. Kids who were breast-fed as infants scored higher on standardized math and reading tests and, in general, did better in school than formula-fed kids.

Breast is best

Let's say you weigh 130 pounds and are growing as fast as a baby. How much do you think you'll weigh within 1 year? The answer: You'd be a 400-pound gorilla.

It's not surprising that a baby needs a huge quantity of high-quality nourishment to maintain a growth rate that triples its size in the first year. And breast milk by far does the best job for baby. Modern nutritional science has been unable to re-create a substitute with the qualities of mother's milk. The American Academy of Pediatrics, long an enthusiastic endorser of breast-feeding, in 1997 came out with the recommendation that mothers breast-feed for 1 year—longer if mother and baby want to.

The human breast is a remarkable organ able to create a product fine-tuned to the baby's nutritional and health needs of the moment. Here are some of the advantages of breast-feeding:

- The milk provides all the nourishment the baby needs for the first 6 months of life.

- Breast milk provides the essential fatty acid, DHA. The baby may not be able to manufacture DHA from linolenic acid fast enough to keep up with brain development, so a supply from mom is essential.

- Colostrum, the clear, sticky milk produced immediately after birth, is full of antibodies designed to protect the infant. The milk thereafter continues to provide baby with antibodies. Breast-fed infants have fewer infectious diseases and bouts of diarrhea than bottle-fed babies.

- Breast milk contains powerful anticancer proteins. Activated in the stomach, they help destroy defective cells, preventing them from turning into cancers.

As for mother's nutrition, she should consume 600 to 800 extra calories a day. Eat the same diet consumed during pregnancy, just in increased quantities. It will contain all the nutrition that goes into the milk. The body has wonderful ways of adapting to lactation. For instance, during the first 3 months the milk draws calcium from mother's bones. When the baby is older and the mother no longer nurses, the bones recover their lost structure.

Infant formulas, an alternative to breast milk

The American Academy of Pediatrics, in ranking mother's milk the best nourishment for babies, ranks at a distant second infant formulas based on cow's milk. Formulas based on soy protein came in third. One reason is that soy protein quality is not on the same level with cow's milk protein. Soy-based infant formulas are made from soy-protein isolate, a processed food product. On a quality level scale of 1 to 4, soy-protein isolate falls to level 4. Perhaps the most controversial feature about soy-protein isolate is the high isoflavone content. As noted in earlier chapters, soy isoflavones mimic the sex female hormone, estrogen.

An infant fed only a soy-based formula may be exposed to a level of estrogen several times higher than a level known to change the menstrual pattern of adult women. There is an uncertainty about the long-term effects of such early exposure to a potent hormone.

Soy-based infant formula, nevertheless, finds favor with parents whose child doesn't seem to tolerate cow's milk. But according to Susan Baker, a professor of pediatrics at Medical University in South Carolina, true lactose intolerance as opposed to a temporary reaction due to an intestinal infection is far rarer than commonly thought.

> " Breast-fed babies have a 60 percent less chance of developing an ear infection and are 80 percent less likely to develop lower respiratory infections. [Breast-feeding] significantly lowers the risk of food and airborne allergies. It means more time cuddling with mother, less crying.
> —American Academy of Pediatrics "

The bottom line for parents is to follow the American Academy of Pediatrics' ranking: breast milk by far the best, cow's milk formula second, and soy-based formula bringing up the rear.

Feeding your infant solid foods

Babies can start on solid food, if ready, at age 4 to 6 months. In choosing the raw foods to prepare baby's food, follow the same principles in choosing adult food—stick with upper-level foods.

The following recommendations (Table 16.3 on the following page) for feeding infants solid food come from drkoop.com Children's Health Center. This is an online Web site with practical information of feeding children of all ages. The site can be accessed at www.drkoop.com.

Be sure to introduce baby to a wide variety of fruits and vegetables. Prepare the food yourself. Lightly cook vegetables and puree or mash them. Raw fruits can be pureed or mashed. You can buy an easy-to-use food mill especially for this purpose. Keep it at the table and whatever the family is eating, baby can eat as well.

In preparing baby's food yourself, you have full control over quality. Commercial baby food may include chemical thickeners, sugar, and salt. Expose your child to the full nutrition and full taste of freshly prepared fruits and vegetables, not a sweetened concoction that has been deteriorating for goodness knows how long in a warehouse and on a supermarket shelf.

Taste preference: Two directions

In introducing baby to new foods, keep in mind that the child is an open and empty notebook ready to

TABLE 16.3: SUGGESTED SOLID FOODS FOR INFANTS

4–6 months	2–3 tablespoons of iron-fortified rice cereal twice a day; introduce other iron-fortified infant cereals gradually, as well as pureed fruits and vegetables, one at a time
6–8 months	Mashed vegetables and fruits
	Infant breads and crackers
	Up to 2–4 ounces of diluted, 100 percent, premium-quality juice fortified with vitamin C (no orange juice until 12 months)
8–10 months	Soft-cooked fruits and vegetables
	Finely cut or blended meats, fish, chicken, cheeses
	Plain yogurt, chopped tofu, egg yolks, cooked and pureed legumes (e.g., beans, peas, lentils)
	Breads, pasta, brown rice
10–12 months	Continue to introduce a wide variety of no-sugar foods; puree, blend, or chop as needed
12 months	Whole cows milk to replace infant formula

(Source: Dr. Koop's Children's Health Center—www.drkoop.com)

This information is not intended to be a substitute for professional medical advice. Consult a qualified healthcare provider for specific advice about your child.

Watch Out!
Nursing mothers should not attempt to lose weight gained during pregnancy. This is a time when any shortfall in nutrition would be reflected in the quality of the milk.

receive written taste preferences. Likes and dislikes are established at an early age. In fact, for breast-fed infants, the flavors of mothers' food come through in the milk and are already channeling the child's taste preferences.

A child's taste preference is set in preschool years and, for modern children, preferences take one of two directions:

■ A well-rounded palate that welcomes the subtleties and variety of tastes inherent in unprocessed fruits, vegetables, whole grains, dairy, and meat products. These are foods ranked at quality levels 1 and 2.

■ A narrow range of tastes centered on salty, sweet, and fat—the processed foods of quality levels 3 and 4.

It seems that of the two directions, the second one is winning—overwhelmingly. Janet Bode, in her book *Food Fight: A Guide to Eating Disorders for Preteens and Their Parents*, describes a survey of 87 Brooklyn, NY, schoolchildren ages 11 to 13. Bode found that the children on average ate 4.7 servings of fruits and vegetables. Pretty good? That's not per day. It's 4.7 servings per week.

Of the 87 kids,

■ Seventeen ate no fruits and vegetables whatsoever, except french fries

■ Nine ate only one serving of fruits and vegetables per week

■ Thirty-nine ate five or fewer servings of fruits and vegetables per week

■ One child ate three servings of fruits and vegetables per day—that was the maximum any child reached

Much of what the children ate that qualifies as a serving of fruits and vegetables came from processed fruit juice. Most of them ate nothing that contains fiber. Moreover, few ate dairy products. Thus, the calcium they missed in vegetables was also missed in dairy. Their preferred beverages were tea, coffee, and soft drinks. Their preferred foods were pizza, burgers, potato chips, and other highly processed foods.

This is only one small study, of course, but many other studies, including a countrywide nutrition survey conducted by the federal government, confirm these disquieting results.

Bright Idea
According to the USDA, kids drink too much soda, more than the water they drink. Kids, however, like the fizz. Mix sparkling water (low sodium) with premium or freshly squeezed fruit juice.

At this early stage in life, the children had already fallen into the five dietary traps described in Chapter 14, "Holistic Nutrition Against Cancer, Heart Disease, and Other Degenerative Diseases." As a reminder, these traps are

1. Refined sugars.
2. Refined and bleached wheat flour.
3. Refined vegetable oils.
4. Chemical burden—pesticide and industrial waste residues, food additives, and chemicals from manufacturing processes and from packaging.
5. Shrunken food diversity.

The five dietary traps lead to premature degeneration of one or more body systems. That degeneration can start early in life. Low-quality nutrition at this age weakens immune defenses and sets the child up for health problems later on.

In a practical sense, by the time the child is 11 or 12, peer pressure becomes important. The kids want to eat what everyone else is eating—burgers and pizza. Nevertheless, if at an early age they have been exposed to a variety of fresh fruits and vegetables, whole grain products, and upper-quality meat and dairy products, that ingrained taste preference should dominate in food choices.

Food preference starts in the home

This brings us back to the preschool age and how to encourage a taste preference for foods that avoid the five dietary traps.

Taste preference starts in the home. Parents set the standard. You can't expect children to eat differently than their parents; if parents shun fruits and vegetables, the children will, too. In that

Watch Out!
TV ads lure kids
to salty, high-fat
snacks. Children
are overwhelmed
by ads telling
them that fries
and high-fat
snacks are good
for them. They
are also encour-
aged to snack
while watching
TV. A study of
160 school kids
in New York
found that the
more children
watched TV, the
more fat they
consumed.

Brooklyn school study, the children said they learned about nutrition from their parents. One assumes their low-level eating pattern reflected their home-eating style.

In any event, let's think positively. Here are suggestions for broadening your child's interest and taste in a variety of foods:

■ Keep a bowl of fresh fruit in a handy, child-level location. For infants and toddlers, place cut pieces of fruit or grapes in front of them at mealtimes.

■ If you give the child fruit juice, freshly squeeze it or buy premium grade. Avoid juice drinks, and don't overdo the juices. Remember that juice provides little or no fiber compared to the whole fruit.

■ Start your children on whole-grain breads and baked goods. They will henceforth find the refined, bleached, and cottony breads tasteless.

■ Start young children with raw pieces of peppers, zucchini, cucumber, cauliflower, broccoli, and other vegetables. Children love dips such as hummus, yogurt, cheeses, and bean puree.

■ Don't start children on french fries. Almost half their calories come from fat, which includes a high percentage of the unnatural trans fats.

■ If meat and dairy are part of the family regimen, start your child on quality products. Quality does not include ice cream, wieners, sausages, commercial hamburger, and luncheon meats. They all fall into the lower quality levels 3 and 4. See Chapters 5 and 6 for more detailed information about quality choices.

- Check for two things on the nutrition label of ready-to-eat breakfast cereals: grams of sugar, and whether or not the grain is whole. Select a breakfast cereal that has zero grams of added sugar and that is made with whole grain. Beware of misleading claims like a honey-nut cereal that has more sugar than honey. Don't believe the package headline that says "lightly sweetened" or "low in fat." Read the label for the exact information.

- Don't let your child pick the breakfast cereal. Supermarkets stock the highly sugared, low-quality cereals on lower shelves—child height. You'll find quality cereals on the upper shelves.

- Add sliced banana, berries, or other fruit to the child's cereal.

- For alternative breakfast suggestions, try poached egg on whole-grain toast or melted cheddar cheese on whole-grain toast.

Here are more tips for lunch:

- Make a sandwich for lunch with whole-grain bread, and a selection of turkey slices, sprouts, onions, and grated carrots and/or zucchini. Use mustard or go light on the mayo. For a hearty eater, include a slice of Swiss-style cheese (not American or processed cheese). Make sure the turkey slices come from solid turkey meat, not a chunked and reformed, emulsified turkey breast.

- Make a vegetarian sandwich with whole-grain bread, hummus or cheeses, lettuce, tomato, sprouts, and onion.

- Make the standard peanut butter and jelly sandwich, made with whole-grain bread, a jam

Unofficially...
Kids who eat a quality breakfast perform better at school. They are more alert, able to concentrate better, and are less prone to seek a vending machine to satisfy their hunger with a salty, high-fat or sugary snack. They save time and enjoy school more because they work more efficiently.

in which the first named ingredient is fruit, and unhomogenized peanut butter (make sure the peanut oil is not replaced with a cheap, "filler" oil).

- When at home, make a tuna salad sandwich with lots of veggies, such as celery, onions, grated carrots, and fresh tomatoes wrapped in a whole-grain tortilla.

- Sauté crumbled tofu with sweet pepper slices or zucchini. Put in whole-grain pita pocket with chunked tomato and lettuce.

- Another pita filling: chopped hard-boiled egg mixed with small amount of mayo, together with grated carrot, pepper slices, and chopped raw spinach.

- More suggestions for pita fillings: peanut butter, cheese, tuna, raisins, celery, grapes, or fruit slices, such as pineapple, pear, and apple.

- Include in your child's lunch box baby carrots or pieces of other raw vegetables.

- Mix cottage cheese with crushed fruit.

- Include trail mix. Mix raisins, chopped dried fruit, pumpkin or sunflower seeds, and raw nuts (depending on age, you can break up pieces). Trail mix is dry, non-messy, and easy to carry in a jacket pocket.

- Broaden your children's taste experiences even more by taking them to Chinese, Indian, or other restaurants with regional cuisines.

For family meals, young children should eat what the parents eat. When parents choose a variety of upper-level foods that avoid the five dietary traps, young children develop a preference for this level of food sophistication.

The sugar, sour, salt, and fat taste direction

Children are easily seduced by the alternative taste direction—sugar, sour, salt, and fat. That bag of potato chips will surely seduce with salt and fat. Tomato ketchup seduces with sweet and sour—sugar and vinegar. These are simple but powerful tastes that override all others. A child eating these foods finds the delicate flavors and odors of unprocessed foods dull by comparison.

For the young child, exposure to foods laden with sugar, salt, sour, and fat establishes the dominant taste preference. The child loses interest in the foods of subtle and varied taste. Fruits and vegetables, the heart of healthy eating, go out the window. From a cell's-eye view, the child's overall nutrition plunges, with three consequences:

1. Immune defenses increasingly become less robust. The child more readily picks up infections that invariably thrive among children in day care or school.

2. Lower facial features of the young child develop through quality nutrition and chewing on firm food. Children eating sugary and generally soft foods tend to develop pinched dental arches with narrow jaws.

3. The child is more likely to become obese.

Processed foods offering seductive flavors present a high percentage of sugar and fat calories. Refined sugar and fat are compact, calorie-dense ingredients. Sugar calories are unaccompanied by fiber, phytochemicals, and the full spectrum of nutrients the body needs to convert calories to energy and build body tissues. The fat calories are just that—calories.

Watch Out!
A 40-pound boy drinking a 12-ounce can of cola receives proportionately as much caffeine as an adult drinking two cups of coffee. Studies show that kids develop the same caffeine addiction as adults. Kids experience withdrawal symptoms when they don't get their timely caffeine fix.

There are two main consequences: The child overeats sugar/fat foods and is more likely to become obese; and the child's immune defenses falter, opening the door to sickness.

The following table shows examples of commercial kid foods.

TABLE 16.4: COMMERCIAL KID FOODS

Food Product	Total Calories	Percent Calories from Sugar	Percent Calories from Fat	Percent Total Calories, Sugar and Fat
Cosmic Chicken Nuggets	460	16	41	57
Circus Show Corn Dog	450	41	30	71
Burger King Whopper	640	5	55	60
Wendy's Kid's Meal	270	10	33	43
KFC, Barbecued Chicken Sandwich	256	28	28	56
Plain donut	198	16	50	66

Values calculated from label information or USDA food composition databases.

Apart from the donut (where you expect to find sugar), the other items in the table above are main-course foods. The addition of sugar helps to condition the child to expect the sweet in every food and to dislike those foods that don't have added sugar.

A plain donut has a sugar/fat combination that amounts to 66 percent of total calories. Would you feed your child nothing but donuts for a meal?

Adolescence

The adolescent growth spurt starts for girls at about age 11 and ends at age 15. For boys the growth spurt starts at about age 12 and continues until age 19. During this period:

- Bone structure doubles in weight for both girls and boys.

- Boys double their muscle mass.

- Girls put on more body fat and at the end of the growth spurt carry about 23 percent of body weight as fat. For boys the figure is about 12 percent.

What does growth mean from a cell's-eye view? Growth lays down new tissues, new cells, and new body systems related to sexuality and maturity. Food demands can be awesome. An active 15-year-old boy often expends on a daily basis 3,000 calories or more. We shouldn't, however, make the mistake of rating a teenager's nutrition in terms of calories. The number of calories tells us how much food is consumed. The critical question: What's the teenager actually eating? Creating new body structures takes more than calories; it takes the full spectrum of nutrients, fiber, and phytochemicals.

Just as teen nutritional demands reach peak intensity, their social lives change. They take jobs. They become more responsible for what they eat. Time becomes more precious. They don't plan meals. Eating becomes reactive—wait until hungry, then reach for the easiest convenience food in the house or head for the nearest fast-food restaurant.

Erratic eating patterns and low-level food choices contribute to a variety of health issues important to teenagers:

- Acne
- Blotchy complexion
- Split hair ends (for girls)
- Excessive weight gain or obesity

- Lack of energy
- Weak resistance to colds and stomach upsets

A teen's fast-food meal

The problem with many teen diets is that they are rich in fat and sugar, calories that provide only energy. The foods do nothing for new bone tissue or smooth skin. Consider a meal at a fast-food restaurant—what it gives and doesn't give a teenager. The following table shows the breakdown of a meal consisting of a cheeseburger, medium order of fries, and a cola soft drink.

Unofficially...
The top school-lunch choices are: tacos, burgers, pizza, and macaroni and cheese. Kids prefer finger food, brightly colored foods, and foods that crunch.

TABLE 16.5: NUTRITIONAL BREAKDOWN OF A MEAL AT A FAST-FOOD RESTAURANT

Food	Calories	Fat, grams	Protein, grams	Carbo-hydrate, grams
Cola drink, 16 ounces	210			58 (100 per-cent sugar)
Double burger with cheese	960	63	52	46
Fries, medium	370	20	5	43
Totals	1,540	83	57	147

(Source: USDA nutrition databases)

The 1,540 calories in this meal supply half the caloric needs of an active teenage boy expending 3,000 calories a day. For a less-active boy or for a teenage girl, whose daily caloric needs are in the low 2,000s, 7 calories out of 10 come from this one meal.

The fast-food meal is skewed towards fat

Let's see how this fast-food meal (listed in the table above) affects a teen's vitality. Here's the percentage breakdown of total calories into fat, protein, and carbohydrate calories:

- Percent calories from fat—49 percent
- Percent calories from protein—15 percent
- Percent calories from carbohydrate—38 percent

First, the good news. The Food and Nutrition Board of the National Academy of Sciences recommends a teenage boy get 70 grams of protein daily, a teenage girl 65 grams. This meal provides 57 grams, which comes close to meeting the total needs for the day. So no problem in this regard.

Now the bad news. Half the calories in this meal come from fat, far in excess of a more desirable rate of about 30 percent. Conversely, the carbohydrate calories are low. They should be at least 55 percent or higher. The skewed high-fat ratio has three consequences:

1. Muscles run mostly on carbohydrate. The only time muscles burn fat in quantity is when the individual engages in intense, endurance activity (see Chapter 11, "Don't Let Bad Food Habits Cancel Fitness Benefits"). Thus, the body is stuck with all this fat tumbling into the digestive system. The only metabolic option open is to dump the fat straight into the person's thighs and midriff.

2. The low carbohydrate ratio of this meal is not good for anyone engaged in physical activity. Muscles need carbohydrates to build glycogen, the fuel muscles burn.

3. The high-fat meal reaches far into the future with long-term health implications. The fatty plaques that build up in heart arteries can start forming in teen years.

One could argue that teenagers balance this meal with fruits and vegetables. But that doesn't happen. Typical teenagers make up the rest of the day's calories by eating packaged snacks and other highly processed foods. There is a marked similarity in all these foods to what makes up a fast-food meal.

The fast-food meal springs all five dietary traps

The fast-food meal falls into not one or two of the dietary traps, but all five. Here's why:

- **Traps 1 and 2, refined sugar and refined and bleached flour.** Carbohydrate in this meal comes from the sugar in the cola drink, the refined wheat flour in the hamburger bun, and the potatoes of the french fries. Thus, 70 percent of the carbohydrate (soft drink and bun) is refined. The consumer is deprived of the full vitamin and mineral spectrum of unrefined carbohydrates. The body strains to metabolize this meal. The stresses appear visibly in acne, poor skin complexion, and greater vulnerability to illness.

  Because of the refined carbohydrate and the high animal fat content, the entire meal supplies only 6 grams of fiber. This amount falls short of the recommended minimum of 25 grams a day.

  Fiber-challenged bowels are sluggish, giving toxins a chance to be absorbed. Low fiber also prevents the normal sweep of excess cholesterol out of the body, contributing to higher blood cholesterol.

- **Trap 3, refined vegetable oils.** French fries deliver 20 grams of fat, all of it fat that soaked in while cooking in the deep-fat fryer. Fast-food restaurants use refined, hydrogenated oils that contain up to 40 percent of the unnatural trans fats. Further, any omega-3 fatty acids in the

Watch Out!
Elite athletes are aware of subpar performance when they eat fast foods. The U.S. swimming team at the 1996 Olympics in Atlanta, Ga., swore off fast-food burgers while training and in competition.

original vegetable oils are destroyed during refining. The meat provides a small amount, but overall, such a meal is woefully short on omega-3 fatty acids, needed to keep brain and nerve tissue in top form.

- **Trap 4, chemical burden.** Industrial waste products, like PCBs and dioxin that contaminate the land, accumulate in animal tissues. Thus, these chemicals are high in the hamburger and cheese of this meal. In addition, food additives in the baked bun and fat breakdown products in the cooking fat of the fries compound the total chemical burden. Amounts aren't enough to make the individual sick; nevertheless, over the long run they contribute to weakened immune defenses.

- **Trap 5, lack of diversity.** Diversity is not alternating a burger with a pizza. A pepperoni, mushroom, and Italian sausage pizza delivers 80 percent of its calories from the same fat and refined white flour as the burger meal. A teenage diet consisting of burgers, pizza, soft drinks, and other packaged foods restricts diversity. To enjoy healthy and productive lives, teens need fruits, vegetables, and whole grains to provide the rich diversity of nutrients. Without diversity, the body is deprived of the full spectrum of vitamins, minerals, fiber, and phytochemicals. The body never reaches full expression of its natural potential.

An unfulfilled potential may not seem evident during teen years. A teenager locked in those five dietary traps may feel fine, excel in sports, and look great. Yet, from a cell's-eye perspective, the young body draws on future vitality. These traps force the body into using resources and energy that should be built into solid tissue for years that lie ahead.

One example: Teenage girls, especially, fail to lay down a sturdy skeleton. Once they reach early adulthood it's too late. They are stuck with substandard bone structure. The fast-food meal described in the table earlier this chapter delivers only 250 milligrams of calcium, far short of the 1,200 milligrams a day the teenager needs. It's not likely the individual will get much more calcium in other foods. Health authorities estimate that teenagers, on average, get only about 450 milligrams a day. You can see why.

Smart nutrition in the teen years

Unofficially...
The Centers for Disease Control says American teenagers have bad health habits. This government agency surveyed 16,000 teens, aged 12 to 17, and found that 1 in 5 smoked; 1 in 5 binge-drank; 1 in 3 did not exercise; and 9 in 10 seldom, if ever, ate fruits or vegetables.

Look upon the desire, almost a craving, for the high-salt, high-sugar, high-fat processed foods as an addiction. As pointed out in the chapter's beginning section, craving starts in preschool years. Parents of young children should be aware of that fact and look ahead to the time when their kids become teenagers. Children exposed to a rounded diet in early years will likely steer clear of the five dietary traps. They will not be terribly interested in fast foods; salty, high-fat snacks; and other processed foods.

Here are tips for smart nutrition for teens:

- The principles of smart nutrition that work for adults work as well for teens. Basically, they are: Eat plenty of fruits and vegetables, whole grains, and modest amounts of upper-level meat and dairy products. Avoid the five dietary traps. Check Chapter 14 for details.

- Many teens prefer vegetarian-style eating. Follow the suggestions in Chapter 9 for eating a balanced diet that supplies all the protein a teen needs. Be sure then to take a vitamin B$_{12}$ supplement.

■ Teens with their big appetites snack almost constantly. Try these foods: apples, pears, oranges, grapes, dried fruits, baby carrots, trail mix, peanut butter on a whole-grain bread or bagel, and bean tacos. The pita fillings described earlier in the chapter are great for teenagers, too.

Many teenagers have weight problems. One in five teens is overweight, a situation that complicates life later on. Fat teenagers become fat adults. They suffer five times the rate of colon cancer as normal-weight adults and are more likely to die before age 70 from heart disease.

Overweight teens should avoid crash diets. By switching from high-fat foods in fast-food restaurants and packaged snacks to eating more fruits and vegetables and whole grains, weight automatically drops.

Finally, teens need exercise. Whether fat or thin, all teenagers should exercise regularly. This advice is not usually necessary for boys; however, teenage girls tend to be less active. Encourage your teen to take up tennis or join a fitness class. They can ski, swim, hike, or whatever, as long as it's something that stretches and exercises the muscles.

Keep in mind that physical activity does more than exercise the muscles. Activity speeds up basal metabolic rate (BMR), making body metabolism more efficient. The big benefit is a trimmer body. Efficient bodies don't collect fat.

And one more word: We have to be realistic. The teen years are ones of unlimited promise. Kids feel they can do anything, slay the dragon, and live forever. The health concerns of their parents seem so remote as to be laughable. That's why in this

Bright Idea
Save time for your children. Teens, although they don't like to admit it, are influenced by what parents do. Parents should eat a balanced diet and, importantly, share at least one family meal a day with their teenage kids.

chapter we put the emphasis on instilling smart eating habits at an early age, when the child is open and curious about food.

Just the facts

- A fetus has only one chance to develop. Underdevelopment due to a shortage of nutrients cannot be made up later.

- Breast milk is by far the best food for the first six months of life. Infant formulas based on cow's milk are a distant second, while soy-based formulas trail in third place.

- For better or worse, a person's taste preferences are established in the preschool years.

- Teenagers easily fall into the dietary trap of eating a narrow range of refined foods. Parents should encourage teenage children to eat more fruits, vegetables, and whole-grain products.

GET THE SCOOP ON...

The defect in official dietary advice ▪ A review of the four quality levels ▪ Dietary needs at life's different stages ▪ Ten dietary tips for seniors

Nutrition Through the Ages: Young Adult to Golden Years

Although nutrition issues often generate controversy, nutrition authorities do agree on the amount of fat and carbohydrates you should eat. The American Cancer Society, the American Dietetic Society, the American Academy of Pediatrics, The National Institutes of Health and the American Heart Association came together in 1999 to endorse a common dietary guideline:

- No more than 30 percent of total calories from fat

- No more that 10 percent of total calories from saturated fat

- 55 percent of calories from complex carbo-hydrates, such as grains, fruits, and vegetables

- Dietary cholesterol limited to 300 milligrams or less a day

Chapter 17

481

- Salt intake no more than 1 teaspoon
  (6 grams)

Smart nutrition subscribes in general to these guidelines. The proportions of fat and carbohydrate are reasonable.

The advice to limit cholesterol to 300 milligrams really tells you to limit your intake of meats and animal-based foods because that's where cholesterol is located. Cholesterol does not occur in the plant world.

The salt limit is a warning to cut down on the amounts of fast foods and other processed food, because that's where you find the most salt. A 12-ounce can of New England clam chowder, for instance, contains 3.5 grams of salt. A fast-food cheeseburger delivers 3.5 grams, more than half the salt you should take in all day.

This advice is useful as far as it goes, but the advice doesn't take you very far. Imagine going into a restaurant and saying to the waitperson: "I'd like a meal with no more than 10 percent saturated fat and no more than 30 percent total fat." The restaurant staff would think you were crazy. And do you ever see anyone in a supermarket going up and down the aisles with calculator in hand, adding up the fat calories of the items they select? Not likely.

The point of the matter is that you order *food* in a restaurant, not fat calories. In the supermarket you select food items because they appeal to you, not because of a chemical analysis of the food. Unless you're prepared to keep the USDA food database (it's a big, fat volume) on your kitchen table and calculate the percentages of fat and carbohydrates in your meals, you'll never know the exact number of which calories you're eating.

> **"**
> The more we depart from the state of nature, the more we lose our natural tastes.
> —Jean-Jacques Rousseau, French philosopher (1762)
> **"**

And it is not always easy to guess. At a meeting of dietitians and other food professionals, the participants were asked to estimate the total number of calories and fat calories in the food they were served for lunch. On average, they underestimated the number of calories by half, and the same for the fat calories.

The moral of this story is that, if even food professionals have difficulty estimating calories and fat in a food they eat, how can the average person guess?

We need a set of guidelines that takes the guesswork out of food choices and at the same time puts your daily diet in the same ballpark as the common advice of those nutrition authorities. What do you actually buy in the supermarket or order in a restaurant? A working guideline has to focus on the food.

Four quality levels—a guideline that works

The guideline featured in this book is based on the concept of *better than*. The idea is that you eat only so much. You are always making food choices. So, why not take the better nutritional choice? This *Unofficial Guide* takes different food groups and ranks the types of foods on a quality level on a scale of one to four. As we've seen, level 1 is tops, and level 4 is at the bottom. For example, here are four quality levels in the vegetable group.

- Quality Level 1: Fresh, raw
- Quality Level 2: Fresh, lightly cooked
- Quality Level 3: Frozen
- Quality Level 4: Canned

Quality refers to nutrition. This scale of quality levels means that, when you have a choice between

Watch Out!
The muffins you buy today aren't the size they were 10 or 15 years ago. They've grown. One of those muffins sold in mall shops can deliver 650 to 900 calories and as much as 48 grams of fat. For an average-size woman, that muffin represents one-third to one-half of her calories for the day.

canned and frozen, the frozen offers a better nutritional value than the canned. Raw vegetables in general offer a better nutritional value than fresh, lightly cooked. In the supermarket, you generally have a choice between fresh produce and frozen. Fresh produce (assuming it is really fresh) would be your better choice.

An element of practicality enters the guideline of quality levels. You probably don't wish to eat all vegetables raw (potatoes, for example), but quality level 1 tells you that a green salad offers top nutrition. The quality levels guideline is a means for judging nutritional value on a relative scale. Thus, canned vegetables, although ranked at level 4, have some nutritional value. It is just that frozen vegetables offer better nutritional value, and so on.

The beauty of having four quality levels is that they are easy to remember, so easy to use. No long lists of specific food items. You can go into a supermarket and make *better than* selections to fit your budget and lifestyle.

Quality level guidelines for all the major food groups are described in detail in Part II of the book and are summarized in a single table in Appendix E.

Criteria for assigning a food to a quality level

What criteria are used in assigning a food (say, frozen vegetables) to quality level 3? For the scale of quality levels to have any validity it must be rooted in scientific knowledge. There are three criteria:

1. The degree of processing. Processing includes home cooking as well as commercial manufacturing processes. All food starts out as a living plant or creature. When a plant food is harvested, the food remains alive in the sense that enzymes continue to work and the plant tissue

consumes oxygen. This is why a plant remains turgid, fresh, and edible for days after harvest. Similarly, meat from a freshly slaughtered animal retains enzymic activity that helps to keep the meat fresh and retain nutritional value. Processing such as heat, freezing, and grinding kills enzymic action, as well as destroying delicate vitamins.

In short, the more a food product is processed, the further that food moves down the quality scale.

2. The amount of nonnutritional chemicals added to the food. Foods may contain pesticide residues and chemical additives used in food processing. All these chemicals burden the body, cutting efficiency. It's like having to deal with a swarm of mosquitoes at a picnic. You manage, but you don't function at top efficiency.

From a cell's-eye perspective, body systems don't work as well. We do know that excessive chemical exposure, for instance, wears down immune defenses. Thus, the more nonnutritional chemicals contaminating a food product, the more the product drops down the quality scale.

3. Fiber. All plant foods at the time of harvest contain fiber. Fiber doesn't offer calories or nutrition in the strictest sense. Fiber, however, plays an important role in the body. It cleanses the bowels and improves the efficiency of nutrient absorption. Fiber sweeps toxins and excess cholesterol from the body. Fiber also slows sugar (glucose) absorption, preventing the rapid dumping of sugar into the blood.

Moneysaver
Food processing costs money. The more a food is processed, the more it costs to produce. You pay for processing in the price of the item, so you can save money by buying food products that are less processed and higher in nutritional quality.

The dumping provokes an insulin response, which results in the conversion of the glucose to fat.

The more fiber removed by food processing, the further down the quality scale the plant-based products drop. With respect to animal products, this criterion doesn't apply, because they don't contain fiber. Animal products have fat, which slows the absorption of glucose, preventing dumping.

In summary, these are three criteria used in developing the guides to quality levels of foods you see in this book.

Where your food choices rank

Judging one's eating habits depends on more than one food choice.

Go over your answers to the questions in the following quiz and see how many upper-level choices (levels 1 and 2) you check.

If most of your choices are numbers 1 and 2, then you are choosing upper-level foods. These foods offer better nutritional quality than foods at levels 3 and 4.

If many of your regular choices are numbers 3 and 4, ask yourself if you would be just as satisfied eating a level 1 or 2 choice. If the answer is yes, then here's an opportunity to upgrade your nutrition.

This quiz concerns single foods or meals. You must also think about nutritional balance for the day. For the remainder of the chapter we do just that, looking at total food patterns. We take examples at four stages of adult life—young adult, pre-pregnancy, mid-life, and golden years. How can you upgrade personal nutrition to meet the needs of an ever-changing body?

A. A typical weekday breakfast is:

1. A bowl of whole-grain cereal with a sliced banana or berries
2. Whole-grain pancakes with a touch of maple syrup
3. A commercial muffin
4. A toaster pop-up pastry

B. My mid-morning snack often is:

1. An apple, orange, or other fruit
2. A handful of raw nuts
3. A granola bar
4. A candy bar

C. When I have a sandwich for lunch, it is likely to be:

1. Whole-grain bread or pita pocket with lettuce, tomato, sprouts, or other raw vegetables, light on the mayo or other dressing
2. Grilled chicken, lettuce, with touch of mayo or mustard spread on whole-grain bread
3. Roast beef, mayo on a white bun
4. Fast-food cheeseburger and fries

D. At salad bars, my plate is loaded with:

1. All fresh items, light amount of oil and vinegar
2. A mixture of fresh items and cooked or pickled items, with oil and vinegar dressing
3. Chopped egg, cheese, and potato or pasta salad
4. Sliced meats and cheese

E. In the afternoon I usually snack on:

1. Carrot sticks, celery, or piece of fruit
2. Whole-grain crackers with hard cheese, or fig cookie
3. White bread and homogenized peanut butter
4. Mall cookie

Bright Idea
Take a snack to work rather than relying on the vending machine at your workplace. Vending machines are your worst enemy when it comes to fighting overweight. They are loaded with fatty and high-calorie foods. Bring fruit or veggies or a small handful of trail mix to work.

Watch Out!
Young men in their 20s who are 20 pounds overweight double their chances of developing osteoarthritis in knee or hip or both. They become candidates for knee or hip replacements at an early age.

F. At dinner the food that covers most of my plate is:

1. Lightly steamed, assorted fresh vegetables
2. A mixture of steamed fresh vegetables and potatoes
3. Roast chicken or grilled steak
4. Sausages or deep-fried chicken or fish

G. My dinner vegetables are most likely:

1. Lightly steamed red, green, and yellow vegetables
2. A mixture of steamed potatoes and two colored vegetables
3. Frozen peas or frozen mixed vegetables
4. French fries and/or canned vegetables

H. When I dine in a restaurant, I usually order:

1. Grilled chicken with mixed vegetables (no fries) and a side green salad (no iceberg)
2. Grilled steak (solid meat, not hamburger), baked potato, and large green salad
3. Pasta with meatballs
4. Deep-fried chicken and fries

I. As a vegetarian, my main meal usually is:

1. Steamed mixed vegetables plus cooked dry beans, green salad
2. Stir-fry vegetables and tofu
3. Taco with canned, refried beans
4. Textured vegetable protein (TVP) burger, fries

J. My dessert at home or in a restaurant usually is:

1. Fresh fruit, sometimes with plain, low-fat yogurt
2. Fruit and hard cheese
3. Yogurt, with cooked fruit
4. Ice cream, cake, or pie

A young adult frets about weight

Janet Headly, age 21, works in an office. She doesn't normally think much about what she eats, but she is concerned about the 30 pounds she's gained. She says she eats no differently now than when she was a teenager, yet she wasn't overweight then. The following table shows Janet's typical 1-day food choices. The table also gives examples of how she can improve her nutrition and at the same time deal with her weight.

TABLE 17.1: FOOD CHOICES OF A 21-YEAR-OLD OVERWEIGHT WOMAN

	Janet Headly, Age 21, Food Choices	Dietary Upgrades, Levels 1 and 2 Choices
Breakfast	Typical white-flour bagel with cream cheese or bakery muffin with coffee	Whole-grain bagel with light coating of quality peanut butter or goat cheese, or whole-grain muffin; freshly squeezed juice
Lunch	Pizza or cheeseburger with fries and cola soft drink or chocolate milk	Sandwich of whole-grain bread, or pita pocket with lettuce, shredded carrots, sprouts, tomato, cucumber slices, cheese (not processed) or turkey slices. Easy on the mayo. Or, the equivalent as a salad and whole-grain roll. Mineral water with slice of fresh lime.
Dinner	Fish sticks, fries, coffee, piece of cake for dessert	Grilled salmon, halibut, or other clean, fresh ocean fish, plus broccoli and carrots and garden salad (such as mixed greens, peppers, onions, grated carrots, other veggies, grapes)
Snacks	Candy bar, jelly beans, coffee, cookies	Whole fruit, raw nuts

Janet Headly's food choices present, to put it mildly, a few nutritional problems.

Bright Idea
Save time for eating. Eating on the run can be stressful, and stress reduces the amount of vitamins and minerals you absorb from food. Thus, even the healthiest of foods lose nutritional value when you eat under stress.

- Janet, at age 21, has recently finished her teenage growth spurt. She still eats a quantity of food she ate during her teen years, but her caloric needs have dropped 500 or 600 calories, the number of calories in her order of french fries with a 12-ounce cola soft drink. She simply eats too much food.

- Her diet bulges with fat and refined carbohydrates, including a lot of sugar. She eats calorie-dense foods, convenient to eat—but also easy to overeat. The fat she eats, in particular, has nowhere to go except straight to thighs and hips.

- Her diet is wretchedly unbalanced, low in vitamins and minerals. The plant food she does consume, refined grains and sugar, provide no fiber. Without fiber to provide bulk, this type of diet places a strain on the intestinal tract, a strain that could lead to heart disease or cancer later in life.

- The lack of fruits and vegetables deprives Janet of the protective effect of phytochemicals. We have much to learn about the benefits of phytochemicals, but we do know that they are staunch antioxidants. Antioxidants protect cells from premature aging and the downhill body processes that lead to cancer.

As far as upgrading Janet's diet to level 1 and 2 foods, we try to stay within her general food preference. The suggestions are "better than" choices.

Breakfast: Change the bagel to whole grain. The cream cheese is almost 100 percent fat. Select soft cheeses like goat or semi-soft like gouda which have less fat and more protein. She should also start the day with fresh juice, or better, a whole fruit.

Lunch: The idea is to upgrade the sandwich to include raw vegetables and eliminate the fries, which are close to 50 percent fat. Replace the high-sugar soft drink with mineral water. This lunch is just as hunger-satisfying, with probably half the calories as Janet's lunch.

Dinner: Fish sticks are a mish-mash of fish bits and chemical additives glued together, breaded, and deep fried in fat. The frying oil for both the fish sticks and fries is hydrogenated, carrying a burden of the unnatural trans fats. From a cell's-eye view, this meal is highly unsatisfactory—plenty of calories, but little in the way of vitamins and minerals needed to digest those calories.

Snacks: Got to get Janet off the sugar, empty-calorie kick. Snack time is a good time to eat fruit or nuts. Nuts, especially walnuts, provide omega-3 fatty acid that also improve skin tone.

A word about coffee. Nothing good can be said about coffee, except that some people need the stimulus to get going in the morning. If you drink coffee, keep it down to a single cup, no more than two, in the morning only. If you need to drink coffee or a cola soft drink frequently during the day, look to what you are eating. The need for a continual stimulus is a sure sign your diet does not provide your body what it needs to create energy. For this reason, coffee doesn't appear on Janet's upgraded diet.

Overall, the suggested "better-than" choices upgrade and balance Janet's diet. She will find that her basal metabolic rate (BMR) jumps as she feels

more energetic. With increased BMR, fewer calories, and a balanced spectrum of nutrients, Janet will
find that her weight drops without conscious effort
to deny her hunger.

A young woman plans for pregnancy

Hilary Vigstedt, age 27, was recently married and
looks towards a pregnancy in about 2 years' time.
She says she wants to be "in peak physical condition"
for that event. Her food choices, however, are going
to undermine that wish.

TABLE 17.2: FOOD CHOICES OF A WOMAN PLANNING FOR PREGNANCY

	Hilary Vigstedt, Age 27, Food Choices	Dietary Upgrades, Level 1 and 2 Choices
Breakfast	Toaster pop-up pastry, juice drink and coffee	Whole-grain cereal with freshly ground flaxseed sprinkled on top, sliced fruit, skim or 1% milk. Or poached egg on whole-grain toast. Freshly squeezed or premium juice.
Lunch	Braised pork chop, baked potato, and pastry for dessert, coffee	Braised pork chop and baked potato plus broccoli, sweet potato, or carrots. Green side salad and fresh fruit for dessert. Mineral water with a slice of fresh lime.
Dinner	Pizza or tacos and coffee, ice cream for dessert	At home, make a homemade vegetable soup. Include a green salad. Fruit and yogurt, or low-fat, low-sugar oatmeal cookie for dessert.
Snacks	Danish and coffee	Fruit, baby carrots

Hilary Vigstedt's food choices will not win any
nutritional prize for these reasons:

- Hilary's diet, like that of Janet's, is laden with
  fat, sugar, and refined white flour. The diet is
  calorie-dense—a lot of calories unaccompanied
  by nutrients.

- Her food, overall, is deficient in vitamins, minerals, fiber, and phytochemicals.

- Her only vegetable choice is a baked potato. There is nothing wrong with a baked potato, except that potatoes count in the grain group. They are placed there because of their high starch content. In effect, her diet for the day has a big fruit and vegetable void.

- Her diet from a cell's-eye view is remarkably dull. The toaster pop-up pastry, luncheon pastry, tacos, pizza crust, and danish are made from the same refined white flour. Where's the diversity? The same dull nutrition.

The pork chop and baked potato are the only bright spots in an series of low-quality choices. The meat provides some vitamins and minerals and other nutrients, including vitamin B_{12}. The potato also provides a spectrum of vitamins and minerals.

Nevertheless, vitamins and minerals supplied by the meat and baked potato do not compensate for an absence of critical nutrients from the rest of Hilary's food choices. This fact, plus the lack of fiber and phytochemicals, undermine Hilary's body metabolism. Her body cells have to strain to process the calories from all that fat and refined carbohydrates. This diet, if anything, diminishes the physical condition Hilary desires.

Hilary's dietary upgrades explained

Here are comments on the dietary upgrades to Hilary's diet.

Breakfast: The toaster pop-up pastry is a highly sugared product. A better choice is a whole-grain cereal which, moreover, provides an opportunity to sprinkle freshly ground flaxseed. The flaxseed garnish

Bright Idea
People prefer to cook hamburger because it is cheap and cooks fast. But once meat is ground, it rapidly loses the nutritional qualities of solid, fresh meat. Delicate vitamins are oxidized by exposure to air, and both vitamins and minerals leak out with the fluid. If you normally eat hamburger, upgrade your nutrition by switching to solid cuts of beef.

adds the critical omega-3 fatty acid. If Hilary takes in enough of the omega-3s, her body will store them for a fetus to draw upon. By going in this direction, her breakfast moves to foods low in added sugar, high in fiber, and diverse in nutrition.

Lunch: Hilary prefers to take her main meal at lunchtime, so the pork chop and baked potato remain with added vegetables and a side salad. Gone are the calorie-rich pastries.

Dinner: This suggestion is for home preparation, a vegetable soup made from fresh vegetables. The soup can be concentrated, more like a stew, and cooked just enough to soften the vegetables. To increase the protein content, add lentils or split peas.

Snacks: The Danish is a sugar/fat combo loaded with calories. It does nothing for the body. As with Janet's snacks, the suggestion is fruit or raw vegetables.

Overall, the dietary upgrades provide a complete spectrum of vitamins, minerals, fiber, and phytochemicals. If Hilary eats comparable meals most days, her body indeed will reach the peak condition she wants, ready for a baby.

Pass a strong immune presence to baby

What about immunities? Immunity is a critical issue for the long-term health of the baby. The mother passes immunities to the child during the fetal stage and, if she nurses, through her milk. For a mother to pass along a strong immune presence to baby, her own immune system must be, to use Hilary's phrase, in peak physical condition.

The immune system is particularly sensitive to a letdown in nutritional quality. This is why individuals who eat a low-level diet suffer more sick days from colds, respiratory infections, and the flu. While such nutrition in general depresses the immune system, scientists have identified nutrients particularly critical to immune function:

- Vitamin A

- Vitamin C

- Vitamin E

- Selenium

- Zinc

Hilary's diet is woefully short of all five nutrients. Without yellow vegetables, her diet provides no beta-carotene, the substance that forms vitamin A in the body. The potato and pork chop provide vitamin C, but not much, and not in the quantity she'd get from raw fruits and raw vegetables in a salad. Vitamin E occurs in whole grains but is lost during refining. Meat contains some selenium and zinc. But like vitamin E, selenium and zinc occur in whole grains, not in refined white flour. So the foods in Hilary's diet made solely from refined wheat flour contribute none of these two minerals.

You might think the simple solution to strengthening the immune system is to take a supplement of these five vitamins and minerals. Not so fast. The lack of these five nutrients is an indicator of a substandard diet. There is much more to creating a powerful immune defense than ingesting these particular nutrients. The deep-seated deficiency in Hilary Vigstedt's diet can only be addressed by upgrading the whole diet.

Unofficially...
Invited to a wedding feast? You may find few foods that fit your upgraded dietary habits. Go ahead and enjoy the feast and social gathering. Don't worry about an occasional day of nutritional craziness. The key to good nutrition, energy, and health is to maintain steady habits over the long run.

Watch Out!
Watch out for high-calorie alcoholic drinks. The ones highest in "empty calories" are mixed drinks with cola, lemon-lime soda, and sweet mixes such as Tom Collins or whiskey sours. In any event, women should drink no more than one drink a day, men two drinks.

There is merit in taking vitamin and mineral supplements, but first take care of the diet. (See Chapter 8, "To Supplement or Not to Supplement Is No Longer the Question," for suggestions on supplementing with vitamins and minerals.) A dietary overhaul ensures that the body's immune system and other body systems reach peak condition and stay there.

A woman in mid-life worries about weight

Ashley Graham, age 44, is concerned about a waist that, in spite of regular exercise, keeps expanding. Her typical food choices have advantages and disadvantages (Table 17.3).

TABLE 17.3: FOOD CHOICES OF WOMAN WITH EXPANDING WAIST

	Ashley Graham, Age Early 40s, Food Choices	Dietary Upgrades, Level 1 and 2 Choices
Breakfast	Shredded wheat, skim milk, and sliced banana. Juice from concentrate. Regular coffee.	Stay with the shredded wheat, skim milk, and banana or try granola with fruit and skim milk. Add 2 tablespoons of freshly ground flaxseed. Upgrade the juice to either premium grade or freshly squeezed juice.
Lunch	Canned oyster stew or large slice of Italian sausage pizza. Canned peaches and decaf coffee.	Large garden salad, either with hunks of chicken or turkey or low-fat cottage cheese. The salad should include a broad assortment of lettuce and vegetables with fruits. Mineral water with a slice of fresh lime.
Dinner	Stir-fry veggies over Minute Rice. Canned pudding or ice cream for dessert.	Put the stir-fry veggies over brown rice. Make a pudding from scratch with eggs and milk, or have fruit with yogurt for dessert.
Snacks	Granola bar, donut.	Fruit, carrot sticks or other vegetables with hummus dip, raw nuts.

- Her breakfast of a whole-wheat cereal and sliced banana is good.

- Her luncheon bowl of oyster stew, however, is a cream soup, high in fat (52 percent of calories). Her alternative Italian sausage pizza is no better—46 percent calories from fat. Commercial pizzas are made with refined white flour and the cheese is often a low-quality, processed cheese. The pizza provides calories but not much nutrition.

- Ashley's dinner of stir-fry vegetables is a good choice, but she accompanies the vegetables with an instant rice, a highly processed product. Compared to brown rice, the instant rice has lost half of its calcium and 90 percent each of its magnesium, potassium, and vitamin B_6. Apart from the shredded wheat for breakfast, the day's carbohydrate comes from fiberless, refined grain products.

- Fruit. She does eat a banana at breakfast, a plus. Yet she eats no raw vegetables during the day, either as salad or something like carrot sticks.

Ashley's upgrades explained

The suggested upgrade for Ashley's breakfast menu leaves the shredded wheat, although an equivalent alternative is granola. The juice is upgraded from a frozen concentrate to freshly squeezed juice. The concentrate is made by evaporating juice at high heat. In addition, the frozen concentrate is often stored for lengthy periods, during which time nutritional value continues to deteriorate. Overall, much of the original nutritional value of the fruit has been lost.

Watch Out!
Don't let your weight creep up with age. As people age they gain weight—on average, a pound a year. This gradual but persistent weight gain is accompanied by increasing levels of blood cholesterol and especially LDL cholesterol (the so-called bad form).

For lunch, Ashley should drop the high-fat meal in favor of a garden salad. Lunchtime for most people is a lighter meal, an opportunity to eat raw vegetables in the form of a salad. Although her canned peaches qualify as a fruit in the USDA Nutrition Guide, canned fruit, by virtue of high heat during processing and added sugar, ranks at quality level 4. A fresh fruit is a "better-than" choice.

For dinner, keep the stir-fry veggies but now include brown rice. Brown rice retains the outer coating where the B vitamins and minerals are located. The brown rice also has more flavor.

The dessert can be more fruit with yogurt, or a pudding made, not from a mix, but with real eggs and milk.

For snacks, drop the candy bars. Granola bars have the same high sugar/fat combo as other candy bars. They are hardly "healthy." Since Ashley includes fruit in her meals, why not include fruit as a snack? Or she could snack on raw vegetables or raw nuts.

Approaching menopause, the body tends to lay down fat

Ashley is approaching that stage of life when hormones change. As estrogen levels drop and other hormones alter, the body tends to put more fat around the middle. In any event, by reducing the fat level in her diet and including more raw foods, Ashley's metabolic rate will go up. In addition, she won't eat as many calories. The upgraded diet, plus the fact Ashley exercises regularly, will stop the expanding waistline. Her weight should not increase and may very well drop.

The biggest mistake Ashley could make is to keep eating more or less the way she does now but temporarily go on a crash diet to lose weight. Such diets are calorie-deprived, and that also means nutrition-deprived. The body loses weight because of starvation. Unfortunately, some of that lost weight is vital body protein.

Practically everyone who goes on a crash weight-loss diet gains the weight back within a year or so. Weight gained back is fat. The lost protein remains lost, diminishing body vigor.

Some anti-aging tips

A classic mistake individuals make is to use their body weight as the sole indicator of dietary success. They can be quite thin and still have a body 10 years older than their chronological age. Real dietary success is measured in total body vitality: deep immune defenses, boundless energy, and snail-paced aging processes.

No, we can't do anything about the onrush of time, and we all have a built-in biological clock that paces our aging. But this clock conceals a big secret. Its pendulum is flexible. You can slow the clock down or speed it up.

Of all the things you do in life, what you eat has the biggest influence on clock speed. Persons who consistently eat a diet of quality level 3 and 4 foods accelerate their internal clocks. They age faster and suffer degenerative diseases earlier in life.

On the other hand, persons who consistently choose foods at the upper quality levels 1 and 2 brake their internal clocks to a snail's pace. Your basic goal, then, is to eat a balanced diet of upper-level foods.

The relation between nutrition and aging pops up in unexpected ways—for instance, hearing.

Watch Out! People who eat polyunsaturated vegetable oils, such as safflower, sunflower, and corn, lower their immune defenses. The problem is that the high linoleic content of these oils suppresses availability of omega-3 fatty acids essential for top immune function. Switch to oils low in polyunsaturates, such as olive or peanut.

Hearing loss affects 28 million Americans and ranks as one of the four most chronic conditions in older people. For some types of hearing loss, diet seems to play a role. Just how diet relates to hearing loss remains uncertain, however. One study of older women with impaired hearing found that they ate low-quality diets compared to age-matched women with normal hearing.

The exact mechanism by which poor nutrition contributes to hearing loss is uncertain. However, hearing acuity normally diminishes with age, and by slowing one's biological clock through good nutrition, hearing ability is bound to benefit.

In addition to eating upper-level foods, here are three more anti-aging tips:

1. Supplement with antioxidant vitamins A, C, and E. Oxygen in cells produces substances called free radicals. Free radicals ricochet around inside cells, banging up cell enzymes and otherwise causing great damage—this is one reason for premature aging. Cells have defenses to control free-radical formation, but those defenses need beefing up. That's where the antioxidant vitamins play a role. Vitamin E, in particular, has been shown to reduce the risk of heart disease in post-menopausal women and the risk of prostate cancer in men. The recommended supplements are: 5,000 IU (International Units) of A or 25,000 IU of beta-carotene (it is converted to vitamin A in the body), 500 to 1,000 milligrams of C, and 200 to 800 IU of E.

   A note of caution: You are beginning to see phytochemicals, such as lycopene, bottled and advertised as antioxidants. Phytochemicals are indeed a valuable weapon against free radicals, but don't rely on pills. Eat your vegetables and fruits, including deeply colored ones.

2. In addition to antioxidant vitamins, take a multivitamin and mineral supplements equivalent to the Daily Value (DV) of each. See Appendix D for the list.

3. After a good diet, physical exercise is the next best brake to slow down your biological clock. Walking is great. Strolling at 3 miles an hour on level ground consumes 240 calories an hour. A brisk walk at 4 miles an hour consumes 360 calories per hour. If walking represents your exercise, shoot for a minimum of four hours a week. Also, if terrain in your neighborhood permits, include hills.

Any form of sport or exercise is good. The important thing is to make it regular. Remember that exercise speeds up your BMR. BMR normally slows down as you get older. Exercise has multiple benefits, including keeping weight under control, bolstering immune defenses, and (in women) stopping bone decay.

A woman in her golden years worries about diabetes

Sally Francoeur is 68 years old. Diabetes runs in her family, and she is concerned that at her age she might become diabetic. Sally's food choices, however, need improving if she wishes to lower her risk of the disease.

Sally Francoeur's food choices chip away at her body tissues, accelerating her biological clock. The

Unofficially...
Walking sharpens your brain. A University of Illinois study recruited 124 sedentary men and women, aged 60 to 75. Participants walked an hour-long loop around the university campus three times a week. The researchers found that the walkers improved by 25 percent their ability to plan, establish schedules, remember choices, and make timely decisions.

TABLE 17.4: FOOD CHOICES OF WOMAN COURTING DIABETES

	Sally Francoeur, Age 68, Food Choices	Dietary Upgrades, Level 1 and 2 Choices
Breakfast	White toast, jam, and coffee.	Cooked oatmeal or whole-grain ready-to-eat cereal with low-fat milk. Sliced fruit or berries.
Lunch	Grilled-cheese sandwich made with processed cheese and white bread.	Grilled-cheese sandwich made with cheddar or other cheese (not processed) and whole-grain bread. Garden salad. Mineral water with slice of fresh lime.
Dinner	Commercial frozen dinner: chicken, vegetables, and gravy. Dessert of canned pudding.	Grilled chicken breast or piece of fresh fish. Selection of steamed, fresh vegetables. If Sally doesn't have a salad with her lunch, dinner should include a side salad. Fruit (and yogurt) for dessert.
Snacks	A can of a "liquid meal."	Smoothie made with fresh fruit and yogurt.

choices fail to provide the nutritional support cells need to stay robust. Her choices are an open invitation to health problems, including the adult-onset diabetes she wishes to avoid. Here's why:

- Sally's diet lacks any raw food. She misses out on the complete spectrum of nutrients that only raw foods provide.

- The white toast, jam, liquid meal, and pudding deliver the naked carbohydrate calories of refined sugar and white flour. The fiber, phytochemicals, and range of vitamins and minerals found in unrefined carbohydrates are not there. This is one reason such a diet erodes her inner vitality.

- Sally eats no fruit, and the only vegetables she gets are the ones in the frozen dinner. These vegetables have been highly processed and frozen, their nutritional value drained.

One positive thing that can be said for Sally's diet is protein. The chicken, cheese, liquid meal, and white bread all provide protein, so in that regard her total protein intake is adequate.

Sally's dietary upgrades explained

For breakfast, Sally needs to introduce raw fruits and vegetables into her regimen. Breakfast is a good place to start, by putting sliced fruit on her cereal. The whole-grain cereal and fruit provides fiber, plus a spectrum of vitamins and minerals found only in fruits and whole grains.

For lunch, Sally likes the grilled-cheese sandwich. The suggested upgrade keeps the grilled-cheese sandwich but uses better quality ingredients. She should include a green salad at lunch or at dinner.

Regarding dinner, most commercial frozen dinners rank at the bottom of a nutritional quality scale. Sally gets much better nutrition from a fresh piece of meat or fish eaten with fresh vegetables, lightly steamed.

Desserts should not be thought of as pure indulgence. The pudding out of a can is the sugar/fat combo, with no nutrition. Sally likes pudding, so why not make a pudding with eggs and milk? It's a tasty dessert with a nutritional bonus.

With a more balanced diet and less highly processed food, Sally's chances of sliding into adult-onset diabetes is lessened. In addition, the "better-than" choices satisfy hunger with fewer calories. Sally may lose some weight, and at the very least she shouldn't gain any more. Weight gain presents an added metabolic burden, increasing chances of adult-onset diabetes.

Bright Idea
Want a healthy heart? Eat nuts. A study of 86,000 women showed that women who ate nuts more than five times a week had one-third the heart problems of women who didn't eat nuts. True, nuts are high in fat, but the mix of fats is beneficial to the heart and body. Nuts, particularly walnuts, have a high level of the desirable omega-3 fatty acid.

The lowdown on liquid meals

The liquid meal Sally drinks as a snack deserves special comment. These meals derive 60 percent or more of their calories from sugar—generally a mixture of sugar, corn syrup, and high-fructose corn syrup. The low-fat versions do not contain an oil, which would normally retard the dumping of sugar from the intestines into the blood. The result: All that refined sugar dumps rapidly into the bloodstream. Because of the rapid dumping, the body has to dispose of the sugar. The body converts it to fat.

The dumping may also provoke a insulin release. The wide fluctuations of insulin levels in the blood caused by the release over the years wears down the body's ability to handle insulin. This is not the food a person concerned about adult-onset diabetes should be eating as a snack.

Liquid meals are advertised as providing vitamins and minerals. Drinking a mixture of sugar water with vitamins and minerals is not the same as eating a natural food. In the food, vitamins and minerals are built into the food's structure. The way vitamins and minerals are absorbed into the body and the way they interact with each other differ vastly from vitamins and minerals floating around in a can of liquid.

Another burden is the load of chemical additives, including the coal-tar dyes like FD&C Red #3, FD&C Yellow #6, and FD&C Blue #1. As one grows older, the body's ability to deal with toxic chemicals such as coal-tar dyes lessens. Why give your liver the added job of detoxifying these chemical additives?

Liquid meals are a poor way of obtaining one's sustenance. On a quality scale of 1 to 4, liquid meals rank at level 4.

Moneysaver
Phytochemicals, plant substances such as lycopene and chlorophyll, help slow down one's biological clock. They protect vital tissue from being oxidized. Entrepreneurs have put lycopene or other phytochemicals in pills, but there is little evidence the pills work. Save your money. Eat fruits and vegetables and get lycopene plus 10,000 other beneficial phytochemicals.

Our bodies are not like an insect's

A theme developed earlier in the book is that our bodies are not like those of adult insects. The adult insect's body is fixed. The components of the body do not change—they last a lifetime, albeit a short lifetime. The adult insect's food need be no more than sugar water (nectar), enough to supply energy.

The human body, by contrast, needs a complex nutrition because it constantly undergoes renewal. Your skin cells last only a couple of days, being replaced by new ones. Your hair and nails never stop growing. Individual proteins in cells have short lives, a day at most, and in some cases only a few minutes. Each protein is replaced with an identical new copy. Red blood cells, which carry oxygen from lungs to tissues, have a maximum life span of 120 days. To replace worn-out ones, your body every hour of the day makes 200,000 new red blood cells.

Body renewal requires energy and the complete range of nutrients. Unlike the adult insect, which can survive on sugar water, we need a balance of

- Protein.
- Carbohydrate.
- Fat, including the essential fatty acids.
- 13 Vitamins.
- 16 Minerals.

And that's not all. For smooth, efficient digestion we need fiber. For protection against oxidation we need the help of the thousands of phytochemicals.

We call elements like vitamins, minerals, and protein nutrients when they are in food, but once in the body they become cell building blocks. You need all those blocks to make 200,000 new red blood cells an hour to remodel your bones, to renew your skin—in fact, to renew every millimeter of our body from scalp to toe.

In short, human nutritional needs are ongoing. Every day is a new day for your body, a new day for renewal, for eating foods that supply *all* the nutrients the body needs for complete renewal.

Nevertheless, we humans do age, and as we do the processes of renewal slow down and don't work as well as they did in earlier years. Because of this drop in efficiency, the body is less able to cope with

- Vitamin and mineral deficits.

- An absence of fiber.

- A lack of antioxidant phytochemicals.

Unfortunately, with aging, as body requirements for a complete spectrum of nutrients goes up, appetite goes down. Individuals don't eat as much as they did formerly. So older folks can't afford to waste calories on foods like refined sugar that do nothing but provide energy. Every calorie must count.

Ten tips for nutrition in the golden years

This book has offered many tips for improving your nutritional outlook. Here are the senior's top 10:

1. Eat upper-level foods, foods that rank at quality levels 1.

2. Eat as much organically grown or raised food as possible. Cut down on toxic chemicals in your food. By buying organic food products you also support a clean, environmentally friendly agriculture.

3. Eat two to five pieces of fresh fruit every day. Eat fruits in season and especially fruits that grow in your region.

4. Eat raw vegetables every day—a green salad or sliced vegetables with a dip.

5. Make vegetables the heart of your dinner, occupying the largest proportion of the dinner plate.

6. Eat breakfast. And eat small meals more frequently. Keep your digestive tract busy at all times.

7. Take vitamin and mineral supplements in addition to—not instead of—upper-level foods.

8. Avoid deep-fried foods.

9. Drink plenty of water. As one gets older, the thirst mechanism falters. The body doesn't work well when short of fluid. You can become dehydrated without realizing it.

10. Exercise regularly. Include weight-lifting exercise as well as aerobic exercise.

> 66
> We command nature only by obeying her.
> —Roger Bacon, 13th-century English friar and philosopher
> 99

Just the facts

▪ Official dietary guidelines talk of percentages of fat, carbohydrate, and protein, but provide no practical advice on what to buy in a supermarket or restaurant.

▪ The criteria for assigning foods to a particular quality level depends mainly on the amount of processing the food has undergone. The more processing, the lower on the quality scale the food falls.

▪ As one progresses through adult years, the body constantly changes, and caloric needs gradually diminish. Many people, however, fail to adjust their food intake, with the result that weight builds over the years.

- Everyone has a built-in biological clock that ticks off the years, governing the speed at which we age. Although you can't stop the clock, you can slow it down with high-quality nutrition. Aging slower, you are less likely to suffer a degenerative disease.

- In senior years, metabolic efficiency drops while the body's need for nutrients goes up. Thus, seniors must be doubly careful to choose foods that supply a full range of vitamins, minerals, fiber, and phytochemicals. Every calorie must count.

Glossary

Aflatoxin A toxin produced by the mold *Aspergillus flavus* which grows on peanuts and grains. It's extremely toxic.

Allergen A substance, usually a protein, that provokes an allergic reaction from the body's immune system.

All-purpose flour A blend of refined, white flours made from a mixture of hard and soft wheats. Can be used for breads, cakes, and pastries. May be bleached or unbleached. Protein content is 8 to 11 percent.

Amaranth An ancient grain.

Amenorrhea Cessation of a woman's menstrual cycle. Happens when body fat drops to about 10 percent of weight.

Anaphylaxis An allergic reaction that occurs rapidly, in which the throat swells and the individual has difficulty in breathing. Can be life-threatening.

Androstenedione A hormone thought to enhance athletic performance. This effect has not been proven and, in fact, the opposite maybe the case.

Ankylosing spondylitis   A stiffening and immobility of the spinal column due to disintegrating vertebrae.

Annatto   The yellow seeds of the annatto plant are ground, producing a powder that is used to color cheese.

Aspergillus flavus   A mold that grows on peanuts or grains and creates a deadly toxin, called **aflatoxin.**

Autoimmune disease   General term for disorders in which the body produces antibodies against its own tissues, resulting in tissue injury.

Basal Metabolic Rate (BMR)   The amount of heat (energy) a person produces when in a complete state of physical and mental rest.

BGH   See **Bovine Growth Hormone.**

Blanched vegetables   Blanching means boiling in water or steaming for 1 to 3 minutes. The purpose is to inactivate enzymes that otherwise would cause the vegetables to spoil faster.

Blood sugar (glucose)   The sugar that circulates in the blood.

BMI   See **Body Mass Index.**

BMR   See **Basal Metabolic Rate.**

Body Mass Index (BMI)   A method of relating the amount of fat a person carries to weight. The BMI is a better measure of one's ideal weight than traditional height-weight tables.

Botulism   Disease caused by a neurotoxin produced by a bacterium, *Clostridium botulinum.* This toxin is the most powerful poison known.

Bovine Growth Hormone (rBGH)   A genetically engineered hormone that, when injected into cows, causes them to produce 10 to 15 percent more milk. It's used in dairy herds in the United States, but is banned in Canada. European countries have declared a moratorium on its use.

Bulgur wheat Consists of hard or soft wheat berries that have been boiled, dried, and then cracked into coarse pieces. The result is a pre-cooked, cracked whole wheat.

Calorie Used in nutrition, a contraction of kilo-calorie. One kilocalorie is defined as the amount of heat needed to raise the temperature of 1 kilo-gram (2.2 pounds) of water 1 degree Centigrade.

Campylobacter jejuni A foodborne bacteria that causes diarrhea and a general illness lasting up to 11 days. The most common source of foodborne illness.

Carbohydrate A class of substances consisting of carbon and water (hydrogen and oxygen). The ratio of carbon to water is always 1:1.

Carnivore An animal that eats other animals; a meat eater.

Carotenoids A class of yellowish plant pigments that includes beta-carotene.

Casein A major protein in milk. When milk curdles it is the casein that precipitates (curds).

Celiac Sprue Individuals with this condition react to gluten and related substances in grains. The lining of the intestine sloughs off, causing malabsorption of foods.

Chlorophyll A green plant pigment that captures sunlight, providing the energy the plant needs to grow.

Cholesterol A waxy substance essential for the formation of the membranes that envelop every cell. The human body makes all the cholesterol it needs.

Cholesterol eaten in food generally suppresses the body's own synthesis. Cholesterol exists only in the animal world. Plants don't make cholesterol.

Chunked and formed meat An artificially shaped meat manufactured by reconstituting chunks of meat. The chunks have been tumbled or massaged, mixed with additives and sometimes finely ground meat, and molded into a shape. The general process is also called **flaked and formed.**

Clostridium botulinum The bacteria that causes botulism. See **Botulism.**

Colostrum A clear sticky milk produced in the first few days after a woman gives birth. It is rich in the antibodies that protect the baby against disease.

Comminuted meat Meat that is ground very fine. Used in making sausages and deli meats.

Couscous This is not a grain but a form of pasta made from semolina flour. It is the traditional dish of North African countries.

Creatine A substance found in muscles. Creatine phosphate is an instant source of muscle energy for a punch or leap. The body makes the creatine it needs.

Cruciferous vegetables A family of vegetables which have flowers shaped like a cross. The botanical name of this family is *Brassica*. Examples are cabbage and broccoli.

Crustaceans Aquatic animals having segmented limbs and an exoskeleton, such as crabs, lobsters, and shrimp.

Diabetes A disease in which the body is unable to lower its level of blood glucose. Normally, insulin is released in response to high blood glucose. In the juvenile form of diabetes, the individual's pancreas does not produce insulin. In the adult-onset form, the individual may still produce insulin, but the body does not respond.

Dietary Supplement Health and Education Act This act, passed in 1994, governs the labeling of supplements. The act does not require the manufacturer to test the supplements in advance or to prove the supplement works. The FDA does not monitor products to ensure they contain what the label says it contains. Responsibility rests with the manufacturer.

Diketopiperazine A chemical substance formed when the artificial sweetener, aspartame, is heated, causing it to break down.

Diverticulitis A condition occurring when pockets (diverticula) form in the muscular walls of the colon. These pockets become inflamed.

Docosahexaenoic Acid (DHA) An essential fatty acid of the omega-3 fatty acid family, containing 22 carbon atoms. It's found mainly in nervous system tissue. Plants make only linolenic acid (an omega-3 fatty acid). Animals convert linolenic to DHA.

Durum flour The same flour as semolina, except it is ground finer. Used to make noodles.

Eicosapentaenoic Acid (EPA) An essential fatty acid of the omega-3 fatty acid family, containing 20 carbon atoms.

Endosperm The food a seed stores for the time when it germinates. In grains the endosperm consists of starch.

Enriched flour Refined and bleached wheat flour that has been supplemented with iron and four vitamins: thiamin, niacin, riboflavin, and folic acid. May be supplemented with calcium.

***Escherichia coli* O157:H7**   A foodborne bacteria that causes, within one to eight days, bloody diarrhea (a sign the intestinal wall is being destroyed) and abdominal cramps. Usually little or no fever is present. The illness lasts five to eight days. Can be fatal in young children.

Essential amino acids   Twenty amino acids are the components of proteins. The human body is unable to make 9 amino acids. These essential amino acids must be obtained from the proteins of the diet.

Essential fatty acids   Fatty acids the human body is unable to make and thus must obtain in the diet. The two principle essential fatty acids are linoleic (omega-6) and linolenic (omega-3). Both contain 18 carbons.

Estrogen   The female sex hormone. There are several natural estrogens secreted by mammals. The main estrogen secreted in a woman's ovary is *estradiol.*

FD&C dyes   The Food Drug and Cosmetic Act of 1938 approved for use in foods a number of coal-tar dyes, given the designation FD&C.

Fiber   The plant substance not digested in the human gut. Fiber can be either insoluble or soluble in water. Soluble fibers like pectin form gels. Only plant foods contain fiber.

Flaked and formed   See **Chunked and formed meat.**

Food Quality Protection Act   An Act passed by Congress in 1996 designed to protect children from excessive exposure to pesticides in their food. The act is unique in requiring the total danger of pesticides to be assessed, rather than a single pesticide in a single food.

Fortified foods   Manufactured food products that have added vitamins and/or minerals. Some brands of fruit juice, for example, are fortified with calcium.

Framingham   A town in eastern Massachusetts. Since 1948 the health of some 5,000 of its residents has been closely monitored.

Free radical   A class of chemical substances formed in cells by the action of oxygen. Free radicals are unstable substances that rapidly decompose, damaging cell structures in the process. The damage can lead to premature aging and diseases like cancer. Antioxidants prevent free radical formation.

Fructose   The principle sugar of fruit and honey.

Functional foods   The industry buzzword for foods purporting to improve performance and confer some health benefit.

Glucose   A simple sugar found in fruit, honey, and corn syrup. It is also the sugar that circulates in the blood.

Gluten   A protein found principally in wheat but in other grains as well. Gluten gives dough its elasticity, enabling the dough to trap carbon dioxide released by the leavening agent (yeast or baking powder).

Glycemic index   A measure of the amount of rise in blood sugar (glucose) when a person ingests a carbohydrate. Drinking a glass of water containing pure glucose causes the greatest rise, and this value is arbitrarily assigned 100. The glycemic index of other foods is measured against glucose.

Glycogen   A polymer of glucose that the body stores in muscles and liver for use as ready fuel.

Glycogen is the animal counterpart of starch in plants.

GRAS   An acronym for *Generally Recognized As Safe.* Many substances used in making commercial foods are by their nature thought to be safe. These substances are granted GRAS status by the FDA without the need for extensive safety testing.

Grits   Coarsely ground grain, especially corn.

Guillian-Barré Syndrome   This syndrome, which occurs in one out every thousand food-poisoning infections, leads to acute neuromuscular paralysis.

Hard wheat   Spring wheat with a high gluten content. Used in bread flours. Protein content is 12 to 14 percent.

Hemochromatosis   This disease is caused by a hereditary condition in which the individual absorbs too much iron.

Hepatitis A   A foodborne virus that can cause symptoms that include fever, tiredness, loss of appetite, nausea, abdominal discomfort, dark urine, and jaundice (yellowing of skin and eyes).

Herbivore   An animal that eats plants.

HMR   See **Home Meal Replacement.**

Home Meal Replacement   A commercial term used to cover a complete meal a person buys to consume at home. The meal may, for example, be a hot meal bought at a restaurant takeout or a frozen meal from a supermarket.

Hypertension (high blood pressure)   Blood pressure is a measure of the force the heart exerts to pump blood through the arteries. Pressure reaches maximum at the top of the beat—systolic pressure—and a minimum when the heart rests—diastolic pressure. Blood pressure is a measure of these two pressures. "Normal" is considered to be 120/80. Hypertension is due to less flexible arteries, causing the force or blood pressure to increase and those numbers to be higher.

Insulin   A protein hormone made and stored in the pancreas. When a person eats a sugar or starch food, the blood glucose level rises. The pancreas releases insulin, which signals the adipose tissue and the liver to absorb excess glucose from the blood.

Insulin resistant   The pancreas produces the hormone insulin in response to elevated blood glucose, but the liver and adipose tissue that normally react to insulin and remove glucose from the blood don't react. The blood glucose level remains dangerously high.

Isoflavones   A class of plant substances that are part of the broader term, phytochemicals. Some isoflavones, particularly those in soybeans, have weak estrogenic activity. They mimic the action of the body's own estrogen.

Kamut   An ancient grain.

Ketone bodies   Substances produced in the body as a result of incomplete fat breakdown. They circulate in the blood and are excreted in the urine. Uncontrolled diabetics and individuals who eat a very low carbohydrate diet form large amounts of ketone bodies.

Ketosis   A condition in which a person is making large amounts of ketone bodies.

Lactase   An enzyme secreted in the gut that breaks lactose into its component sugars, glucose and galactose.

Lactoalbumins   A class of proteins found in milk.

Lactose   The sugar found in milk. It consist of two simple sugars, glucose and galactose.

Lactose intolerance   A genetic situation in which the individual loses the ability to produce lactase after about age 3. Without lactase it is impossible to digest the milk sugar, lactose.

Legumes   A plant family whose members grow in symbiotic relation with nitrogen-fixing bacteria. Because the bacteria use nitrogen from the air, legumes don't require nitrogen from the soil. Legumes include alfalfa, clover, lentils, peas, and all members of the bean family.

Lipoproteins   A class of substances that circulate in the blood and which consist of protein and fat (lipid). Lipoproteins are subdivided into LDL (low-density lipoproteins) and HDL (high-density lipoproteins).

Listeria monocytogenes   A foodborne bacteria. An infected person usually has fever, muscle aches, and sometimes gastrointestinal symptoms such as nausea or diarrhea. If infection spreads to the nervous system, symptoms such as headache, stiff neck, confusion, loss of balance, or convulsions can occur. Can be fatal.

Lycopene   This phytochemical is a member of the carotene family. It is believed to be a potent antioxidant. It is particularly rich in tomatoes, watermelon, and pink grapefruit. Lycopene is stable in high temperatures, and thus canned tomatoes are a good source.

Macrobiotic   The macrobiotic diet is a strict version of a vegan diet (no meat or animal products) that favors grains.

Mad cow disease The medical name for this disease is *bovine spongiform encephalopathy (BSE)*. BSE attacks the brain, causing it to disintegrate into a spongy mass—hence the name. The animal goes mad before dying. A similar disease with the same symptoms occurs in humans—*Creuztfeldt-Jacob disease*.

Masa Mexican corn flour, made by boiling the corn in a 5 percent lime solution. The lime releases the vitamin niacin, which otherwise remains locked in an unusable form, and alters the amino acid composition in a more favorable way.

Metabolism The collective chemical activity taking place in living cells. This process includes rebuilding of body tissues, conduction of nerve impulses, and production of muscular energy.

Mineral This term refers to nonorganic substances like iron, calcium, and zinc.

Minute Rice Precooked rice grains are slashed. When put in boiling water, water penetrates the cuts and the rice cooks rapidly.

Miso A fermented soybean product.

Monosodium Glutamate (MSG) MSG is a taste enhancer, which like salt enhances existing flavors of a food. MSG is used extensively in processed foods to enhance otherwise bland tastes.

Natto A fermented soybean product.

Nutraceutical A commercial term used to define substances extracted from a natural source and either put into a supplement or added to a food product in order to confer some health benefit.

Nutrient A general term used for substances the body is unable to make and thus must obtain from the diet. Nutrients include vitamins, minerals, essential amino acids, and essential fatty acids, as well as carbohydrate, fat, and protein.

Omnivore   An animal that eats both plant and animal foods.

Organic flour   A nonstandardized flour, so its definition varies. Made from wheat grown without chemical pesticides. It may also mean that no toxic fumigants have been applied during storage and no preservatives added to packaging or food product. The word "organic" does not specify whether or not the flour has been refined.

Osteoporosis   A disease in which the internal structure of the bones disintegrates, lessening bone density and increasing the chance of fracture.

Ovo-lacto vegetarian   One who eats no meat but eats eggs and dairy products. This is the most common form of vegetarianism.

Pasteurization   A process in which a food product is heated sufficiently enough to kill disease-causing bacteria.

Pellagra   A disease caused by a deficiency of the vitamin niacin. This disease is characterized by weakness, severe roughness of the skin, and dementia (mental illness).

Pemmican   A dried meat made by native Americans. They cut buffalo and deer meat into strips, sun-dry it, and pound it with crushed blueberries, cranberries, or wild cherries. The berries contain natural antimicrobial agents.

Penicillium   A class of molds used to ripen cheeses on their surface, such as Brie and Camembert.

Phytate   A class of plant substances found mainly in the bran (outer coat) of wheat and other grains.

Phytates tie up (chelate) minerals and prevent their absorption by the intestine.

Phytochemicals This general term defines any substance found in a plant. With respect to nutrition, the term is used to define substances that are not nutrients but are still useful to the body. Many phytochemicals, for example, are powerful antioxidants.

Phytoestrogens This term refers to plant substances that mimic the action of the female sex hormone, estrogen.

Placenta An organ created in the uterus during pregnancy. The placenta transfers nutrients from the mother's blood to the blood of the fetus, and waste products in the reverse direction.

Polychlorinated Biphenyls (PCBs) A toxic chemical that, while no longer manufactured, persists in the environment because of its unusual stability. It accumulates in the fatty tissues of food animals and in the body fat of people. Excessive amounts can lead to mental retardation and behavioral problems.

Polydextrose A chemically treated starch that mimics the "mouth feel" of fat. It's used in low-fat products to simulate fat.

Polyphenols A specific class of phytochemicals that occur mainly in red wine and chocolate. They are potent antioxidants.

Protein A class of substances which, unlike fat and carbohydrates, contains nitrogen. Many body structures are composed of proteins, such as hair, muscles, enzymes, and antibodies.

Quinoa An ancient grain. Pronounced KEEN-wa.

Rennet (or Rennin)   An enzyme isolated from the stomach lining of calves. It is added to milk in the initial phase of cheese making, causing the casein of milk to curdle.

Rickets   A deficiency disease caused by lack of vitamin D. In children, the long bones do not develop adequately and the child becomes bow-legged.

Salmonella   A foodborne bacteria that causes diarrhea, fever, and abdominal cramps 12 to 72 hours after infection. The illness usually lasts 4 to 7 days.

Scurvy   A disease caused by a deficiency of vitamin C (ascorbic acid), characterized by muscular weakness and a loss of connective tissue. Teeth fall out and body tissues disintegrate, followed by death.

Seitan   Wheat gluten made into a dough which can be simmered with tamari, soy sauce, and sea vegetables.

Semolina   A coarsely ground and refined flour of durum wheat, which is a hard, spring wheat. The dough is not as elastic as dough from other spring wheats, and is more suitable for extrusion. It is usually enriched, and is used to make couscous and pasta. Nutritionally, it is in the same class as enriched, white wheat flour.

Shigella   A foodborne bacteria causing, within 1 to 7 days, diarrhea, fever, vomiting, abdominal cramps, and bloody mucus in stool. Lasts 4 to 7 days, although it may take several months for bowel habits to return to normal.

Soft wheat   A winter wheat with a low gluten content. Unsuitable for bread making, soft wheat is used to make cakes, cookies, crackers, and pastries. Protein content is 7 to 9 percent.

Spelt   A high gluten grain that can be used to make leavened bread.

Stroke   This condition results from a blockage in an artery of the brain. Can lead to brain damage and death.

Sublingual   "Under the tongue." Many pills and supplements are best taken sublingually.

Sucrose   A sugar consisting of glucose and fructose. Table sugar is sucrose.

Sulphoraphane   A phytochemical found in broccoli and believed to be the major chemical responsible for broccoli's anticancer properties.

Tempeh   A fermented soybean product.

Testosterone   The male sex hormone produced in the testes.

Textured Vegetable Protein (TVP)   This food product is manufactured from soybean protein. It can be textured to give the "mouth feel" of meat or fish. It does not offer the balanced nutrition that a meat or fish offers.

Tocopherol   The chemical name for vitamin E. The most active form is d-alpha tocopherol.

Tomalley   The soft green liver of a cooked lobster.

Toxicologist   A scientist who specializes in studying the nature of poisons and their effects on people.

Toxin   A poisonous substance produced by a bacteria or plant.

Trace mineral   A mineral the human body uses in minute amounts, such as copper and chromium.

Trans fats   Trans fatty acids, components of trans fats, are unnatural forms of natural fatty acids. They form during the hydrogenation of oils to make margarine and vegetable shortening. Their consumption has been linked to a number of diseases, including heart disease.

Transgenic Transgenic plants and animals result from cross-breeding, in which a gene from one species is inserted into another species (genetic engineering). A gene from a bacteria that makes a toxin deadly to corn borers, for instance, is inserted into corn. The corn now makes the toxin, which kills the corn borers.

TVP See **Textured Vegetable Protein.**

Unbleached flour Refined wheat flour that has not been subjected to chemical bleaching. It may be aged to allow natural bleaching by the oxygen of the air.

Unbolted flour Bolting means to pass flour through a sieve. Because it has not gone through the sifting process, unbolted flour still contains the grain's bran.

Vegan One who excludes all meat and animal products (dairy and eggs). Many vegans also exclude honey.

Vitamin An vital organic substance the body is unable to make. Vitamins must be obtained from the diet.

Resource Guide

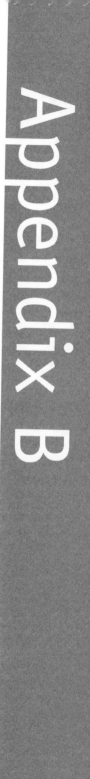

Allergies and food
Addresses

The American Academy of Allergy, Asthma, and Immunology
611 East Wells St.
Milwaukee, WI 53202
www.aaaai.org

The Food Allergy Network
10400 Eaton Pl., Suite 107
Fairfax, VA 22030-2208
Phone: 703-691-3179
www.foodallergy.org

The International Information Council Foundation
ificinfo.health.org

Mothers of Asthmatics
3554 Chain Bridge Rd., Suite 200
Fairfax, VA 22030
Phone: 703-385-4403

Books

Gottschall, Elaine. *Breaking the Vicious Cycle. Intestinal Health Through Diet.* Kirkton, Ontario: Kirkton Press, 1994.

Rapp, Doris, M.D. *Is This Your Child?* Helps parents with allergic children eliminate problem foods. Describes a rotation diet for allergic children.

Radetsky, Peter. *The Twentieth Century. The Explosion in Environmental Allergies—from Sick Buildings to Multiple Chemical Sensitivities* (Little Brown).

Cancer and nutrition

5 A Day Program
National Cancer Institute
EPN 232
6130 Executive Blvd., MSC 7330
Bethesda, MD 20892-7330
Phone: 800-4CANCER

Diabetes

American Diabetes Association
1701 North Beauregard St.
Alexandria, VA 22311
Phone: 800-342-2383
www.diabetes.org

Food safety

Books

Ashford, Nicholas, and Claudia Miller. *Chemical Exposure at Low Levels and High Stakes.* 2nd Edition. New York: Van Nostrand, Rheinhold, 1998.

Needleman, Herbert and Philip Landgran. *Raising Your Children Toxic Free: How to Keep Your Child Safe from Lead, Asbestos, Pesticides and Other Environmental Hazards.* New York: Farrar, Straus and Giroux, 1994.

Sarjeant, Doris, and Karen Evans. *Hard to Swallow, the Truth About Food Additives.* Burnaby, Canada: Alive Books, 1999.

Steinman, David. *Diet for a Poisoned Planet. How to Choose Safe Foods for You and Your Family.* New York: Ballantine Books, 1990.

Web sites

The Environmental Protection Agency (EPA) maintains a Web site that provides safety information and lists of pesticides with the legal tolerance levels used on specific crops.
www.epa.gov/pesticides/food

Consumers Union Website
www.ecologic-ipm.com

The Food and Drug Administration's Bad Bug Book is available at the FDA Web site. The book is a useful description of bacteria and viruses that can contaminate food and make you sick.
vm.cfsan.fda.gov/~mow/intro.ht

The U.S. Department of Agriculture offers food safety information about meat, poultry, and eggs.
www.usda.gov/agency/fsis/consedu
www.nal.usda.gov/pubs_dbs
Phone: 800-535-4555

Physical fitness and diet
Books

Katch, Frank and William McArdle. *Introduction to Nutrition, Exercise, and Health.* Philadelphia: Lea and Febiger, 1993.

Web sites

CNN Interactive, diet and fitness site
cnn.com/health/diet.fitness/

The Internet Society for Sports Science and *Sports Science,* a peer-reviewed journal, posts information on diet and sports.
www.sportsci.org/

Organic and whole foods
Book
Kilham, Christopher. *The Bread and Circus Whole Food Bible. How to Select and Prepare Safe, Healthful Foods.* Reading, Mass.: Addison Wesley, 1991.

Mail-order companies
Crusoe Island Natural Foods
267 Route 89 South
Savannah, NY 13146
Phone: 800-724-2233
www.crusoeisland.com
webmaster@crusoeisland.com

Diamond Organics All Organic Food
P.O. Box 2159
Freedom, CA 95019
Phone: 888-ORGANIC

Govinda's
2651 Ariane Dr.
San Diego, CA 92117
Phone: 800-900-0108
Govinda's specializes in handmade bars with organic ingredients.

Fiddler's Green Farm
P.O. Box 254
Belfast, ME 04915
Phone: 800-729-7935
fiddler@mint.net

Fiddler's Green Farm offers certified organic pancake and baking mixes, cereals, and jams.

Indian Harvest Specialfoods, Inc.
P.O. Box 428
Bemidji, MN 56619-0428
Phone: 880-294-2433
www.indianharvest.com
Indian Harvest is a good source for heritage beans and wild rice.

King Arthur Flour
The Baker's Catalog
P.O. Box 876
Norwich, VT 05055-0876
Phone: 800-827-6836
www.kingarthurflour.com
King Arthur sells bread flours and bread-making accessories.

Maine Coast Sea Vegetables
Franklin, ME 04634
www.seaveg.com
info@seaveg.com

Morgan Mills
East Union, ME 04862
Phone: 207-785-4900
You'll find organically grown grain products at Morgan Mills.

Walnut Acres Organic Farms
Penns Creek, PA 17862-0800
Phone: 800-433-3998
Walnut Acres offers a wide selection of certified organic grains, grain products, canned goods, organic meats, and preserves.

Supplements: Vitamins, minerals, and herbs

Book

Foster, Steven and Varro Tyler. *Tyler's Honest Herbal: A Sensible Guide to the Use Of Herbs and Related Products.* Haworth Herbal Press, 1999.

Web sites

The American Botanical Council hosts an educational site concerning herbs.
www.herbalgram.org

The National Institutes of Health, Office of Dietary Supplements, offers a database of technical articles on herbs and other dietary supplements. Abstracts only.
odp.od.nih.gov/ods/

The FDA posts a Frequently Asked Questions (FAQs) section about Dietary Supplements.
www.fda.gov/default.htm (Click FAQ, then Food, then Supplements.)

Vegetarianism

Books

Barnard, Neal, M.D. *Food for Life. How the New Four Food Groups Can Save Your Life.* New York: Crown Publishers, 1993.

Kushi, Michio and Aveline Kushi. *Macrobiotic Diet.* New York: Japan Publications, 1985.

Vegetarian cookbooks

Katzen, Mollie. *Enchanted Broccoli Forest.* Berkley, Calif.: Ten Speed Press, 1995.

Katzen, Mollie. *Vegetable Heaven.* New York: Hyperion, 1997.

Madison, Deborah. *Vegetarian Cooking for Everyone.* New York: Broadway Books, 1997.

New Recipes From Moosewood Restaurant, The Moosewood Collective. Berkley, Calif.: Ten Speed Press, 1987.

Wolfert, Paula. *Mediterranean Grains and Greens.* New York: HarperCollins, 1998.

Web sites

The American Dietetic Association has posted its position paper on vegetarianism at its Web site. www.eatright.org/adap1197.html

International Vegetarian Union
www.ivu.org

Vegetarian Times
www.vegetariantimes.com

The Vegetarian Resource Group
P.O. Box 1463
Baltimore, MD 21203
Phone: 410-366-VEGE
www.vrg.org/

The Vegetarian Kitchen lists lots of good recipes. www.vegkitchen.com

Another site loaded with recipes is Veggie Heaven. www.veggieheaven.com

Macrobiotic Library
www.macrobiotics.org

General Web sites

American Dietetic Association
Phone: 800-366-1655
www.eatright.org

Canada's National Institute of Nutrition
A well-organized site, loaded with information.
www.nin.ca

Center for Science in the Public Interest. Publisher of the Nutrition Action Health Letter. Excellent

site for behind-the-scenes information on foods.
www.cspinet.org

CNN Interactive Food Site. A variety of facts about foods.
cnn.com/HEALTH/indepth.food/

Dairy Council of California
www.dairycouncilofca.org

Drkoop.com. A commercial Web site, which includes information on diet and health.
www.drkoop.com/

National Agriculture Library
www.nalusda.gov/pubs_dbs

National Pork Producers Council
www.nppc.org

Nutrition Village
Good Web site for information on phytochemicals, designer foods, and much more.
www.naturalland.com/nv.htm

Shape Up America!
A joint venture of industry and nonprofit organizations devoted to combating obesity.
www.shapeup.org

Tufts University Nutrition Navigator
This Web site brings up over 200 other Web sites related to nutrition.
navigator.tufts.edu

United States Department of Agriculture (USDA)
www.usda.gov

USDA Nutrient Database
www.nal.usda.gov/fnic/foodcomp/

United Soy Producers
www.talksoy.com

Wheat Foods Council
Good source of information on everything about wheat.
www.wheatfoods.org

Recommended Reading List

Barer-Stein, Thelma. *You Eat What You Are*. Buffalo: Firefly Books, 1999.

Cleave, T.L. *The Saccharine Disease*. Bristol, U.K.: Wright, 1974.

Crawford, Michael and David Marsh. *The Driving Force: Food in Evolution and the Future*. London: Mandarin Books, 1989.

D'Adamo, Peter with Catherine Whitney. *Eat Right for Your Type*. New York: Putnam, 1996.

DesMaisons, Kathleen. *Potatoes not Prozac*. New York: Simon and Schuster, 1998.

Eaton, Boyd, Marjorie Shostak, and Melvin Konner. *The Paleolithic Prescription*. New York: Harper and Row, 1988.

Erasmus, Udo. *Fats that Heal, Fats that Kill*. Burnaby, Canada: Alive Books, 1993.

Goldbeck, Nikki, and David Goldbeck. *The Goldbeck's Guide to Good Food*. New York: New American Library, 1987.

Havala, Suzanne, and Robert Pritikin. *The Complete Idiot's Guide to Being a Vegetarian.* New York: Macmillan, 1999.

Ho, Mae-Wan. *Genetic Engineering, Dreams or Nightmares?* New Delhi: Research Foundation for Science, Technology, and Ecology, 1997.

Holmes, Randee. *Additive Alert.* Toronto: Pollution Probe Foundation, 1994.

Jacobson, Michael and Sarah Fritschner. *The Completely Revised and Updated Fast Food Guide.* New York: Workman Publishing, 1991.

McGee, Harold. *On Food and Cooking.* Mount Vernon, N.Y.: Consumers Union, 1984.

Northrup, Christiane. *Women's Bodies, Women's Wisdom: Creating Physical and Emotional Health and Healing.* New York: Bantam, 1998.

Pitchford, Paul. *Healing with Whole Foods: Oriental Traditions and Modern Nutrition.* Berkeley, Calif.: Atlantic Books, 1993.

Sarjeant, Doris and Karen Evans. *Hard to Swallow.* Burnaby, Canada: Alive Books, 1999.

Schell, Orville. *Modern Meat: Antibiotics, Hormones, and the Pharmaceutical Farm.* New York: Random House, 1984.

Staten, Vince. *Can You Trust a Tomato in January?* New York: Simon and Schuster, 1993.

The Surgeon General's Report on Nutrition and Health. New York: Warner Books, 1989.

Werbach, Melvyn. *Nutritional Influences on Illness.* New Canaan, Conn.: Keats Publishing, 1988.

Williams, Roger. *The Wonderful World Within You.* 20th Anniversary Edition. Wichita, Kans.: Bio-Communications Press, 1998.

Yellowlees, Walter. *A Doctor in the Wilderness.* London: Janus Publishing, 1993.

Important Documents

Federal government agencies that regulate food

United States Department of Agriculture (USDA)

- Agricultural Marketing Service, AMS
- Animal and Plant Health Inspection Service (APHIS)
- Agricultural Research Service (ARS)
- Food Safety Inspection Service (FSIS)
- Grain Inspection, Packers, and Stockyards Administration (GIPSA)

U.S. Department of Health and Human Services

- Food and Drug Administration (FDA)
- Centers for Disease Control (CDC)
- Environmental Protection Agency (EPA)
- Federal Trade Commission (FTC)
- National Oceanic and Atmospheric Administration (NOAA)
- National Marine Fisheries Service (NMFS)

United States Treasury

- Customs Service
- Bureau of Alcohol, Tobacco, and Firearms (BATF)

USDA and FDA dietary guidelines for Americans

- Eat a variety of foods.
- Balance the food you eat with physical activity.
- Choose a diet with plenty of grain products, fruits, and vegetables.
- Choose a diet low in saturated fat and cholesterol.
- Choose a diet moderate in sugars.
- Choose a diet moderate in salt and sodium.
- If you drink alcoholic beverages, do so in moderation.

Serving sizes of food categories in USDA Food Guide Pyramid

Food Category	Amount in a meal or snack	Recommended number of servings
Grains	1 slice of bread	6–11
	$1/2$ cup of cooked pasta	
	5–6 small crackers	
	$3/4$ cup of dry breakfast cereal	
Fruits	1 medium size piece of fruit	2–4
Vegetables	$1/2$ cup of chopped vegegetable, equivalent to a medium-size carrot or potato	3–5
	1 cup of a chopped leafy vegetables	
	$3/4$ cup of vegetable juice	

Food Category	Amount in a meal or snack	Recommended number of servings
Meat, fish, eggs, dry beans, nuts	3 ounces of meat, a piece about the size of your palm	2–3
	1 egg	
	1/2 cup of cooked dry beans	
	1/3 cup of nuts	
Dairy	1 cup of milk	2–3

The National Cancer Institute recommendations for fruit and vegetables

Eat a minimum of five servings a day to reduce your risk of cancer. A serving consists of:

- 1 medium fruit or 1/2 cup small or cut-up fruit.
- 3/4 cup (180 milliliters) of 100 percent juice.
- 1/4 cup dried fruit.
- 1/2 cup raw nonleafy or cooked vegetables.
- 1 cup raw leafy vegetables (such as lettuce).
- 1/2 cup cooked beans or peas (such as lentils, pinto beans, and kidney beans).

Daily Values (DV) for nutrition labeling

The Daily Values used on nutrition labels are calculated as follows:

- Fat based on 30 percent of calories
- Saturated fat based on 10 percent of calories
- Carbohydrates based on 60 percent of calories
- Protein based on 10 percent of calories (applies to adults and children over age 4)
- Fiber based on 11.5 grams of fiber per 1,000 calories

The Daily Values in the following table are based on a person eating 2,000 calories per day. A normal-size, moderately active woman would consume about 2,000 calories a day.

Mandatory Components on Nutrition Label	Daily Values
Total fat	65 g
Saturated fat	20 g
Cholesterol	300 mg
Sodium	2,400 mg
Total carbohydrate	300 g
Dietary fiber	25 g
Vitamin A	5,000 IU
Vitamin C	60 mg
Calcium	1,000 mg
Iron	18 mg
Voluntary Listing On Nutrition Label	**Daily Values**
Vitamin D	400 IU
Vitamin E	30 IU
Vitamin K	80 mcg
Thiamin	1.5 mg
Riboflavin	1.7 mg
Niacin	20 mg
Vitamin B_6	2 mg
Folic acid	400 mcg
Vitamin B_{12}	6 mcg
Biotin	300 mcg
Pantothenic acid	10 mg
Phosphorus	1,000 mg
Iodine	150 mcg
Magnesium	400 mg
Zinc	15 mg
Selenium	70 mcg
Copper	2 mg
Manganese	2 mg

Voluntary Listing On Nutrition Label	Daily Values
Chromium	120 mcg
Molybdenum	75 mcg
Chloride	3,400 mg
Potassium	3,500 mg

Abbreviations: g=gram, mg=milligram, mcg=microgram, IU=International Unit (1 gram=1,000 milligrams; 1 gram=1,000,000 micrograms)

(Source: Code of Federal Regulations, Food and Drugs, Title 21, Part 101.9, Nutrition Labeling of Food)

The 10 health claims authorized by the FDA for food product packaging

- Low calcium intake is one risk factor for osteoporosis, a condition of lowered bone mass or density. Lifelong adequate calcium intake helps maintain bone health by increasing as much as genetically possible the amount of bone formed in the teens and early adult life and by helping to slow the rate of bone loss that occurs later in life.

- Sodium is a risk factor for coronary heart disease and stroke deaths. The most common source of sodium is table salt. Diets low in sodium may help lower blood pressure and related risks in many people. Guidelines recommend daily sodium intakes of not more than 2,400 mg. Typical U.S. intakes are 3,000 to 6,000 mg.

- Diets high in fat increase the risk of some types of cancer, such as cancers of the breast, colon, and prostate. While scientists don't know how total fat intake affects cancer development, low-fat diets reduce the risk. Experts recommend that Americans consume 30 percent or less of daily calories as fat. Typical U.S. intakes are 37 percent.

- Diets high in saturated fat and cholesterol increase total and low-density (bad) blood cholesterol levels, and thus the risk of coronary heart disease. Diets low in saturated fat and cholesterol decrease the risk. Guidelines recommend that American diets contain less than 10 percent of calories from saturated fat and less than 300 mg cholesterol daily. The average American adult diet has 13 percent saturated fat and 300 to 400 mg cholesterol a day.

- Diets low in fat and rich in fiber-containing grain products, fruits, and vegetables may reduce the risk of some types of cancer. The exact role of total dietary fiber, fiber components, and other nutrients and substances in these foods is not fully understood.

- Diets low in saturated fat and cholesterol and rich in fruits, vegetables, and grain products that contain fiber, particularly soluble fiber, may reduce the risk of coronary heart disease. (It is impossible to adequately distinguish the effects of fiber, including soluble fiber, from those of other food components.)

- Diets low in fat and rich in fruits and vegetables may reduce the risk of some cancers. Fruits and vegetables are low-fat foods and may contain fiber or vitamin A (as beta-carotene) and vitamin C. (The effects of these vitamins cannot be adequately distinguished from those of other fruit or vegetable components.)

- Defects of the neural tube (a structure that develops into the brain and spinal cord) occur within the first 6 weeks after conception, often before the pregnancy is known. The U.S. Public Health Service recommends that all women of childbearing age in the United States consume 0.4 mg (400 mcg) of folic acid daily to reduce their risk of having a baby affected with spina bifida or other neural tube defects.

- Between-meal eating of foods high in sugar and starches may promote tooth decay. Sugarless candies made with certain sugar alcohols do not.

- Dietary soluble fiber, such as that found in whole oats and psyllium seed husk, when included in a diet low in saturated fat and cholesterol, may affect blood lipid levels, such as cholesterol, and thus lower the risk of heart disease. However, because soluble dietary fibers constitute a family of very heterogeneous substances that vary greatly in their effect on the risk of heart disease, the FDA has determined that sources of soluble fiber for this health claim need to be considered case by case. To date, FDA has reviewed and authorized two sources of soluble fiber eligible for this claim: whole oats and psyllium seed husk.

Peak season for fruits grown in North America

Tropical fruits like bananas are available year around. Fruits from South America, New Zealand, and Australia may complement the northern growing seasons.

PEAK SEASONS FOR FRUITS GROWN
IN NORTH AMERICA

Fruit	Peak Season
Apples	October–March
Apricots	June–July
Blueberries	July–August
Cherries	June–July
Coconuts	October–December
Cranberries	October–December
Grapefruit	September–April
Grapes	July–November
Mangoes	May–August
Cantaloupe	June–August
Honeydew	June–September
Nectarines	July–August
Oranges	December–June
Papayas	May–June
Peaches	June–September
Pears	September–November
Pineapple	March–June
Plums	July–August
Raspberries	June–August
Strawberries	April–June
Tangerines	November–January
Watermelons	May–August

Habitat of commercial fish

FISH ARRANGED FROM THE LEAST FAT TO THE MOST

Freshwater	Ocean, Nearshore	Ocean, Offshore
Yellow perch	Pink salmon	Cod
Bass	Chum salmon	Haddock
Perch	Sockeye salmon	Yellowfin tuna
Brook trout	Sardines	Flounder or sole
Rainbow trout	Herring	Ocean perch
Whitefish		Pacific halibut
Lake trout		Albacore tuna

Recommended maximum storage times for common foods

PRODUCT	STORAGE PERIOD	
	In Refrigerator	In Freezer
Fresh meat:		
Beef: Ground	1–2 days	3–4 months
Steaks and roasts	3–5 days	6–12 months
Pork: Chops	3–5 days	3–4 months
Ground	1–2 days	1–2 months
Roasts	3–5 days	4–8 months
Cured meats:		
Lunch meat	3–5 days	1–2 months
Sausage	1–2 days	1–2 months
Gravy	1–2 days	3 months
Fish:		
Lean (such as cod)	1–2 days	up to 6 months
Fatty (such as blue, perch, salmon)	1–2 days	2–3 months
Chicken: Whole	1–2 days	12 months
Parts	1–2 days	9 months
Giblets	1–2 days	3–4 months
Dairy products: Swiss, brick, processed cheese	3–4 weeks	*
Milk	5 days	1 month
Eggs: Fresh in shell	3–5 weeks	–
Hard-boiled	1 week	–

Cheese can be frozen, but freezing will affect the texture and taste.

(Source: Publication No. [FDA] 99-2244)

Classes of chemical additives permitted in food

Chemical additives are used in food processing for three reasons:

1. They enable food ingredients to withstand the temperature and prolonged processing on an industrial scale where food is made by the ton.

2. They add color, flavor, and texture to processed foods that have little or none.

3. Chemical additives enable food products to remain on the shelf or in the warehouse for years without losing crispness, color, or flavor.

The following are the different classes of food additives.

Anticaking agents

Anticaking agents are added to salt, icing sugar, and dry mixes to keep them free flowing, otherwise they would cake from the humidity. Examples:

- Calcium aluminum silicate
- Calcium stearate
- Magnesium silicate

Bleaching, maturing, and dough-conditioning agents

These chemicals are used to bleach flour in order to impart a chalk-white color. Some of the agents also oxidize the protein, gluten, making it stiffer. This process is called maturing. Maturing agents allow the baker to use cheaper flour of lower gluten content. Examples:

- Acetone peroxide
- Chlorine
- Potassium persulfate

Coloring agents

Coloring agents range from natural colors, like annatto and the red color from beets, to the synthetic coal-tar dyes (FD&C series). Examples:

- Carbon black (also named vegetable carbon)
- Trisodium 3-carboxy-5-hydroxy-1-p-sulfophenyl-4-p-sulfo-phenylazopyrazole (Tartrazine, FD&C Yellow #5)
- Silver metal

Emulsifying, gelling, stabilizing, and thickening agents

Thickening chemicals are used to give soups, sauces, salad dressing, and other foods an appealing, thick character. They are also used to give cheap ice cream its smoothness, and they are used as glazes. Examples:

- Calcium hypophosphite
- Gum arabic (obtained from acacia trees that grow in Sudan)
- Hydroxypropyl methyl cellulose

Food enzymes

Food enzymes are biologically active proteins that cause a change in the food. Amylase, for instance, is added to bread, juices, and baked goods. It causes starch to break down to sugar, making the product sweeter. Examples:

- Cellulase (breaks down cellulose fiber)
- Invertase (breaks sucrose into its two component sugars, glucose and fructose)
- Protease (breaks down proteins)

Firming agents

Firming agents absorb water. They are added to pickles, canned tomatoes, canned fruits, and flours to make them harder. In the case of the canned fruits, they reduce mushiness. Examples:

- Aluminum sodium sulfate
- Calcium chloride
- Calcium phosphate, dibasic

Glazing and polishing agents

Glazing and polishing agents give many foods their shine. They are also used to coat produce, such as peppers and apples, to protect against moisture loss. Examples:

- Beeswax
- Carnauba wax
- Shellac

Sweeteners

Sweeteners are a class of chemicals, other than sugars, that impart a sweet taste to foods. Examples:

- Aspartame
- Maltitol
- Sorbitol

Acidulants and pH adjusting agents

Acidulants and pH adjusting agents are used to change the acidity of a food. Vinegar (acetic acid), for example, is used to make pickles and meats more acid. Alkalis, such as baking soda (sodium bicarbonate), counter excess acidity in foods. Examples:

- Ammonium phosphate, dibasic
- Citric acid
- Sodium potassium tartrate

Preservatives—antimicrobials

Antimicrobials are chemicals that poison living organisms (in this case bacteria or molds that might grow in the food product). They are added to practically all manufactured foods. Examples:

- Potassium benzoate
- Propyl paraben (propyl p-hydroxybenzoate)
- Sulfites

Preservatives—antioxidants

Antioxidants are chemicals that prevent the oxidation of fats in foods (rancidity). They are added to lard, margarine, breakfast cereals, chewing gum, meat products, and essentially any product that contains fat. Examples:

- Ascorbic acid (vitamin C)
- Butylated hydoxyanisole (BHA)
- Propyl gallate

Sequestering agents

Sequestering agents bind metals. Traces of metals from the processing machinery enter food products and can be a problem, promoting discoloring and changing the flavors. The metal is still present in the food but is locked up in the sequestering agent. These chemicals are used in beer, salad dressing, sandwich spread, canned fish, margarine, and soft drinks. Examples:

- Ammonium citrate, dibasic
- EDTA, ethylenediamine tetraacetic acid
- Sodium tripolyphosphate

Starch-modifying chemicals

Natural starch, such as corn starch or wheat flour, used in home cooking to thicken gravies, soups, and puddings, would disintegrate in the intense heat and prolonged storage periods of industrial food processing. Food manufacturers treat starch with chemical agents that modify the character of the starch, making it resistant to breakdown. Some two dozen different chemicals are used to modify starch, none of which appear on the food label. You see only the words "modified food starch" in the ingredients list. Examples of chemicals used to modify starch:

- Epichlorhydrin
- Hydrogen peroxide
- Phosphorus oxychloride

Yeast foods

Yeast foods are used in baked goods whose dough is leavened with yeast. These chemicals are nutrients the yeast needs to grow fast. Examples:

- Ammonium chloride
- Calcium chloride
- Manganese sulfate

Solvents used for extraction and as carriers

Chemical solvents are used to extract the essence from spices and caffeine from coffee beans. The solvents are also used to dissolve artificial dyes—that is, carry the dye into the food to ensure even mixing. Examples:

- Acetone
- Castor oil
- Isopropyl alcohol (Isopropanol)

Guides to Nutritional Quality Levels

For your convenience, all the nutritional quality tables in Part II (Chapters 2 to 6) are combined into the table below.

As a reminder, the four quality levels are on a relative scale. No attempt is made to label a food good or bad, or to use the popular term "junk food." I prefer the term "better than" (or "worse than"). Foods at level 4 have a certain nutrition value. Canned vegetables, for instance, have some nutritional value. But when you have the choice, frozen vegetables offer better nutritional value than canned vegetables, and fresh vegetables lightly cooked are better than frozen vegetables.

As described in the chapters, you have to exercise common sense in using the quality levels. "Fresh" produce means truly fresh. When you have a choice between frozen vegetables and wilted lettuce or softened carrots, take the frozen.

In general, a food or food product that is certified organic ranks one quality level higher. For example, canned vegetables organically grown rank on level 3 instead of level 4. Breads made from certified organic flours rank one level higher than the corresponding nonorganic products.

The concept of the four nutritional quality levels is simple. A food or food product at a higher level offers better nutrition, fewer chemical additives, and less industrial processing than a product on a lower level.

Finally, the nutritional quality levels are designed as an aid to choosing foods. The more foods you choose at the upper quality levels (levels 1 and 2) that fit into your lifestyle, the better your overall nutrition will be.

Food Category	Level 1	Level 2	Level 3	Level 4
Vegetables	Fresh, raw* (preferably organic)	Fresh, lightly cooked	Frozen	Canned
Fruits	Fresh raw (preferably organic)	Frozen	Dried	Canned
Fruit juices	Freshly squeezed	Premium juice in dated carton or bottle	Juice reconstituted from frozen concentrate	Juice drinks
Breads	Whole wheat, whole wheat with other whole grains (preferably organic)	Whole wheat mixed with unbleached white flour	Frozen-dough breads containing whole grain, artisanal breads made from unbleached white flour	Frozen-dough breads and commercial cottony breads made with enriched white flour
Pasta	Fresh, whole grain	Dry, whole grain	Fresh, semolina flour	Dry, semolina flour
Corn and corn flours	Sweet corn on the cob, fresh	Whole corn flour (unbolted), masa, blue corn flour	Corn flour (cornmeal), degermed grits	Corn flakes breakfast cereal
Dried beans	Organic dried beans, lentils, peas, soaked and home cooked	Nonorganic beans, lentils, peas, soaked and home cooked	Commercial beans canned in water	Commercial beans canned in brine (salt), molasses, or tomato sauce, pork and beans
Nuts	Nuts in the shell, raw	Nuts, preshelled, raw	Nuts, dry roasted	Nuts roasted in oil
Peanut butter	Peanuts, freshly ground	Peanuts, ground (nothing added) and packed in their own oil	Peanut butter, homogenized	Peanut oil replaced with cheap, hydrogenated oil, sugar added, and the product homogenized

Food Category	Level 1	Level 2	Level 3	Level 4
Olive oil	Extra virgin, mechanically expressed, low temperature	Virgin, or extra virgin blended with solvent-extracted olive oil	Pure, solvent extracted and refined, no specification to virginity	Pomace, cheap oil extracted from cake left over from higher quality extractions
Vegetable oils	Mechanically expressed (cold) and unrefined	Cold pressed, unrefined	Refined oils	Refined and hydrogenated oils
Meat	Meat from free-range, organically raised animals	Lean steaks; pork chops, broiled or grilled; beef and pork roasts, baked	Frozen meats, commercial hamburger, baked ham	Bacon, weiners, sausages, luncheon meats, flaked (chunked) and formed meats; low-fat meats
Poultry	Free-range, organically raised chickens and turkeys, grilled, broiled, or roasted	Fresh chicken and turkey, grilled, broiled, or roasted	Frozen chicken and turkey, whole or parts	Deli-style turkey breast. Rolled turkey breast, flaked chicken breasts with grill marks, battered and deep-fried chicken
Eggs	Fresh eggs, free-range, "organic" hens	Commercial eggs (look for those rich in the omega-3 fatty acids)	Liquid eggs, dried eggs	Egg substitutes, frozen liquid eggs (restaurants use liquid eggs to make omelets)
Fish	Wild sea fish, fresh, broiled, grilled, baked	Farm fish, fresh, broiled, grilled, baked (caution: some fish are contaminated)	Frozen fish, shrimp, and crab	Fish sticks, fake crab, canned fish
Fluid milk	Milk from organically raised cows	Pasteurized, nonhomogenized milk	Pasteurized and homogenized	Ultrapasteurized, canned or condensed

*Raw vegetables are those you would put into a salad. Some vegetables, like potatoes and kale, need to be cooked.

The *Unofficial Guide*™ Reader Questionnaire

If you would like to express your opinion about smart nutrition or this guide, please complete this questionnaire and mail it to:

The *Unofficial Guide*™ Reader Questionnaire
IDG Lifestyle Group
1633 Broadway, floor 7
New York, NY 10019-6785

Gender: ___ M ___ F

Age: ___ Under 31 ___ 31–40 ___ 41–50
___ Over 50

Education: ___ High school ___ College
___ Graduate/Professional

What is your occupation?

_____

How did you hear about this guide?
___ Friend or relative
___ Newspaper, magazine, or Internet
___ Radio or TV
___ Recommended at bookstore
___ Recommended by librarian
___ Picked it up on my own
___ Familiar with the *Unofficial Guide*™ travel series

Did you go to the bookstore specifically for a book on smart nutrition? Yes ___ No ___

Have you used any other *Unofficial Guides*™?
Yes ___ No ___

If Yes, which ones?

_____

_____

_____

What other book(s) on smart nutrition have you purchased? _____

_____

_____

Was this book:

___ more helpful than other(s)

___ less helpful than other(s)

Do you think this book was worth its price?

Yes ___   No ___

Did this book cover all topics related to smart nutrition adequately?

Yes ___   No ___

Please explain your answer:

_____

_____

_____

Were there any specific sections in this book that were of particular help to you?   Yes ___   No ___

Please explain your answer:

_____

_____

_____

On a scale of 1 to 10, with 10 being the best rating, how would you rate this guide? ___

What other titles would you like to see published in the *Unofficial Guide*™ series?

_____

_____

Are Unofficial Guides™ **readily available in your area?**   Yes ___   No ___

Other comments:

_____

_____

_____

_____

Get the inside scoop...with the *Unofficial Guides*™!

Health and Fitness

The Unofficial Guide to Alternative Medicine
ISBN: 0-02-862526-9 Price: $15.95

The Unofficial Guide to Conquering Impotence
ISBN: 0-02-862870-5 Price: $15.95

The Unofficial Guide to Coping with Menopause
ISBN: 0-02-862694-x Price: $15.95

The Unofficial Guide to Cosmetic Surgery
ISBN: 0-02-862522-6 Price: $15.95

The Unofficial Guide to Dieting Safely
ISBN: 0-02-862521-8 Price: $15.95

The Unofficial Guide to Having a Baby
ISBN: 0-02-862695-8 Price: $15.95

The Unofficial Guide to Living with Diabetes
ISBN: 0-02-862919-1 Price: $15.95

The Unofficial Guide to Overcoming Arthritis
ISBN: 0-02-862714-8 Price: $15.95

The Unofficial Guide to Overcoming Infertility
ISBN: 0-02-862916-7 Price: $15.95

Career Planning

The Unofficial Guide to Acing the Interview
ISBN: 0-02-862924-8 Price: $15.95

The Unofficial Guide to Earning What You Deserve
ISBN: 0-02-862523-4 Price: $15.95

The Unofficial Guide to Hiring and Firing People
ISBN: 0-02-862523-4 Price: $15.95

Business and Personal Finance

The Unofficial Guide to Investing
ISBN: 0-02-862458-0 Price: $15.95

All books in the *Unofficial Guide*™ series are available at your local bookseller.